Illegal Drugs

A Complete Guide to Their
History, Chemistry, Use and Abuse

PAUL M. GAHLINGER, M.D., PH.D.

sagebrush
PRESS

THE SAGEBRUSH MEDICAL GUIDES

The Sagebrush Medical Guides aim to describe everything about an unusual health topic. Open this book anywhere you like. You don't need to read it cover to cover. From the basic facts to the precise details, the contents are useful to students, parents, health and legal professionals, and anyone else interested in the subject.

Illegal Drugs is the first volume in the Sagebrush Medical Guides. It covers all 178 drugs that are illegal in the United States, and describes every aspect of illegal drugs.

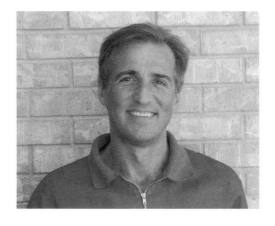

ABOUT THE AUTHOR

Paul M. Gahlinger, M.D., Ph.D., M.P.H., FACOEM, is Adjunct Professor in the Faculty of Medicine, University of Utah, Salt Lake City. His research interests have taken him to over 85 countries, from Africa and Antarctica to consulting for NASA at the Kennedy Space Center. A certified substance-abuse Medical Review Officer and FAA Aviation Medical Examiner, he has studied the effects of drugs in various work settings and in the space program. He is the author of *Northern Manitoba from Forest to Tundra, The Cockpit: A Flight of Escape and Discovery,* and co-author (with J.H. Abramson) of *Computer Programs for Epidemiologists.*

Res non per se at per usum, bona aut mala est

Nothing of itself is good or evil; only the manner of its use makes it so.

Printed in the U.S.

Library of Congress Cataloguing-in-Publication Data

Gahlinger, Paul M.
    The Sagebrush medical guide to illegal drugs / Paul
M. Gahlinger. -- 1st ed.
    p. cm.
    Includes bibliographical references and index.

    1. Narcotics. 2. Drug abuse.   I. Title.

RC566.G34 2001   616.86'3
                              QBI00-1016

ISBN 0-9703130-1-2

The purpose of this book is to provide information about illegal drugs. This information is descriptive only and is not intended to be, and nor should it be considered, a substitute for competent medical care, counseling, or legal advice. While every attempt has been made to ensure accuracy, some errors may persist. The author and publisher assume no responsibility whatsoever for any use the reader may make of the information provided herein.

The unauthorized possession, sale, or manufacture of an illegal drug is a crime, which can result in penalties including imprisonment.

The information given here is intended to help readers understand illegal drugs. All of this information is readily available from government, academic, and popular sources—indeed, references to these sources are included to validate the text and direct readers to printed and electronic literature. In order to avoid any possible encouragement of drug manufacture or use, specific recipes for drug manufacture are not provided and Internet sites that give this information are not specified.

This book includes many drug names that are registered trademarks. For ease in reading, the trademark symbols ™ or ® are not used; instead, all terms known, or suspected to be, trademarks or service marks are appropriately capitalized. Generic drug names are given in lower-case. For example, the brand name Valium is capitalized, but its generic name diazepam is not capitalized. Trade and generic names are often used interchangeably.

Contents

Preface   i

PART I   **Forbidden Fruit**   **1**

Chapter 1   **Flesh of the Gods—or the Devil's Poison?**   **3**

The Discovery of Drugs   5
     Substances and spirits   6
     The dose makes the poison   8
     Use and abuse: the four types of drug   9
     Controlled substances   10
     How are drugs named?   11

Why Are Some Drugs Illegal?   11
     Danger to self   12
     Danger to others   12
     Danger to society   12
     Drug terms   13

Will the "Drug Problem" Ever be Solved?   14

Chapter 2   **The Long, Strange History of Psychoactive Drugs**   **17**

Opium: The Pleasures of Poppy Juice   19
     The first drug problem   20
     American inventions: the pipe and the syringe   21
     Opium Wars   23
     The "soldier's disease": morphine in the American Civil War   25
     A better morphine: codeine and heroin   26
     Addiction alarms   27

Marijuana: The Ancient Herb   30
     The big numb   30
     A woman's drug   31
     Hashish assassins?   31
     The sacred becomes profane   32
     Rope and dope   32
     Marihuana becomes marijuana   34
     Marijuana as medicine   34
     Modern recreational use   35

Cocaine: The Sacred Leaf   37
     Gift from the gods   37
     From coca to cocaine   38
     The drink of kings and popes   39
     Freudian slip   40
     Things don't go better with coke   41

Hallucinogens: Mind, Myth, and Madness   43
     Eleusian mysteries   43
     Fear of witches   44

Do hallucinogens cause hallucinations? 46
Set and setting 47
Military takes notice 48
Psychedelic therapy 49
Counterculture crackdown 50

Chapter 3   The War on Drugs   55
A Century of Increasing Drug Control 57
1906: Pure Food and Drug Act 58
1909: Smoking Opium Exclusion Act 58
1915: Harrison Narcotic Act 59
1917: The first War On Drugs 59
1920: Prohibition 60
1937: Marihuana Tax Act 61
1965: Drug Abuse Control Amendments 63
1970: Comprehensive Drug Abuse Prevention & Control Act 63
1972: Nixon's War on Drugs 64
1981: Reagan's War on Drugs 65
1984: Comprehensive Crime Control Act 67
1986: Anti-Drug Abuse Act 67
1986: Controlled Substances Analogue Enforcement Act 68
1993: Clinton's War on Drugs 69
2001: Bush's War on Drugs 71
How is a Drug Made Illegal? 72
How does a substance become a "drug of abuse"? 72
Five Schedules of Controlled Substances 72
Drugs Illegal in the United States 76
Schedule I Controlled Substances 76
Schedule II Controlled Substances 78
Federal and State Drug Laws 80
Types of drug crime 80
Federal drug penalties: marijuana 82
Federal drug penalties: other drugs 83
"But officer ...!" 84

Chapter 4   Drug Use and Abuse   87
The Notion of Substance Abuse 89
Types of illegal drug use 89
Drug Use Illnesses 90
Single-dose problems 90
Intravenous drug use 91
Overdose 93
Long-term problems 93
Withdrawal 94
Pregnancy 95
Addiction 95
Substance dependence 95
Stages of addiction 98
Stages of recovery 99
Twelve-step programs 100

Drug Resistance Educational Programs   101
    Fads and fashions   101
    Top ten reasons why people use illegal drugs   102
    Top ten reasons why people do not use illegal drugs   104

Chapter 5   **Drugs at Work: Employee Drug Testing**   **107**
Hazards of Drug Use in Industry   109
    Federal Regulations: the NIDA 5   112
Workplace Drug Monitoring   113
    Americans with Disabilities Act   113
    Drug testing programs   114
    How are people tested for drugs?   115
    Chain of custody   116
    Tampered specimens   117
    Laboratory analysis   118
Can Drug Tests Be Fooled?   119
    Adulteration products   119
    Diluted urine   121
    Legal medications that can cause positive drug tests   122
What Happens When A Drug Test Is Positive?   124

Chapter 6   **Chemicals and the Brain**   **127**
Quickest Way to the Brain   129
    How are drugs taken?   129
    Blood-brain barrier   131
    Mental road map   132
The Anatomy of a Neuron   134
    Mind and matter   134
    Electrical signals   134
Sending and Receiving Signals: Neurotransmitters   137
    Locks and keys   137
    Excitement and inhibition   137
    Acetylcholine   138
    Dopamine   139
    Epinephrine   139
    GABA and Glutamate   140
    Norepinephrine   140
    Opioids and endorphins   140
    Serotonin   141
    Drugs and their neurotransmitters   142
Natural, Synthetic, and Designer Drugs   142
    Natural drugs   143
    Synthetic drugs   143
    Designer drugs   144
    Testing drug purity   146
A Little Chemistry (Just Enough to Make Sense of It All)   148
    Simple molecules   148
    Breaking down a drug name   149
    Opiates and opioids   151

The amphetamine family   151
The indole hallucinogens   156
Metabolism of Drugs   157
Types of Tolerance   158
A Final Word: The Secret of Psychoactive Drugs   159
Contact high   160
Non-drug altered states of consciousness   160

Chapter 7   Just Say Know   163
Illegal Drug Use Today   165
By their drugs so shall ye know them   165
National drug surveys   166
Street terms and slang words   169
The Business of Illegal Drugs   173
Basic economics: supply and demand   173
Youth employment   174
Prostitution   175
Smuggling   175
World drug trade   176
Psychoactive Drugs That Are Not Illegal   177
Alcohol   177
Amanita muscaria   178
Amyl nitrate   178
Ayahuasca   179
Betel nuts   179
Broom   180
Caffeine   180
Calamus   181
California Poppy   182
Catnip   182
Coleus   182
Damiana   182
Datura   182
Dextromethorphan   183
Doña ana   183
Ephedra   184
Hawaiian baby wood rose   184
Henbane   184
Hops   185
Hydrangea   185
Inhalants   185
Kava kava   186
Ketamine   187
Lobelia   188
Mandrake   188
Morning Glory   188
Nitrous oxide   189
Nutmeg   189
Salvia divinorum   190

San Pedro 191
Tobacco 191
Trihexylphenidyl 193
Virola 193
Food for Thought 193

PART II Illegal Drugs From A to Z **195**

Alphabetical List of Drugs Illegal in the United States **197**

Amphetamines **203**
Speed: The Story of Amphetamines 205
From ephedra to amphetamine 205
Ice 208
The rise of Ritalin 208
Other amphetamine-like drugs 209
You can never be too thin 210
Who Is Using Amphetamines? 211
Meth labs 213
Pure speed? 215
Chemical Characteristics 216
Testing for amphetamines 217
Legal and illegal amphetamines 218
Withdrawal Signs 218
Long-term Health Problems 219
What To Do If There Is An Overdose 220

Barbiturates **223**
Dolls and Devils: The Story of Barbiturates 225
Three types of barbiturates 225
Valley of the Dolls 226
Downside of the downers 226
Who Is Using Barbiturates? 227
The choice of suicides 227
Chemical Characteristics 227
Testing for barbiturates 229
Withdrawal Signs 229
Long-term Health Problems 229
What To Do If There Is An Overdose 230

Cathinone **231**
Nine Lives of Cat: The Story of Cathinone 233
Migration of people and their drugs 234
Methcathinone 234
Who Is Using Cathinone? 235
Cat contaminants 236

Chemical Characteristics 236
Withdrawal Signs 237
Long-term Health Problems 237
What To Do If There Is An Overdose 237

Cocaine 239

Flake: The Story of Cocaine 241
   Chewing coca 242
   Coca becomes powder cocaine 242
   Powder cocaine becomes freebase 243
   Freebase becomes crack 244
Who Is Using Cocaine? 245
   Traditional use: *Coqueros* 246
   Medical use 246
   Recreational use 247
   The Colombian cartels 248
   From field to flake: the making of cocaine 249
   Economics of crack 250
   Pure coke? 251
Chemical Characteristics 253
   Cocaine and alcohol 254
   Testing for cocaine 254
Withdrawal Signs 255
Long-term Health Problems 256
   Cocaine nose 257
   Cocaine lungs 257
   Cocaine and the heart 257
   Cocaine and the brain 258
   Cocaine paranoia 258
   Cocaine babies 259
What To Do If There Is An Overdose 259

DMT, Bufotenine, and Psilocybin 263

Businessman's High: The Story of DMT 265
Who Is Using DMT? 266
Smoking Toad: The Story of Bufotenine 266
   Toxins and toadstools 267
   Mayan toad statues 267
   Toad licking in Australia 268
   Toad smoking in America 269
Who Is Using Bufotenine? 270
Magic Mushrooms: The Story of Psilocybin 270
Who is Using Psilocybin? 272
Chemical Characteristics 273
   DMT 273
   Bufotenine 274
   Psilocybin 274
Withdrawal Signs 275

Long-term Health Problems   275
What To Do If There Is An Overdose   275

Flunitrazepam   277

Roofies, Rape, and Robbery: The Story of Flunitrazepam   279
  The "forget-me" pill   280
  Easy prey   280
  La Rocha becomes illegal   280
Who Is Using Flunitrazepam?   281
  Why are roofies popular?   282
Chemical Characteristics   282
  Testing   283
Withdrawal Signs   283
Long-term Health Problems   284
What To Do If There Is An Overdose   284

GHB   285

Dancehall Depressant: The Story of GHB   287
  Body builders   288
  Raves   288
  GBL   289
  BD   289
Who Is Using GHB?   290
  Making GHB   290
  Medical uses   291
Chemical Characteristics   292
  Effects on the nervous system   293
  GHB and sleep   293
  Glasgow Coma Scale   294
  Effects on the heart   295
  Effects on the lungs   295
  Other effects   295
  Testing   296
Withdrawal Signs   296
Long-term Health Problems   296
What To Do If There Is An Overdose   297
  Emergency Department care   298

Ibogaine   299

Out of Africa: The Story of Ibogaine   301
  Anti-addiction potential   303
Who Is Using Ibogaine?   304
Chemical Characteristics   304
  Effects   305
Withdrawal Signs   305
Long-term Health Problems   305
What To Do If There Is An Overdose   305

LSD   **307**
    Acid: The Story of LSD   309
    Who Is Using LSD?   310
        Pure LSD?   312
    Chemical Characteristics   312
    Withdrawal Signs   314
    Long-term Health Problems   314
        Flashbacks   315
    What To Do If There Is An Overdose   316

Marijuana   **319**
    Up in Smoke: The Story of Marijuana   321
        Joints and blunts   322
        Acapulco Gold and Maui Wowie   322
        Sinsemilla   323
        Hashish   324
        Hash oil   325
        Superweed   325
        Medical marijuana   325
        Marinol: a medical substitute   327
        The debate continues   327
    Who Is Using Marijuana?   328
        Going Dutch   329
        Medical use   329
        NORML   330
    Chemical Characteristics   330
        Effects   331
        Marijuana and the brain   332
        Drug testing   333
    Withdrawal Signs   333
        Reverse tolerance   334
    Long-term Health Problems   334
        Marijuana and the immune system   334
        Other health problems   335
        Is marijuana addictive?   335
    What To Do If There Is An Overdose   335

MDMA   **337**
    Adam, Eve, and Ecstasy: The Story of MDMA   339
        From amphetamines to MDA   339
        Empathy agent   339
        Designer drugs   340
        Alphabet (and chemical) soup   342
        2C-B   343
    Who Is Using MDMA?   344
        Is that pill Ecstasy?   345
    Chemical Characteristics   346
        Effects   346

Ecstasy and sex 347
Nerve destruction 347
Withdrawal Signs 348
Terrible Tuesdays 348
Long-term Health Problems 348
Brain damage 349
What To Do If There Is An Overdose 349

Methaqualone and Glutethimide 351
'Luding Out: The Story of Methaqualone and Glutethimide 353
Who Is Using Methaqualone & Glutethimide? 355
Chemical Characteristics 355
Withdrawal Signs 356
Long-term Health Problems 357
What To Do If There Is An Overdose 357

Opiates 359
The First Narcotics: The Story of Opiates 361
Opium 361
Morphine 362
Codeine 363
Heroin 364
Medically Used and Abused Opiate Derivatives 365
Hydrocodone 365
Hydromorphone 366
Ketobimidone 366
Oxycodone 366
Thebaine 366
Tilidine 367
Opioids: Synthetic Narcotics 367
Anileridine 367
Etorphine 367
Fentanyl 367
LAAM 368
Meperidine 369
Methadone 369
Propoxyphene 370
Other illegal opioids 370
Who Is Using Opiates? 372
Purity of heroin 372
Another form of China White 375
Chemical Characteristics 375
Effects 376
Testing for opiates 377
Poppy seed positive 378
Withdrawal Signs 379
Treating opiate addiction 380
Ultra-rapid detox 381

Long-term Health Problems   382
What To Do If There Is An Overdose   383

PCP   **385**
Angel Dust: The Story of PCP   387
Who Is Using PCP?   388
Chemical Characteristics   389
    Testing for PCP   390
Withdrawal Signs   390
Long-term Health Problems   391
What To Do If There Is An Overdose   391

Peyote and Mescaline   **393**
Divine Cactus: The Story of Peyote and Mescaline   395
    Varieties of hallucinogenic cacti   396
    The flesh of God   397
    Mescaline   400
    Native American Church   401
    Why is peyote illegal?   405
Who Is Using Peyote and Mescaline?   408
    Inside an NAC peyote ceremony   409
    Mescaline use   410
Chemical Characteristics   410
Withdrawal Signs   411
Long-term Health Problems   411
What To Do If There Is An Overdose   412

PART III   **413**
Self-help Resources   414
    Drug identification   414
    Further information   414
    Drug abuse prevention and treatment coordinators 416
    DEA division offices   420
    National Guard counterdrug coordinators   421
    Drug demand reduction administrators   423
Notes and References   427
Index   443

Preface

A few years ago, I visited a friend in Lucerne, Switzerland. Rudi is a social worker whose specialty is heroin addicts. One evening, I helped him run a needle-exchange operation out of a large white van parked downtown. In only a few hours, we handed out 2,000 syringes. Although I should know better, I was incredulous to find that even the orderly Swiss with their postcard-perfect cities have so many drug addicts.

The next day, Rudi invited me to attend a meeting at the city hall to discuss the drug problem. The meeting was a formal affair, attended by the heads of the government, universities and industries to consider drug abuse programs. While Rudi networked with the politicians, the hostess brought me a glass of Dôle, a full-bodied red wine famous in the region. She then gave me a glass of Humagne, smiling sweetly, and assured me that it had a slightly more robust flavor. When she urged me to try the whites as well, I begged off, saying I had already had quite enough. But she was proud of the local wines and chided me for not sampling them, so I had a glass of Fendant, a glass of Muscat, and another of the Ermitage. By the time the meeting began, I had trouble focusing. Rudi grabbed my elbow and steered me to our seats.

A few minutes later, the moderator said, "We are pleased to have an American here tonight. Dr. Gahlinger, perhaps you could say a few words about your impressions of the drug problem in our city."

I shot a puzzled look at Rudi, who was doing his best to suppress a grin. There was no way out. I got up unsteadily, walked to the front of the room, and turned to face the audience of about 80 people. I desperately hoped that I could speak coherently.

"Thank you for your interest in my impressions," I began. Just as I was starting to get warmed up I shifted my left leg, which seemed to have gone to sleep, and stumbled a bit, catching myself from falling over. I hoped to God no one noticed. "The main problem with drugs in America is somewhat different," I said, and launched into a comparison between crack cocaine and heroin use. Since they asked me to speak, I felt that I ought to say something useful and went on to talk about the two real drug problems in our society: tobacco and ... *uh-oh*, ... I didn't like where this was going. I abruptly concluded—"The drug problem is extremely complex and has no easy solutions. Thank you"—and walked stiffly back to my seat, my face burning, followed by a wave of polite applause.

When we got out into the street, a merciful half hour later, I was ready to strangle Rudi. He threw up his arms, laughing. "I swear I didn't know they were going to call on you. But you did okay, I must say. Everyone was just waiting for you to fall over."

That experience left me with a lot to think about. It was hypocritical for me to talk about drug abuse while I was intoxicated myself, and it gave me a new perspective on the drug problem.

"The American Disease"
The United States has 4 percent of the world's population, but consumes 65 percent of the world's supply of hard drugs.

Why, I wondered, are some of the most injurious, addictive and mind-altering substances in the world—tobacco and alcohol—legal, when other drugs are illegal? Why is a drug legal in some countries and illegal in others? Why is marijuana smoking much less common in Holland, where it is not punished, than in the United States, where it is punished severely? And why do people continue to use illegal drugs even when they face prison sentences longer than those for murder?

Prison sentences in United States for murder (all degrees) and marijuana (large amount)[1]

Murder	6.3 years, average served Parole allowed
Marijuana	10 years, mandatory minimum No parole allowed

The average sentence for a first time, non-violent drug offender is longer than for rape, child molestation, bank robbery, or manslaughter.

In the United States, 178 substances have been declared illegal. These substances are believed to be so dangerous that they are controlled at the highest level for medical use—or forbidden outright, even for medical research. Remarkably, many of these are not physically harmful and have never caused a death. Yet, every year in the United States, tobacco kills 430,000 people. Another 200,000 people are killed by alcohol. In 1999, two million people were hospitalized and as many as 140,000 died from side effects or reactions to prescription drugs. Every year, legal drug use results in about 15 percent of all hospital admissions, with $136 billion in medical costs. It seems odd, then, to make such a big distinction between legal and illegal drugs.

In my research, I found that most people lean toward one of two attitudes to illegal drugs. The first is that it is a health issue. Non-medical drug use is considered an illness. It is called abuse to show that it is sick and wrong. People who hold this view often believe that drugs are inherently evil. They are a threat to the well-being of individuals and society. In this sense, drugs are like an infectious disease that must be stamped out by whatever means—even all-out war.

The second common attitude is that illegal drugs are the forbidden fruit. Risky behavior of any type has its own appeal; it is bold, adventurous, sensuous, and fun. These people believe that drug prohibition is unnecessarily severe. They argue that they should be allowed to use recreational drugs if they can do so in a responsible manner, in the same way that they are allowed to engage in other dangerous sports and pastimes.

 "Why do we not speak of 'ski abuse' or a 'chainsaw problem'? Because we expect people who use such equipment to familiarize themselves with their use, and avoid injuring themselves or others."—Thomas Szasz, Our Rights to Drugs, 1992

Both of these attitudes tend to be very strong, so that the topic of drugs, like sex and religion, has become difficult to discuss in an objective, rational manner. And as with sex and religion, there is plenty of hypocrisy. The first "drug czar," William Bennett, was addicted to tobacco while head of the Office of National Drug Control Policy, and some politicians rail against drug abuse and call for mandatory imprisonment even as they try to hide their own illegal drug use as "a private matter."

 Congressman Newt Gingrich, the Speaker of the House, proposed legislation that would impose the death penalty for people caught carrying as little as 2 ounces of marijuana. He excused his own past marijuana use by explaining that pot smoking "was a sign that we were alive and in graduate school in that era."

Many young people, in particular, take drugs as a way of demonstrating their individuality. They are making a statement, "I am responsible for my own decisions." The problem is that they know very little about the drugs they are taking. They are not helped by people who try to discourage drug abuse, but have little to say except that drugs are bad because they are illegal. The result is a general level of ignorance that does not diminish use and increases harm.

My purpose in writing this book is simple: to provide knowledge. Psychoactive drugs are, and have always been, a feature of every society and should be recognized as such. Since recreational drug use is inevitable, threats of ever-increasing penalties, scare tactics, and "just say no" lectures will do little to stop it. The simple fact is that humans like to alter their consciousness. The goal, then, is not to stop all drug use (which is impossible), but to reduce harm. This is best done by education.

As a physician, I know that psychoactive drugs are dangerous but can also be useful for specific purposes. I have seen morphine kill people and, during my years in the Emergency Department, I have seen it save countless lives. I have seen people destroy themselves with cocaine, and I have applied cocaine to stop bleeding in patients who might have hemorrhaged to death without it. In the hospice, I have seen terminally ill patients with terrible suffering relieved by heroin—and for these people, I am thankful that such a drug exists. Clearly, these drugs have the potential for both great benefit and great harm.

Everyone has a bias, and I readily admit my own. I believe the War on Drugs has been a failure: drug supply interdiction and the imprisonment of over a million Americans have not been effective in reducing drug use. And yet, these substances should be restricted. Like firearms or rattlesnakes,

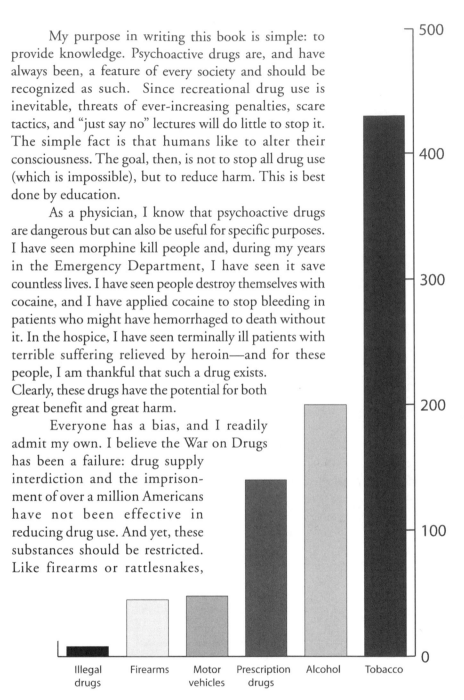

Thousands of deaths caused each year in the United States

drugs can cause a lot of harm in foolish hands, but this does not mean that they have no use or should be illegal. In my opinion, the best solution to the drug problem begins with education.

The research for this book was helped enormously by too many people to list here. I was very fortunate to have advice from DEA officers and administrators, substance abuse counselors, leaders of the Native American Church, and drug users and addicts of every type—each of whom was encouraging and supportive of my effort. In particular, I would like to thank the faculty and my students in the Departments of Pharmacology and Family and Preventive Medicine, University of Utah, for comments on the manuscript. Finally, this book would not exist without the extraordinary help and encouragement of Lesley Baxter, the editor and design consultant at Sagebrush Press.

I am very grateful to the U.S. Drug Enforcement Administration for allowing me to take photographs of drug evidence and museum materials, and for permission to reproduce illustrations from their extensive archives.

In the process of trying to verify information from the literature, I was appalled at how much of it proved to be wrong. Many authors simply repeat errors, adding links to a chain of misinformation that eventually becomes accepted as fact and contributes to the widespread misunderstandings about drugs. Despite my attempts to be accurate, inevitably some errors will remain; I would be very appreciative to readers who could point out corrections for future editions.

It is my hope that this book will be useful to everyone looking for an objective understanding of illegal drugs.

> "It should be our earnest intention to insure that drugs
> not be employed to debase mankind, but to serve it."
> —John F. Kennedy

PART I

Forbidden Fruit

"Psychedelic drugs are a way of entering the
country of lunatics, lovers, poets, and mystics."
—*Sadie Plant, Writing On Drugs* [1]

"When drugs change their users, they change everything."
——*Lester Grinspoon and James B. Bakalar, Psychedelic Drugs Reconsidered* [2]

Adam and Eve, Lucas Cranach the Elder, 1526

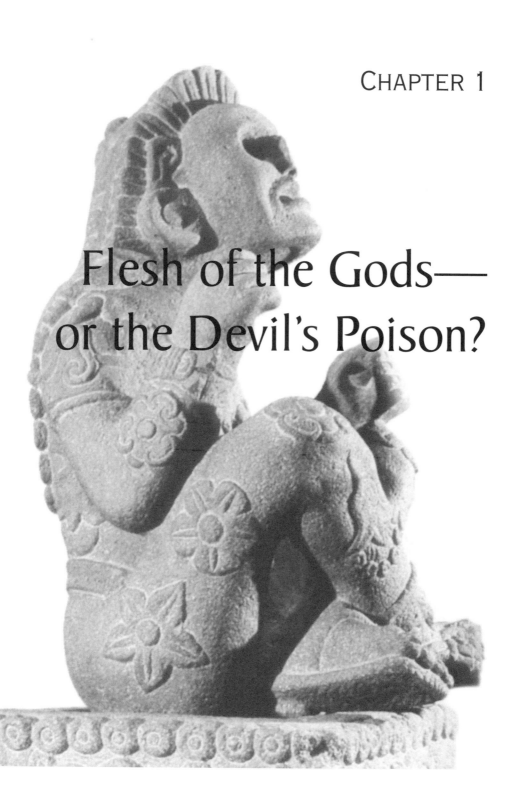

CHAPTER 1

Flesh of the Gods—
or the Devil's Poison?

"The desire to take medicine is perhaps the greatest feature which distinguishes man from animals."—*Sir William Osler* [3]

Aztec god Xochipilli, the "prince of flowers", surrounded by hallucinogenic plants

The Discovery of Drugs

The origin of drug use is quite simple. Humans are inquisitive creatures. If something can be done—no matter how bizarre, silly, or dangerous—somebody, somewhere, will try to do it. If a substance can possibly be eaten, it is certain that somebody will have tried to eat it. Why, for example, would anyone lick the slime off an ugly toad? And why, when it was found that swallowing this slime caused horrendous sickness and nightmare visions, would someone decide to smoke the secretions instead? Yet that is exactly what happened (see *Bufotenine*), and it led to the discovery of yet another mind-altering substance.

Eating unknown substances for no good reason can be very hazardous, but it is just one manifestation of the bold, adventurous attitude that has been largely responsible for the success of the human species. Early Americans discovered over 80 different mind-altering plants. How did they find these? Were they told by God or a spirit, or by the plant itself, as their legends say? More likely, they found them out of simple curiosity and experimentation; the same persistent curiosity and relentless experimentation that led to the tremendous variety of foods in the world.

 Of the half million or so known species of plants, about 150 have been used for hallucinatory effects.

Even animals, both domesticated and wild, will seek out intoxicating foods, such as fermented fruits and psychoactive plants.[4] The archeological record shows that mind-altering drugs have been used by all people who have had access to them. Early humans discovered that eating some plants gave a feeling of relaxation, happiness, drowsiness, or peace. Some gave a feeling of increased energy, alertness, and stamina. And some caused strange sensations, terrifying visions, or a profoundly different awareness.

Drugs were used by the Neanderthal people long before modern humans had evolved, as shown by archeological remains discovered in the Shanidar cave in Iraq dated to 50,000 years ago. As people wandered into new lands and climates, they discovered many more of these substances—some came to be enjoyed, some feared, and some reserved only for religious use. Whether they are used for medicine, pleasure, religion, or curiosity, drugs have become an integral part of human life.

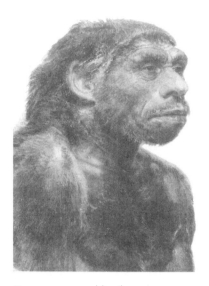

Drugs were used by the Neanderthal people 50,000 years ago

SUBSTANCES AND SPIRITS

Psychoactive drugs have always been closely associated with religion. In early belief systems, any substance with the ability to prevent or cure disease was considered sacred. The ancient texts from many lands—India, China, Egypt, Greece, and the Americas—are filled with references to drugs. The sacred scriptures of India, for example, contain over 1,000 hymns in praise of *Soma*, the psychedelic mushroom. Some biblical scholars claim that the Bible makes mention of marijuana, and that *Manna* of the Exodus may have been a hallucinogenic mushroom.

Since drugs that healed were evidence of God, drugs with the ability to cause illness—poisons— came to be considered the work of the devil. This is reflected in folk names for plants. The hallucinogenic flower *Datura*, for example, is known as "devil's weed," "devil's apple," "*yerba del Diablo*," and similar names in other languages.

As knowledge of both beneficial and harmful drugs grew, people with particular knowledge of these drugs also specialized. Medicinal drugs were studied by herbalists and apothecaries, later to become physicians (from the Greek *physikos*, "science of nature"; doctor is from the Latin *docere*, "to teach") and pharmacists (from the Greek *pharmakon*, "drug"). In every society, beneficial drugs became the specialty of healers, mind-altering drugs became the specialty of shamans or priests, and poisons became the specialty of sorcerers and witches (and today's toxicologists).

Religious practices and psychoactive drugs can produce both mind-altering states and ecstasy—from the Greek word *ekstasis*, the flight of the soul from the body.

For psychoactive drugs, social and religious rituals arose as a way of controlling their use. By allowing these drugs to be used only on certain occasions, or by certain people, the general population could be protected from harm.

Spirit refers to the vital principle, whether in humans or in a substance. From the Latin *spiritus*, "breath," this ghostly essence was also recognized in the smoke or distilled fluid of plant materials.

A plant with mind-altering effects was often considered to have a supernatural force. It was not the plant that caused the mental effects, but its spirit—a person might benefit from the plant's spirit just by holding the material in the hand, placing it on the forehead, or carrying it in an amulet. Over time, the spirit was discovered to reside not in the whole plant, but in a specific part of it. For example, the most powerful part of the opium poppy was found to be in the bulb. Later, it was determined to be not in the entire bulb, but in the dried sap, and then, finally, in an alcohol tincture of this gummy substance. By this process, the active material was extracted, purified, and increasingly refined. Crude herbs became teas and tinctures, powders and oils. With each step, the purity was enhanced, the potency increased, and the plant was transformed into a more effective drug.

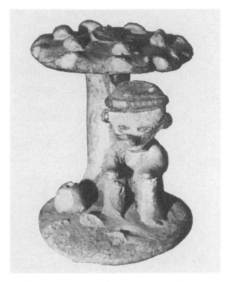

Hallucinogenic mushrooms were known to the Aztecs as Teonanacatl, "divine flesh." This miniature found in Nayarit, Mexico, dated 100 AD, shows a shaman underneath Amanita muscaria.

The process continues in modern drug research. Plants, crude drugs, and herbal compounds are broken down into their constituent chemicals. Each chemical is then analyzed, compared to known chemicals, and its molecular structure determined. Novel or interesting chemicals can then be extracted and purified for further study. Once the structure of a chemical is known, it can be synthesized in the laboratory without further need for the original source. New variations of this synthetic chemical can then be studied for yet more powerful effects.

A drug evolves

Drug	Material	Type	Date discovered
Opium poppy	whole plant	herb	~ 10000 BC
Poppy bulb	plant part	herb	~ 4000 BC
Bulb sap	part extract	herb	~ 3000 BC
Gum opium	dried extract	herb	~ 1000 BC
Laudanum	tincture of dried extract	pharmaceutical	1524
Morphine	chemical from tincture	pharmaceutical	1803
Heroin (diacetyl-morphine)	modified chemical	pharmaceutical	1874
Fentanyl	synthesized opioid	pharmaceutical	1953
3-methyl-fentanyl ("China White")	fentanyl analogue	designer drug	1979

THE DOSE MAKES THE POISON

According to pharmacological science, a drug is defined as "a chemical substance used in the treatment, cure, prevention, or diagnosis of disease or used to otherwise enhance physical or mental well-being."[5] In more common usage, a drug is any substance that in small amounts produces noticeable changes in the body or mind.

Pill comes from the Latin *pillula* meaning "little ball." It refers to a practice that originated in ancient Egypt when drugs were mashed up with bread or clay into a ball to make them easier to swallow.

If a drug helps the body, it is considered a medicine. If it injures the body, it is called a poison. In fact, the difference between a medication and a poison is not that simple. Toxin, from the Greek for "poison arrow," indicates a biologically harmful chemical. Deciding whether a substance is a good drug or a toxin, however, is like deciding whether a particular sound is music or noise—it depends on whether you want to hear it. There are drugs whose purpose it is to cause vomiting or even to kill parts of the body, but their beneficial value outweighs their harm and so they are considered to be medications. There are other substances whose only effect is to induce a dreamy state of mind, but these might be classified as poisons. All drugs become harmful in high enough doses, and many poisonous substances can be useful drugs in very low doses.[6]

A drug is any substance that changes mental state or bodily function.[7] The words drug and dope come from the old Dutch *droog*, "dried powder," and *doop*, "sauce."

A drug's potency dictates how much is needed to cause an effect. For example, at least an ounce or so of alcohol (roughly the amount in a double shot of liquor, a glass of wine, or a pint of beer) must be taken to produce a noticeable change in a person's behavior, while as little as 25 micrograms of LSD will have an equally strong effect. LSD is therefore about one million times more potent than alcohol. A more potent drug is more likely to be poisonous because an excessive dose is more likely to be taken.

"To ask whether one drug is more dangerous than another is like asking whether it is more dangerous to fly a plane than to sail a boat: the question cannot be answered without a great deal more information about the nature of the voyage and the skills, temperaments, and intentions of the travelers."—*Psychedelic Drugs Reconsidered* [8]

Illegal drugs are not necessarily those that are most poisonous, but those that result in other hazards such as addiction or inappropriate behavior. If a drug causes someone to act in ways that are offensive to others, it presents a threat not only to the individual but to the whole society. To protect the well-being of society, these drugs are prohibited.

 "All substances are poisons; there is none which is not a poison. The right dose differentiates a poison and a remedy."
—Paracelsus (1493-1541)

 "In wise hands, poison is medicine. In foolish hands, medicine is a poison."—Casanova (1725-1798), expert in human behavior

USE AND ABUSE: THE FOUR TYPES OF DRUG

For practical purposes, any drug may be considered as belonging to one of four types:

No medical value, no abuse

These drugs do not have a well-established medicinal value, but pose little danger of abuse. Many readily available herbal remedies and homeopathic treatments fall into this category. Their manufacturers are not allowed to claim on the label that the drug has any medicinal value.

Medical value, no abuse

Drugs that have medicinal value, but are not commonly abused. These medications include the majority of over-the-counter remedies and prescription medications. A physician's prescription may be required to avoid incorrect use, not abuse. Anticancer drugs, for example, have little risk of abuse, but can cause severe illness if used inappropriately.

Medical value, high abuse

Drugs that have medicinal value, but also have a high risk of abuse. These drugs are specified in the Controlled Substances Act (CSA, see *Chapter 3*). To prescribe them, a physician requires a license from the Drug Enforcement Administration. Controlled substances are listed in five Schedules, based on their abuse potential. Those listed in Schedule V have the lowest risk of abuse and include medicines such as cough syrup with dextromethorphan. Drugs in Schedules IV and III have an increasing likelihood of abuse. Schedule II drugs have a very high abuse potential but also have some use as medicines, and include drugs such as cocaine and morphine.

No medical value, high abuse

Drugs that have no accepted medicinal value, and a high risk of abuse. These drugs are listed in Schedule I of the CSA. They are illegal except for use in extremely limited circumstances, such as authorized research. Schedule I drugs include heroin, LSD, and marijuana.

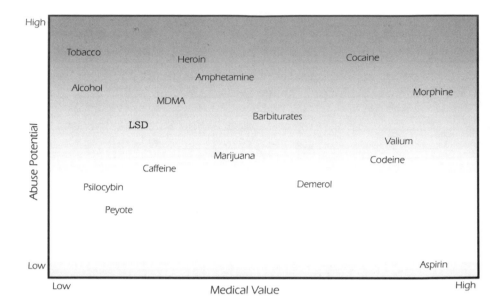

CONTROLLED SUBSTANCES

All drugs illegal in the United States can be considered psychoactive drugs, because all of them affect the central nervous system. In the Controlled Substances Act, they are organized into four basic categories:

Opiates and opioids

Opiates are drugs derived from opium. They are among the oldest drugs in existence and were the first to be seen as a major public health threat. They include heroin, morphine, and codeine.

Opioids are completely synthetic drugs and are not derived from opium. However, they are similar to the opiates in their chemical structure and biological effects. Common opioids include meperidine (Demerol), and fentanyl.

For convenience, the term opiates usually refers to both opiates and opioids. There are many variations and derivatives of opiates—this category accounts for 122 of the 178 drugs that are illegal in the United States.

 Hallucinogens consist of a number of different and unrelated drugs that can alter perceptions. They rarely, however, produce true hallucinations.

Hallucinogens

These drugs are sometimes called psychedelics or psychomimetics. They are grouped in this category because their chief feature is to cause altered perceptions. Well-known members include LSD, PCP, psilocybin, mescaline, and marijuana.

Hallucinogen is the designation used by the U.S. Government and also the most common term in medical research. There are several objections to the term. By referring primarily to visual distortions or other changes in sensation, the importance of mood and thought changes is understated. Some drugs classified as hallucinogens (such as MDA, DOET, etc.) can enhance self-awareness and intensify feelings without producing sensory changes at all.

Stimulants
This is a general category of drugs that excite the central nervous system. Often referred to as "uppers," they include cocaine, amphetamine, and MDMA.

Depressants
These drugs inhibit the central nervous system. They include sedatives (with calming and relaxing effects) and hypnotics (sleeping pills) and are often referred to as "downers." Barbiturates and GHB fall into this category.

HOW ARE DRUGS NAMED?

A drug can have many names. The chemical name describes the molecule. The generic name is a shorter, simpler name that is assigned to the substance by conventional agreement. The trade name is the trademark for a drug registered by the company that produces it, and it often varies between countries because of trademark laws. Finally, the drug can have popular or street names, which differ among people, places, and times.

Confusing? Consider a typical drug such as amphetamine, which is a generic name for the substance. It is known to chemists as phenyl-isopropylamine, its chemical name. Pharmaceutical companies sold it under trade names such as Benzedrine and Obetrol. Later, when it became a popular recreational drug, it was called by street names such as speed, bennies, and pep pills.

Why Are Some Drugs Illegal?

There are 178 drugs classified as illegal in the United States. Most of these are obscure chemicals that the public, physicians, and even substance abuse professionals have never heard of. A few of the better-known illegal drugs are highly addictive substances, such as heroin, cocaine, and methamphetamine. Many others are materials used in the manufacture of drugs, and may be listed only by their chemical names. Some drugs are illegal largely for historical or political reasons and there is little evidence of their abuse or, indeed, of any use at all. Peyote, for example, has no history of significant abuse, and ibogaine is virtually unknown in the United States.

All 178 illegal drugs are considered to cause severe harm: to the user, to others, or to society. Much of the supposed danger of these drugs is often disputed. Because they are illegal, however, it is almost impossible to conduct the research necessary to prove that they may be used safely.

 Because of strict security requirements, it is very difficult for scientists to obtain permission to carry out research involving illegal drugs.

DANGER TO SELF

A dangerous drug is one that is toxic—injuring the body or mind—or causes harm to the functioning of a person. However, toxic drugs are not always regulated by the Government and may not be illegal. For example, solvent inhalers, such as gasoline, glue, and paint thinners, are extremely toxic when used to get high, but they are not illegal because they also have many practical uses. Alcohol, tobacco, and caffeine can also be very toxic, but they are not illegal because they are an accepted part of American culture.

 In 1996, an estimated 10 to 12 million Americans suffered from alcoholism, and about 55 million smokers were addicted to tobacco. Alcohol kills about 200,000 people a year in the United States, and tobacco kills about 430,000 per year. In comparison, 5,000 to 8,000 are killed by all illegal drugs combined.

The drugs that have been made illegal are not only hazardous, but also have no long-standing social use, and a high abuse potential.

DANGER TO OTHERS

Illegal drugs are restricted because they are a threat not only to the health of the individuals using them, but also to their families and to the rest of society. This is especially so of addictive drugs. The greatest danger of these drugs is not to the physical health of addicts, but to their mental state. Addiction results in unpredictable or compulsive behavior that can bring enormous suffering to an addict's family, friends, and co-workers.

DANGER TO SOCIETY

Some drugs, it is argued, are illegal because they are mainly a political threat. This has been true for all psychoactive drugs throughout history. Drugs that change thoughts or behavior can make people less respectful of regulations and traditions. The drug users therefore become harder to control. These drugs may be physically harmless, but a threat to society if they lead to a breakdown in social harmony. In the 1960s, many hallucinogenic drugs were declared illegal because of this concern.

Alcohol and tobacco, for example, are far more dangerous to health than any of the illegal drugs, but they are socially tolerable. In fact, alcohol is often considered to enhance sociability, and tobacco also has a strong, although more subtle, social appeal. In contrast, most of the illegal drugs cause people to withdraw. Opiates and depressants produce an isolating numbness, hallucinogens bring psychotic dissociation, and stimulants can cause violent antisocial behavior. For this reason, despite the very few deaths from illegal drugs, they are feared more than the much more physically dangerous tobacco and alcohol.

 "Wine makes men happy and sociable; hashish isolates them."
—*Charles Baudelaire (1821-1867), French poet and critic*

 "As long as one has this stuff, one doesn't want friends."
—*Oscar Wilde (1854-1900), writing about opium*

DRUG TERMS

What is meant by an *illegal* drug? Drugs may be restricted at any level of government or authority: national, state, county, down to an individual institution or work site. For example, even possession of an aspirin may be a punishable offence in a school or prison. In this book, illegal drugs are those classified as Schedule I and II substances in the CSA. Without proper authorization, possession of these drugs is a felony offence under Federal law. At this time, $40 billion is spent by the U.S. Government each year to control these drugs.

 Illicit drugs are not necessarily illegal. Illicit use is when a drug is taken outside its regulated or medically prescribed use.

It is often thought that illegal drugs are the same as narcotics, recreational drugs, psychoactive drugs or psychedelics. In fact, these are different categories of drug, although there is much overlap among them. Not all are illegal.

 According to Ronald Reagan's Presidential Executive Order 12564, illegal drugs refers to substances in Schedule I and Schedule II of the CSA.

Drugs of abuse is a common term to refer to recreational drugs, but really means any drug, legal or illegal, that is used in an irresponsible or harmful way. Not all recreational drugs (such as caffeine) are abused, and medicines (such as common pain relief medications) are often abused.

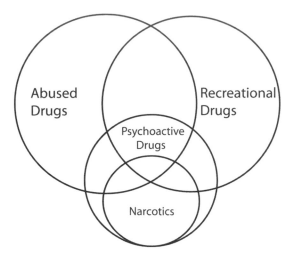

Abused, psychoactive, recreational, and narcotic drugs are not all the same, but there is much overlap among these categories.

Psychoactive drugs are those that affect the central nervous system and therefore stimulate or dull the senses, promote a feeling of euphoria, or alter perception. Many are used recreationally, but not all of them are illegal (see *Chapter 7*). Alcohol is a common psychoactive drug, but if used responsibly would not be considered to be abused.

Recreational drugs are drugs taken for non-medical purposes, usually for pleasure, and not all are illegal. Tobacco and caffeine are the most common recreational drugs.

Narcotic, by its medical definition, refers specifically to drugs related to opium or its synthetic forms. The word comes from the Greek *narkotikos*, meaning "to numb." Because narcotics were the first drugs to be controlled by international agreement, the term is often used loosely to refer to all illegal drugs. Many illegal drugs are not opiates, however, and some opiates have no significant psychoactive effects and are not illegal.

 More than 4,000 plants yield psychoactive substances. About 60 have been in constant use for thousands of years.[9]

Will the "Drug Problem" Ever be Solved?

No.

It is inevitable that people will want to take substances that are forbidden. The only question is to what extent the health of both the drug-user and the rest of society can be protected.

Drug use is a public health problem. It should be viewed in the same manner as any other health problem, such as infectious disease, motor vehicle accidents, or firearm injuries. In each case, there are issues of tradition, of personal freedom and responsibility, and a real or perceived threat to others in society.

Every society that has ever existed has used mind-altering drugs, although not all individuals in a society may choose to participate. The only possible exception has been the traditional Inuit (formerly called Eskimo) of the far North, and some isolated Pacific Islanders, who had no access to these substances. Once these people did have access to drugs, beginning with alcohol, they adopted them quickly and have suffered a devastatingly high rate of alcoholism and drug abuse problems ever since.

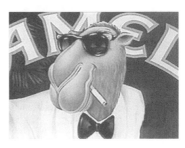

After the highly successful R.J. Reynolds tobacco advertisements, more kids recognized Joe Camel than Mickey Mouse.

The question then becomes not whether drugs will be used, but which drugs will be used. Different societies, different ethnic or social groups within a society, and even different age groups within a social group, all have their preferences. In an imaginary typical American family, dad likes to drink Scotch to unwind after work, mom can't get going in the morning without a cup of coffee, their eldest son smokes a joint with his buddies, their daughter smokes tobacco and is taking Ma Huang to stay as thin as possible, and the younger kids are increasingly likely to be on Ritalin. None of them would consider using any of each other's drugs, and probably all of them think they are only engaging in a harmless practice.

 95% of the adult US population is currently using some type of psychoactive drug, including prescription drugs.

It may be true that people simply want some drugs, any drugs, to provide a little buzz, a little variety in life. If one is not available, another will do. As the French say, "*On s'occupe à quelque chose,*" which roughly translates to, "Everyone is into something." Once they are accustomed to a drug, however, they are likely to stay with it. Despite the "gateway" theory that using one drug is a slippery slope to using many others, it has been shown that most people develop a preference, usually during adolescence, and stick to it. This is why alcohol and tobacco companies target the young so aggressively.

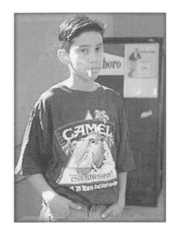

It also appears that forbidding one drug may well increase the use of another. In the high school population since 1991, educational intervention and extreme penalties have caused a decline in the usage of some drugs, such as barbiturates and cocaine, but similar effects are gained from GHB and MDMA (Ecstasy), respectively, and the use of these new drugs has dramatically risen as if to compensate.[10]

Internationally, recreational drugs tend to be more popular in industrialized countries, and the more aggressive and economically successful the nation, the wider its use of drugs. Perhaps the very qualities that contribute to the strength of a people—innovation, independence, and exploration—also encourage them to rebel against drug laws. If something is forbidden, that alone seems to be reason enough for some individuals to try it. Is it surprising, then, that countries with the technology to challenge human limits to explore outer space are also those most likely to use artificial means to explore inner space?

CHAPTER 2

The Long, Strange History of Psychoactive Drugs

"… in an hour, O heavens! … Here was a panacea for all human woes;
here was the secret of happiness."—*Thomas De Quincey,
Confessions of an English Opium Eater, 1821*

Opium: The Pleasures of Poppy Juice

The known history of drugs begins with the opiates, the true narcotics. The first evidence of their use was discovered in Mesopotamia, roughly at the site of the biblical Garden of Eden, and dates to 4,000 BC—about the time, coincidentally, that fundamentalist Christians believe the world was created.

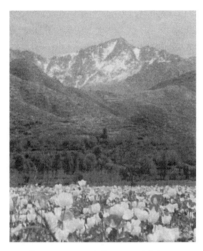

Opium poppy farm in Afghanistan

Six thousand years later, opiates are the world's greatest narcotic problem and control of these drugs influences global politics. Even so, the opiates have kept their place in the medicine chest and are stocked in every hospital and carried in every ambulance.

Opium is the milky white fluid that drips from the cut bulb of the ripening opium poppy. It was boiled to a sticky gum and chewed, burned and inhaled, or mixed with fermented liquids and drunk. Opium preparations are described in the Thebes papyrus of 1552 BC, which recommends their use in over 700 remedies. Hippocrates, the Father of Medicine, wrote about poppy juice and its value to take away pain. In the *Odyssey*, written about 800 BC, Homer spoke about an opium mixture he called *nepenthe*, given by Helen of Troy to Telemachus "to lull all pain and bring forgetfulness of grief."

 More than 6,000 years ago, the Sumerians, living in present-day Iran, cultivated the opium poppy. They named it *hal gil*, "the joy plant."

Romans, and their enemies, viewed opium not only as a painkiller but also as a poison—especially as a pleasant means of suicide. The Carthaginian General Hannibal kept a dose in his ring and used it to end his life in 183 BC.

 Opium comes from the Greek word *opòs*, meaning juice or sap.

In 1524, Paracelsus, the Swiss physician often regarded as the Father of Scientific Medicine, returned from Constantinople to Western Europe with a new concoction, a tincture of opium in alcohol. He called it *laudanum*, "to be

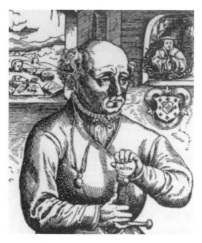

Paracelsus (1493-1541), discovered laudanum

praised." Because opium has an extremely bitter taste, the tincture was mixed with honey, nutmeg, cardamom, cinnamon, or other spices. In Europe, laudanum was commonly prepared by dissolving opium in red wine or port. It was soon used throughout the continent, becoming the cure for every ailment and sometimes for no ailment at all. Victorian literature is filled with references to laudanum, from the tales of Sherlock Holmes to Scrooge, who drank it in Charles Dickens' *A Christmas Carol.*

Before 1800, opium was available in America as laudanum (in alcohol), or as "black drop," containing no alcohol. It was also an ingredient in countless multi-drug preparations. Opium was valued not only for its calming effects but also as a specific remedy for gastrointestinal illnesses such as cholera, food poisoning and parasites, all of which were very common in the Americas.

 "When the payne is grete, then it is nedefull to put thereto a lytell Opium."—*Jerome of Brunswick, 1525*

THE FIRST DRUG PROBLEM

Although opium medicines were widely available throughout the world by the mid-19th century, abuse and addiction seldom aroused much concern. It is not that people were unaware of the trouble opium could cause. Thousands of years earlier, ancient Egyptian medical texts had referred to opium as both a medicine and a poison and warned of its habit-forming nature.[1] By the Victorian era, opium addiction was well known. It was considered to be an uncomfortable, but not especially dangerous, personal characteristic, like addiction to tobacco. It was simply not given a great deal of thought.

 Benjamin Franklin died while addicted to opium, which he had started taking for his gout. At the time, opium dependence was considered to be mostly harmless, like addiction to tobacco.

Addiction was given wider attention with the publication in 1821 of Thomas de Quincey's *Confessions of an English Opium Eater.* The son of a well-to-do family, de Quincey discovered opium as a 17-year-old college student. He struggled with addiction for the rest of his life, first extolling the wonders of opium—"Divine Poppy-juice, as indispensable as breathing"—and then terrified by the nightmares and paranoia that followed, believing he was buried alive and "kissed cancerous kisses by crocodiles."

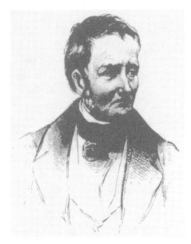

Despite opium's widespread use, addiction did not become a major social problem. Taken by mouth, as a syrup, tincture, or hard substance, it had a relatively mild and sustained effect. In contrast, most addictive drugs tend to have a rapid, short-lasting effect, which stimulates the user to take more in an effort to regain the fleeting euphoria. Because of its oral use, only the consistent and long-term ingesting of opium created dependency, and addicts such as de Quincey were relatively few. This was to change in the middle of the 19th century because of two American inventions: one old, one new.

Thomas de Quincey (1785-1859)

AMERICAN INVENTIONS: THE PIPE AND THE SYRINGE

As opium spread throughout the early United States, opiate use in turn was transformed by two instruments: the smoking pipe and the hypodermic syringe. Both of these provided a much more rapid and intense way of experiencing the drug, and led to a dramatic increase in abuse and addiction.

 The global drug epidemic was largely created by the smoking pipe and the hypodermic syringe.

In ancient times, intoxication by smoke was common, not only in the Americas but in Europe and Asia. It involved leaning over a fire or sitting in a smoke-filled room or tent to inhale the fumes and vapors. Marijuana was used this way for thousands of years, and it is likely that the smoke of many other substances was deliberately inhaled.

The invention of the pipe brought an enormously more efficient way of inhaling a drug. It is not clear exactly when or where it originated, but it did not exist outside the Americas until the voyage of Columbus in 1492. Archeologists believe that the pipe was first developed by the Indians of the Ohio River Valley sometime around the 2nd century BC, and then spread throughout the continent.

The cigarette has a history slightly independent of the pipe. Aztecs and other native peoples from Mexico to South America were known to roll crushed tobacco leaves in wrappers of corn and other vegetables. The conquistadors brought this novelty back to Spain, and called the rolled tobacco leaves *cigars*. By the 16th century, beggars in Seville had begun to pick up discarded cigar butts, shred them, and roll them in scraps of paper. These cheap *cigarillos* spread throughout the continent. During the Napoleonic Wars, the French soldiers named them *cigarettes*.

The pipe was—and still is—a sacred instrument to Native Americans. The bowl symbolizes the female element of the earth; the long stem inserted into the bowl symbolizes the male element. The bowl cups and holds the smoking mixture in a tender embrace, allowing the spirit of the material to turn into a diaphanous smoke that passes into the user. Smoke was the spirit made visible.

A great number of plants were smoked. The smoke of white sage and cedar was used to bless and sanctify a living space. Tobacco, the "grandfather," was the most sacred and important of all. The tobacco pipe was an object of profound veneration. It was smoked in personal prayer and on all ceremonial occasions. It served as a means of communication between humans and the spiritual world.

Columbus's views of the pipe were probably somewhat more prosaic. He took pipes and tobacco (as well as a number of captured slaves) back to Europe to show off what he had found. In Britain, tobacco was at first distrusted and subsequently outlawed by King James I. Eventually, however, as more people acquired the smoking habit, the practice was allowed and tobacco became one of the most common European drugs.

 When Columbus set sail on his first voyage to reach the Indies, he was told to bring back opium. He brought back tobacco instead.

The advantage of using the pipe with other drugs was also quickly noticed. Smoking was a radically more effective method of taking a drug than the previous method of taking it by mouth. When a drug is swallowed, it first goes to the stomach, where it is dissolved in acids. After the stomach, it is further dissolved by other intestinal fluids before being absorbed into the blood stream. Most intestinal blood goes to the liver, whose job it is to detoxify the absorbed substances. Unfortunately for the user, much of the effect of a swallowed drug is lost at every stage of this process (and it doesn't do much good to the liver, either) before the precious substance ever reaches the brain. In contrast, a drug from smoke is absorbed within seconds. It passes almost immediately from the lungs into blood that goes straight to the brain. The effect of smoking a mixture is even faster than injecting it directly into the bloodstream (see *Chapter 6*). Smoking a drug also has other effects that are pharmacologically important. The heat of combustion breaks down a drug preparation—destroying some components, freeing others, and even creating new intoxicating compounds that were not present in the original substance.

Smoking opium was slow to gain popularity. While tobacco gives a pleasant smoke, burned opium produces a dry, harsh and bitter smoke. On the other hand, smoked opium gave a far more rapid and intense effect to those willing to tolerate the bitter fumes. The problem was partially solved when the Chinese replaced the short-handled tobacco pipe with a longer-handled pipe—more like the traditional North American pipe. The typical opium pipe had

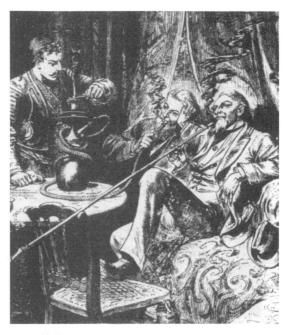

The introduction of the pipe to Europe and Asia in the 16th century started the practice of smoking opium. Until then, opium was primarily ingested.

an 18 to 24 inch-long hollow shaft of bamboo or ebony, which allowed the hot, irritating smoke to cool before it was inhaled. Yet further refinement of the opium pipe led to the development of the water pipe, the *hookah*, in which the smoke was bubbled through a chamber of water, wine, or other liquids. Water pipes helped cool the smoke, filtered some of the objectionable elements, and added a soothing softness or aroma to the smoke. Not surprisingly, the new pipes were a big hit with the opium addicts.

OPIUM WARS

Opium was brought to China by Arabic traders over the Silk Route during the 8th-century T'ang dynasty. It was used mainly as a medicinal herb. By 1746, descriptions began to appear of smoking opium—and accompanying alarms of addiction.

Some of this opium was traded from Indonesia, where Chinese merchants were active, but most of it came from India. By the 1830s, the opium habit was associated with so much crime and corruption that the Chinese Government reacted, banning its use and importation. Stores of opium were confiscated and warehouses were closed down. Community health slogans were painted everywhere to warn people of the dangers of opium. But government repression and public education were not enough to shut down the opium industry. By the end of the century, half of the adult male population of China was addicted and the economy and morale of the country was devastated.

The Chinese character *Yin* means to crave opium. From it came the English word yen, a desire or craving.

To understand the Chinese struggle with opium, it is necessary to consider an entirely different drug: tea. Every country has its recreational drugs. For the British Empire, which at the height of the Victorian era controlled fully two-thirds of the entire globe, the drug of choice was tea.

Tea came from China, and England imported vast quantities of the dried leaves. Unfortunately, the trade was largely in one direction as the Chinese had little demand for English products. The result was a steady drain of British silver to pay for the tea. Then, as India came under British domination, a solution became obvious for the British trade imbalance. In a three-way exchange, Britain sold manufactured goods to India, India exported opium and cotton to China, and China shipped tea to Britain. The arrangement worked well for Britain and India, but the Chinese were considerably less enthusiastic. Their sale of tea to the British had brought in a net surplus, but soon it was no longer enough to balance the growing demand for opium. It was China's turn to face a loss of silver reserves, as money flowed out of the country to pay for the imported drugs.

"Oh! Monstrous folly! Oh! Stupidity unparalleled! … Ye take your money and purchase **DEATH!**"—*Chinese proclamation against opium, 1839*

China's response was to try to remain isolated and self-sufficient by preventing foreigners from trading directly into the interior of the country. Unlike India, which was entirely dominated by the British, China attempted to retain control over its economy and confined foreign trade to the port of Canton. British merchants had always chafed at this restriction because it limited their sales of textiles to the coast, away from the lucrative markets of the interior. When China extended the ban to include opium, it was the last straw.

In June 1840, a British fleet arrived at the mouth of the Canton River to begin the first Opium War, or, as the British preferred to call it, The War for Free Trade. By 1842, the fleet had fought its way up the Yangtze and the city of Shanghai fell to the British guns. China capitulated and signed the Treaty of Nanking, which essentially gave the British unrestricted access to the country and immunity from its laws, and full possession of the port of Hong Kong. It was not enough. Using an upsurge of peasant rebellions as an excuse, Britain and France allied to attack China once again in the second Opium War from 1856 to 1860, demanding further concessions. The Chinese once again were overwhelmed by the foreign firepower.

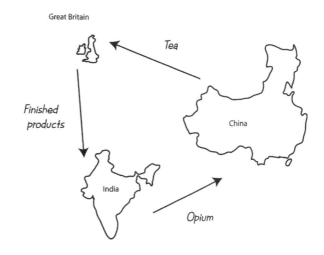

The end of the Opium Wars led to a defeated and demoralized China and an epidemic of opium addiction. By 1900, 25 percent of the China's population—half of the adult male population—was addicted to opium.[2] The bitterness lasted over these humiliating defeats to European capitalists, and came to play a key role in the Communist revolution of the 20th century.

 Hong Kong (from *heang-keang*, "fragrant waters") was one of the many spoils of the first Opium War.

THE "SOLDIER'S DISEASE": MORPHINE IN THE AMERICAN CIVIL WAR

By the 19th century, opium was a popular drug, not only in Europe and Asia but in the United States as well. It was readily available in a wide variety of patent medicines throughout the country and even in remote settlements.

In 1803, a 20-year-old German pharmacist's assistant named Friedrich Sertürner isolated the active principle from opium, which he found to be ten times stronger than crude opium. He called it morphine, after Morpheus, the son of Hypnos (also called Somnus) the

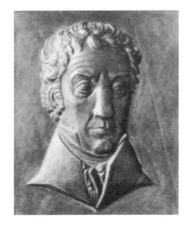

Friedrich Sertürner, discoverer of morphine. It was the first active principle ever extracted from a plant, and marked the beginning of the modern era of drug treatment.

Greek god of sleep. Rosengarten & Co. of Philadelphia (who later evolved into what is now Merck, Sharpe & Dohme), began manufacturing morphine salts in 1832 and quickly became one of the largest distributors. By 1868, both morphine and opium were cheaper than alcohol.

A further development forever changed the use of morphine and many other psychoactive drugs. In 1848, the first practical hypodermic needle was invented.[3] This device was followed, not long after, by the first morphine addict—the wife of the inventor.

Morphine became very popular in the suffering of the Civil War, during which a surgeon's skill was often measured by how quickly he could saw off the gangrenous limb of a screaming patient. As drops, tinctures, or injections, morphine alleviated the physical suffering of the injured. It is likely that morphine helped numb the psychological pain of the war as well. By the end of the war, morphine addiction was called the "soldier's disease," and it is estimated that over 400,000 veterans were addicted.

After the Civil War, morphine and opium became widely available and were cheaper than alcohol.

A BETTER MORPHINE: CODEINE AND HEROIN

Further research on opium showed that there was another natural component that was useful as a painkiller, although it was not as potent as morphine. This compound was isolated as methylmorphine, in 1832, and became known as codeine.

Many attempts were made to modify morphine to produce a more effective, but less addictive, painkiller. In 1874, Alder Wright, a chemist at St. Mary's Hospital in London, boiled morphine with acetic anhydride. The result, diacetylmorphine, was indeed a more effective painkiller. Unfortunately, it would also prove to be vastly more addictive.

Diacetylmorphine was put aside for the next 20 years, until Wright's description came to the attention of Carl Duisberg, of the German chemical company Bayer. The greatest health problem of the 19th century was tuberculosis, responsible for one-fifth of all deaths. Most of the victims were young and in the prime of life. Tuberculosis was spread by coughing, and a tremendous effort was underway to discover more effective cough suppressants. Duisberg believed he had found one in diacetylmorphine, which had the additional benefit of being a very effective pain reliever. Bayer scientists found that the new drug gave a sense of strength and euphoria that made one feel like a hero. They called it heroin.

In 1898, heroin was marketed as a cough treatment. It was followed a year later by another new Bayer medication, aspirin. The new drugs soon found their way into many other medications for almost any illness and even as a general "tonic." Most of these were patent medicines, meaning that their secret ingredients were protected by a patented recipe. Patent medicines were sold in a great variety of pills, powders, potions, and elixirs, often with misleading descriptions or no indication whatsoever of their contents.

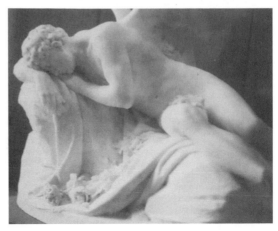

In Greek legend, Morpheus, son of the sleep god Hypnos, was the god of dreams. He is shown here with poppy flowers strewn around him.

ADDICTION ALARMS

When Chinese immigrants came to California in the 1850s to work in the gold mines and then on the railroads, they brought opium smoking with them. In 1876, a new wave of immigrants, sailors, and travelers introduced opium smoking to New York, Chicago, St. Louis, and New Orleans. By the 1890s, opium dens were a common feature in most American towns and cities, frequented not only by the Chinese but also others, especially artists and musicians. Tours of San Francisco's opium dens, known as *hongs*, became a popular attraction, and excited writers such as Rudyard Kipling and Mark Twain. By 1896, it was estimated that there were 300 opium dens in San Francisco, and many more than that in New York.

The typical opium den contained benches or, in the better ones, upholstered couches, where the smoker could relax on his side to hold the long pipe. As the drug took effect, the addict would recline in this position, immobilized in a frozen stupor for hours at a time. Not surprisingly, many addicts developed sore hips. Smoking opium came to be called "on the hip" and then just "hip." Eventually, hip referred to anyone who was avant-garde. In the 1960s, the young people who aspired to be hip—to be involved with music, art, and psychoactive drugs—kept the term and were known as "hippies."

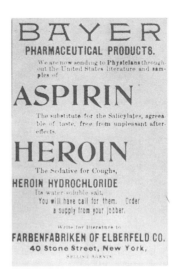

BAYER
PHARMACEUTICAL PRODUCTS.

We are now sending to **Physicians** throughout the United States literature and samples of

ASPIRIN

The substitute for the Salicylates, agreeable of taste, free from unpleasant after-effects.

HEROIN

The Sedative for Coughs,

HEROIN HYDROCHLORIDE

Its water-soluble salt.

You will have call for them. Order a supply from your jobber.

Write for literature to

FARBENFABRIKEN OF ELBERFELD CO.
40 Stone Street, New York,

Opium addicts, lying on their sides smoking long pipes, developed sore hips. Drug users called it being "on the hip," which was shortened to hip, and finally gave the name to the 1960s hippies.

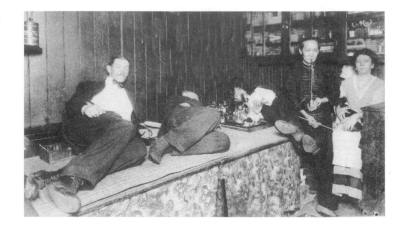

While Chinese immigrants preferred to smoke opium, the rest of the country was becoming increasingly intoxicated on ingested or injected patent medicines. Hundreds of different proprietary medicines could be bought at any store, traveling fair, or by mail order. Most of these contained some type of narcotic, including morphine, cocaine, laudanum, or heroin, which might be conveniently supplied with a syringe. Even the "cures" for the opium habit often contained large amounts of opiates.

A growing alarm began to spread about American drug addiction. In the 1890s, the economy plunged into a great depression, and addiction to alcohol and narcotic drugs reached epidemic proportions. The Anti-Saloon League, which focused on alcohol, was founded in 1893 and eventually led the Temperance Movement to the prohibition of alcohol in 1919. Meanwhile,

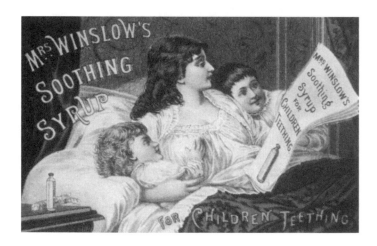

Many children became addicted to the popular narcotic, and deaths from overdose were common.

many others were concerned about the overuse of patent medicines. Drugstore sales of narcotic baby medicines such as Mrs. Winslow's Soothing Syrup or Hooper's Anodyne, the Infant's Friend were so popular that deaths from overdose became a common news item.

As in every human society, fears about dangerous habits were directed not at the true problem but at a scapegoat minority. Immigration from China had been encouraged to help build the railways, but now Chinese immigrants were seen as a threat to the labor force. Active persecution of the Chinese began, particularly on the West Coast, with movements to deport them back to China and with laws forbidding further immigration. Dr. Hamilton Wright, an influential Government lobbyist, railed against Chinese subversion of American society with their opium dens.

China did not ignore this maltreatment of its nationals in the United States. In 1906, China instituted a campaign against domestic opium use and at the same time threatened to boycott American goods to stop the discrimination. The United States, meanwhile, was having difficulty managing uncontrollable corruption and drug smuggling in a new possession, the Philippines, which the United States had won from Spain in 1898. Partly to appease the Chinese by aiding their anti-opium efforts, partly to deal with the Philippines, and finally, to curb the opium-using American Chinese population, the U.S. convened a meeting of regional powers. On February 1, 1909, the representatives of 13 countries met in Shanghai as The International Opium Commission. A follow-up meeting in The Hague produced a signed convention on January 23, 1912, the first international agreement requiring each country to control its narcotics trade.

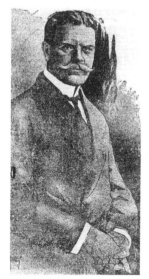

"One of the most unfortunate phases of the habit of smoking opium in this country [is] the large number of women ... co-habiting with Chinese in the Chinatowns of our various cities."
—Dr. Hamilton Wright, the "Father of American Narcotic Laws" [4]

 "Our move to help China in her opium reform gave us more prestige in China than any of our recent friendly acts."
—Diplomatic report to the President

This began a process whereby the United States took a global leadership in controlling the international narcotics trade, even while its own domestic use of addictive drugs was rampant. One hundred years later, the situation has not changed.

Marijuana: The Ancient Herb

*An old story from Iran tells of three men
—an alcoholic, an opium addict, and a hashish eater—
who arrived at the gates of the holy city of Isfahan, locked for the night.
The alcoholic said, "Let us break down the gate."
The opium addict said, "Let us lie down and sleep until morning."
The hashishin said, "Let us pass through the keyhole."*

THE BIG NUMB

Cannabis was one of the earliest cultivated plants, and is now perhaps the most widely grown species in the world. It originated as a wild plant in central Asia, where knowledge of its mind-altering properties has probably existed for tens of thousands of years.

The first written record of marijuana can be found in the Vedas, a collection of holy books set down in India from 2000 to 1400 BC. According to the Atharva-Veda, the god Shiva took pity on humans and brought cannabis from the Himalayas to give health and pleasure. These sacred psalms revered marijuana as freeing the soul from distress and anxiety. By the 10th century AD, a liquid cannabis preparation called *bhang* was described as the food of the gods. A special reverence for marijuana has continued in India to the present day.

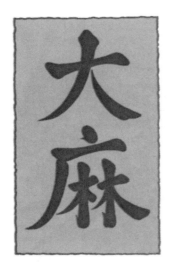

Da Ma, "big numb"

Marijuana was also well established as a medicine in ancient China. The Pen Tsao Ching is credited as the first herbal encyclopedia, written about 100 AD but composed by the emperor Shen-Nung in 2737 BC. It describes the use and cultivation of marijuana to cure illnesses and to alleviate pain. Marijuana remained a common medical herb in China for the next two millennia; Marco Polo wrote of its use on his journey in the 15th century. It has always been known throughout the country as the "big numb."

From the Orient, the use of marijuana spread to the Middle East and throughout Africa. Zulu warriors smoked it before going into battle; humans sacrificed in Fang rituals were given marijuana to prepare them for death, and the Bashilange forced suspected criminals to smoke marijuana until they either confessed or lost consciousness.

By the 5th century BC, marijuana use had also evidently spread to Europe. A funerary urn from that time, discovered in Germany in 1896, was found to contain well-preserved cannabis seeds. Certainly, marijuana was common by the Middle Ages, when it was used both medicinally for a large variety of complaints, as well as recreationally.

 "Poppies, hemp, and darnel were scavenged, dried, and ground up to produce a medieval hash brownie known as 'crazy bread.'"[5]

A WOMAN'S DRUG

Marijuana has always been considered a feminine drug, softening, dulling, and comforting the senses. The Tao, set down in China in 600 BC, dismissed the herb as having too much yin, the passive, female life force. In ancient Japan, women burned marijuana to drive away evil spirits that threatened the family. Marijuana was used in Japanese wedding ceremonies, and hung on trees or in the home to ensure that lovers would remain faithful. In medieval Europe, it was used to hasten the wedding day of young women; in Ireland, to help a woman foretell her future husband. One of the more common uses around the world has been to alleviate menstrual discomfort and the pain of childbirth.

 Marijuana is a Mexican name, from the folk story of María Juana. In Mexico, marijuana is considered a feminine drug—as it has been throughout history in all countries.

HASHISH ASSASSINS?

Hashish, the resin from the cannabis plant, is more concentrated and potent than marijuana. The name comes from the Arabic word for grass. It was developed about 100 AD in northern Africa. From there, it became popular throughout the Islamic world, from Morocco to Afghanistan. It is frequently mentioned in Islamic literature, for example "The Tale of the Hashish Eater," one of the stories by Scheherazade in *A Thousand and One Nights*, written about 1100 AD. In Iran, the Sufi religious sect used hashish to achieve spiritual insight.

 "Hashish, like all other solitary delights, makes the individual useless to mankind, and also makes society unnecessary to the individual."
—*Charles Baudelaire, Les Paradis artificiels (Artificial Paradises), 1867*

Hashish came to Europe when Napoleon conquered Egypt and his soldiers discovered the drug. By the 1840s, it had become popular in the coffee houses of Paris and London.

One of the most persistent myths of hashish is that it gave rise to the word *assassin*, supposedly because of a group of 11th-century terrorists who used hashish in their murderous deeds. The story began with a vague account by Marco Polo and was embellished much later by French and American writers eager to present hashish as a drug menace. It has been thoroughly discredited.[6] Assassin does appear to be derived from the *hashishiyya*, an Islamic sect who made liberal use of the substance, but it is unlikely that they were a bunch of drug-crazed hit men. If anything, users of hashish were more often criticized for their dreamy passivity.

In America, hashish was served at the Turkish Booth at the Centennial Exposition of 1876 in Chicago. Perhaps because it was only available as an expensive import, however, it never became as popular as the home-grown forms of marijuana.

THE SACRED BECOMES PROFANE

In Europe, marijuana and hashish were tolerated so long as they were used only as medicine or in religious rituals. Early writings described wealthy Romans serving up marijuana seed pastries to their guests, but this was an exception. When marijuana began to be used like alcohol—more for fun than as medicine—the public became concerned. By the late 1300s, hashish users were seen as morally corrupt. Caricatures showed the cannabis user bursting into laughter, staggering around, and acting with sexual abandon. In 1484, Pope Innocent VIII condemned the use of cannabis as a tool of the Satanic Mass. Public outrage against recreational marijuana led to pressure on European governments to restrict the drug. The dislike extended as far as Egypt, where fighting between the civic authorities and cannabis farmers defending their fields turned into full-blown battles. Even medicinal use came into question. In the 1800s, marijuana extracts continued to be given for migraine headaches and many other problems, but publications claimed that it made men sterile and warned against its use.

 Did Shakespeare smoke marijuana? A recent analysis of pipe fragments from his home showed traces of cannabis.

ROPE AND DOPE

While the use of marijuana as a drug gradually lost favor, the cannabis plant became much more important for other purposes. During the European Renaissance of the 16th century, the rise of the great powers created a huge demand for fabric, rope, and paper. Cannabis, grown as hemp, supplied all three.

For hundreds of years, cannabis hemp was the dominant fabric. Its strength and durability were superior to cotton, linen, and wool. Large supplies of hemp were used for sails and rope in the building of the military and commercial sailing fleets. It was estimated that a single warship required 80 tons of rough hemp to supply her with the necessary tackle.[7] The need in Britain was so great that King Henry VIII issued a royal edict in 1533 commanding farmers to set aside part of their land to grow cannabis. It was not enough to satisfy demand in the fast-growing maritime power. A hundred years later, Parliament passed legislation granting citizenship to any foreign settler in England or Wales who would grow cannabis. But even this was not sufficient.

 Canvas is a tough cloth with a long history. It was used to make the sails of the ships of ancient Greece and Rome; it was also the fabric for many great paintings. The word comes from the Dutch for cannabis, from which it was made.

For a solution to the hemp shortage, England turned to the overseas colonies. Hemp was first cultivated in Canada in 1606, and Virginia in 1611. The Pilgrims took the crop with them to New England in 1632. As soon as the land was settled, King James I ordered cannabis to be grown in his namesake settlement, Jamestown. The new colonists preferred to grow food—or tobacco, which brought a much higher price—than support the old monarchy, but they had little choice; they also needed hemp for cloth and fiber. In 1639, the Virginia Company required each colonist to plant a certain number of cannabis plants, while landowners in Massachusetts had to plant cannabis by order of their own General Court. In 1761, King George III sent a proclamation requiring the colonists to further increase their production of hemp. By the time of Independence, about 90 percent of American clothing was made from cannabis, as were most other textiles and papers, including the first flags of the United States and even the parchment of the Declaration of Independence and the Constitution. George Washington and Thomas Jefferson each cultivated thousands of acres of cannabis, not only for hemp but as a medicinal herb (Washington used marijuana to soothe his toothaches and inflamed gums). By 1850, cannabis was grown on 8,327 plantations and made into more than 25,000 products.[8]

In the mid-19th century, cotton gradually began to replace hemp for clothing. This was due to the development of the cotton gin, which allowed cotton to be much more easily harvested than the labor-intensive cannabis, and also to the loss of cheap slave labor after emancipation following the Civil War. The end of the era of sailing ships and the advent of cotton as a preferred fabric gradually led to a reduced need for hemp fiber and a decline in cannabis cultivation, until the plant remained only as a widespread weed.

MARIHUANA BECOMES MARIJUANA

Until the 1880s, almost all paper was made from hemp cannabis. It was well known that paper made from hemp was superior to paper from wood pulp, and even now bank notes are still printed on cannabis paper. Furthermore, a larger quantity of cellulose can be produced from an acre of cannabis than an acre of trees.[9] Cannabis, therefore, is naturally superior and more economical to manufacture paper than is wood pulp.

Why, then, did wood pulp become the preferred source for paper? One reason is William Randolph Hearst, the great newspaper publisher of the time, and the owner of millions of acres of the northwestern forestry companies that produced the newsprint. He lobbied to make marijuana illegal to protect Hearst Paper and Timber in which he had invested heavily. Hearst was determined to make cannabis unpopular, by any means possible, in order to protect his wood paper industry.

Prior to the 1930s, marijuana had been called cannabis, hemp, or marihuana (as it continues to be named in the legal code). In an effort to brand marijuana as a foreign substance, the despised Mexican "devil weed," Hearst made his newspapers change the name of cannabis and marihuana to the more Spanish-sounding marijuana.

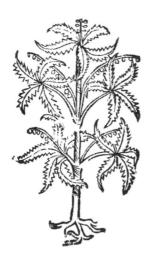

Woodcut from the European herbal Ortus sanitatis de herbis et plantis, 1517

Caput.lxxvi.

MARIJUANA AS MEDICINE

From the time of its initial discovery, marijuana has been used as medicine. The first European reference was found in a Roman herbal of 70 AD, in which cannabis is recommended for earaches. The physician Claudius Galen (AD 130-200) prescribed marijuana for flatulence and all types of pain, but also warned that it might cause impotence. Marijuana was used by folk healers in Poland, Russia, and Lithuania for toothaches and other afflictions. By the 17th and 18th centuries, popular medical use extended to a wide variety of conditions, including depression, cough, jaundice, inflammation, tumors, arthritis, gout, venereal disease, incontinence, cramps, insomnia, epilepsy, and asthma. It was recommended by everyone from the personal physician of Queen Victoria to peasants treating sick farm animals.

Between 1839 and 1900, over 100 medical studies of cannabis were published. A British surgeon and professor of chemistry at the Medical College of Calcutta, W. B. O'Shaughnessy, was intrigued by the many applications of cannabis and worked with a pharmacist named Squire to develop a medicinal extract for easy use. Squire's Extract became one of the most popular remedies of the Victorian era, often used by the Queen herself. The French psychiatrist Dr. Jacques-Joseph Moreau took its use a step further and published a book on his research with cannabis in treating depression, hypomania, and other chronic mental illness. Cannabis was subsequently prescribed for the treatment of epilepsy, delirium tremens, alcohol abuse and other drug addiction.

By the early 1900s, marijuana was a common part of the U.S. medical pharmacopoeia with about 30 varieties of cannabis extract available. Parke-Davis marketed marijuana preparations under the trade names Casadein, Colic Mixture, Veterinary, and Utravol. Eli Lilly sold cannabis extracts as Dr. Brown Sedative Tablets, Syrup Tolu Compound, and Syrup Lobelia. Cannabis was also sold as Piso's Cure, One Day Cough Cure, and Neurosine, and the Squibb Company developed Chlorodyne, a mixture of morphine and marijuana. All of these medications were sold as an extract, in powder, tablet or liquid form, and occasionally as cigarettes for use in the treatment of asthma.

The 1937 Marihuana Tax Act effectively made cannabis illegal, and it became very difficult for doctors to prescribe it. In 1941, it was removed from the U.S. Pharmacopoeia and the National Formulary.

It was not until 1964 that two Israeli chemists, Y. Gaoni and R. Mechoulam, found a way to isolate and synthesize the active ingredient, delta-9-THC.[10] THC is now manufactured and marketed for medical use under the trade name Marinol. Marijuana is otherwise illegal under Federal law, without recognized medical use, although many states are beginning to challenge this restriction.

MODERN RECREATIONAL USE

By the middle of the 19th century, cannabis had become very popular among writers, poets, and artists in Europe. Members of the famous Hashish Club in France, *Le Club des Hachichins*, were some of the greatest literary figures of the day, including Dumas, Nerval, Hugo, Boissard, Delacroix, Gautier, and Baudelaire. Marijuana was also popular at English universities, and was openly used by Oscar Wilde, Elizabeth Barrett Browning, Havelock Ellis, William Wordsworth and Samuel Taylor Coleridge. In the United States Edgar Allan Poe was an early adherent.

Marijuana use gradually fell out of favor in the United States, perhaps because it was overtaken by other drugs, but

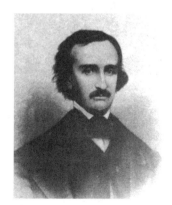

Edgar Allan Poe (1809-1849), father of the modern detective story, and marijuana enthusiast

the *bambalacha* continued to be popular in Latin America. The Spanish had taken hemp to their colonies—to Chile in 1545, Peru in 1554—where it became a common recreational drug.

The modern era of marijuana smoking in the U.S. began with Mexican farm laborers and American sailors in the early 1900s. From these groups, it spread into the Harlem jazz music scene, where it was known as tea.

 "When you're with another tea smoker it makes you feel a special sense of kinship."—*Louis Armstrong*

 "Musicians. And I'm not speaking about good musicians, but the jazz type."—*Drug Commissioner Harry Anslinger testifying to the Senate about who was using marijuana, 1948*

One especially active marijuana peddler to the musicians went by the name of Detroit Red. A burglar, pimp, and all-around criminal, he ended up in prison. It was there, in 1950, that Detroit Red converted to the Black Muslim religion and renamed himself Malcolm X. Much of his spiritual fervor and strict moral code was not a reaction to marijuana, but to heroin, which was far more destructive to the black community. Addiction, he realized, was another form of enslavement.

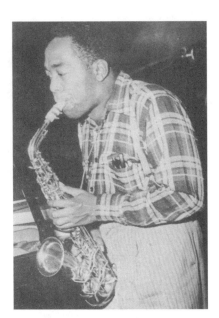

"Quite simply, before Parker, the saxophone was played one way and after him it was played differently."[11] *Charlie "Bird" Parker (1920-1955)*

Despite this concern, a gradual shift took place in the preferred drug of jazz musicians, from marijuana to heroin. This was largely due to one man: Charlie Parker.

Parker thrilled and confounded the music world. Other jazzmen imitated him—they copied his soaring melodies, his dark glasses, his grunge clothing, and then his heroin addiction. "There was no doubt about it," said tenor saxophonist Sonny Rollins, "he was definitely the messiah."

Parker's death at age 34 was a testimony to the hard times of the heroin addict. The irony is that he died of alcoholism, drinking heavily in an attempt to overcome his heroin addiction. He was followed by the great jazz singer Billie Holiday. In 1947, she was busted for heroin and spent eight months at a West Virginia work prison. On her release, she switched to alcohol, a much more respectable drug. She was dead at age 41 from alcohol-induced heart and liver failure.

The post-war white beatniks were fascinated by black jazz music, and took on their drugs as well. Heroin and marijuana became the "hard" and "soft" drugs of the 60s, when their paths diverged and marijuana rode the beatnik popularity into the university culture.

"Jazz was born in a whiskey barrel, grew up on marijuana and is about to expire on heroin."—Artie Shaw

Cocaine: The Sacred Leaf

GIFT FROM THE GODS

When the Spaniards first came to South America in the 16th century, they were fortunate to arrive while the Inca empire was in the midst of a civil war. Had they arrived at any other time, some historians believe, they would have been quickly wiped out. But sheer luck—as well as a considerable amount of courage, boldness, and treachery—allowed a small group of conquistadors to destroy one of the greatest of the ancient civilizations. The conquerors took away vast stores of gold and silver that established Spain as a global power. They took away another product too—one that proved to have an even greater global impact that has lasted to the present day.

Cocaine "can supply the place of food, make the coward brave, the silent eloquent and ... render the sufferer insensitive to pain." —Parke-Davis Company, 1885

Knowledge of coca chewing was first brought to Europe by one of the great explorers, Amerigo Vespucci (after whom America was named), who had found the mouth of the Amazon and determined that South America was a separate continent. On his second voyage in 1499, he described the native Indians chewing a green leaf mixed with a white powder. The leaf was from the coca plant, a shrub growing in the highlands of the Andes. The white powder was made from ground seashells. Centuries later, it was discovered that the leaves contained cocaine, and the shells provided lime to make the leaf mixture sufficiently alkaline to allow its cocaine to be absorbed.

Coca, said the Indians, was brought from heaven by Manco Capac, the son of the Sun God, and the first Inca Emperor. It was "a gift from the gods to

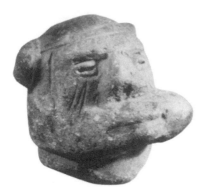

This statue from ancient Peru shows coca chewing

satisfy the hungry, fortify the weary, and make the unfortunate forget their sorrows."[12] It was given to humans by the gods out of compassion, to help people live in the cold, high-altitude plains of the Andes.

In the Inca language Aymara, the word coca, *khoka*, simply means "tree." The leaves were considered sacred and central to life, embodying the spirit of Mama Coca, the nurturing and protective force of nature.

Along with potatoes, coca was one of the first plants domesticated in South America. Archeological discoveries show that coca chewing was well established in Equador by 2500 BC. Native Andeans chewed coca leaves all day long and most carried a small, decorated leather pouch for the leaves and lime powder. Some brewed the leaves into tea.

Coca leaves were an integral part of trade between villages, serving almost as money. The leaf created a bond between the inhabitants of the Inca empire, as it was grown in the lowlands and exchanged for meat and minerals from the highlands. By the time of the Spanish Conquest, coca had evolved into four cultivated varieties, and had spread throughout the Andean region.

The Spaniards were suspicious of coca chewing and first tried to ban it. They soon discovered, however, that without the stimulating effects of coca, the Indians could not undertake heavy labor in the high-altitude silver mines.

16th-century woodcut showing Inca coca trading

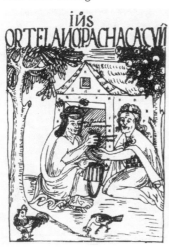

The coca leaf contains more than just cocaine. It is rich in B vitamins and has compounds that allow the body to stabilize blood sugar. Later analyses of coca leaves showed that they contain more iron and calcium than any of the food crops grown in the Andes. In fact, it is likely that without coca the Indians would not even have been able to survive on their potato diet. The Spanish Government relented, and coca chewing remains a central feature of life in Andean villages to this day.

FROM COCA TO COCAINE

For centuries, little notice was taken of coca outside South America. Leaves shipped to Europe lost their potency during the long sea voyages and aroused little interest, unlike coffee and tobacco, which had become increasingly popular. That changed in 1859, when Paolo Mantegazza, an Italian neurologist, published an essay raving about the wonderful qualities of coca, claiming that it gave him "pleasure by far superior to all other physical sensations previously known to me."[13]

Mantegazza's essay was widely read and people took notice. Within a year, a German graduate student, Albert Nieman, isolated pure cocaine hydrochloride from coca. By the 1880s, the white powder was known to be a useful local anesthetic, and in 1884 Dr. Karl Koller began to use it in eye surgery. Cocaine is particularly useful in surgery on the face, eyes, nose, and throat because it constricts blood vessels and limits bleeding and swelling, and the new drug was quickly adopted by physicians. The general public, however, was much more interested in its other properties.

 "I would prefer a life of ten years with coca to one of a hundred thousand without it."—*Paolo Mantegazza, Italian neurologist, 1859*

THE DRINK OF KINGS AND POPES

Extracts of coca leaves were marketed in Europe and the United States in the form of wines, chewing gum, teas, elixirs, and lozenges. The most popular was *Vin Tonique Mariani à la Coca du Pérou*. Mariani wine was a red Bordeaux combined with an extract of coca leaves. It was produced in Paris and dispensed by a physician's prescription for almost any complaint whatsoever. Before long, Mariani was the most popular prescribed remedy in the world, praised by kings, queens, and people of renown

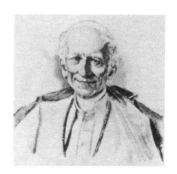

Pope Leo XIII, cocaine enthusiast

from Thomas A. Edison to Ulysses S. Grant, who depended on it for the energy to write his memoirs. Pope Leo XIII was so impressed by the wine, he had a special Vatican medal issued in its praise.[14]

In 1884, purified cocaine became commercially available in the United States. The following year, the Parke-Davis Company marketed coca cigarettes, cocaine for injection and cocaine for sniffing. Other pharmaceutical companies sold cocaine kits complete with everything to take the drug, including hypodermic syringes. The most common excuse for using cocaine was for mild allergies, and most hay fever remedies contained

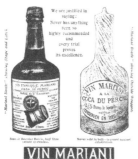

VIN MARIANI
*Nourishes - Fortifies
Refreshes
Aids Digestion - Strengthens the System.*
Unequaled as a tonic-stimulant for fatigued or overworked body and brain.

Prevents Malaria, Influenza and Wasting Diseases.

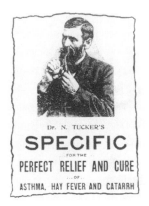

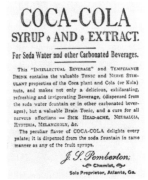

Snorting cocaine: the recommended cure for asthma and hay fever.

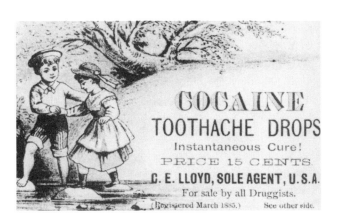

An early advertisement for Coca-Cola.

cocaine as their major ingredient. By 1887, the Hay Fever Association declared cocaine to be its official remedy.

Meanwhile, the Temperance Movement in the United States was picking up steam, creating a popular demand for non-alcoholic drinks. In the mid-1880s, Atlanta became the first major American city to prohibit the sale of alcohol. A local pharmacist, John S. Pemberton, saw an opportunity. In 1886, he developed a water-based syrup that contained extracts of coca leaves and flavoring from the kola nut. The name of his "temperance drink" and "intellectual beverage"[15] was Coca-Cola.

FREUDIAN SLIP

Like many physicians of the day, Sigmund Freud was impressed by the stimulating properties of cocaine, and raved about it in *Über Coca* and other essays. He gave it to his patients, his sister and fiancée, his colleagues, and enjoyed it himself.

Within a few years of his discovery, Freud changed his mind when he began to see the effects of abuse and addiction. He was especially appalled by the experiences of his close friend Ernst von Fleishl, to whom he had prescribed cocaine. When von Fleishl suffered hallucinations of white snakes writhing on his body and ultimately died of cocaine poisoning, Freud came to regret his earlier enthusiasm. He repudiated not only cocaine, but turned his back on *all* drugs and invented a new form of drug-free therapy—the talking cure, psychoanalysis.

From 1886 to 1903, Coca-Cola contained about five milligrams of cocaine, equal to about half a "line" of pure powder. Today, it contains caffeine instead of cocaine, but still has the same coca leaf flavoring.

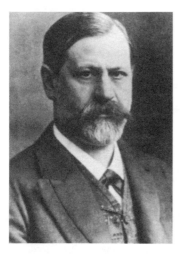

Left, Freud developed psychoanalysis as a reaction to the effects of cocaine and other drug treatment of mental illness

Right, Dr. Halstead, America's first cocaine addict

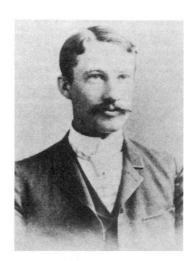

A Tale of Two Addictions

Dr. William Halstead, a highly admired surgeon and founder of the prestigious Johns Hopkins Medical School, had become addicted to cocaine. While Dr. von Fleishl took cocaine to cure his morphine habit, Dr. Halstead used morphine to cure his cocaine addiction.[16]

THINGS DON'T GO BETTER WITH COKE

Concern over the recreational use of cocaine gradually increased around the turn of the century. In 1891, Emil Kraepelin, who developed the modern classification of mental illnesses, added "cocainism" to his list of addictive disorders. Cocaine also began to lose popularity as a medical treatment as the dangers of overuse were realized.

As always, public alarm about drug abuse was not targeted at the root of the problem—the widespread use of cocaine in patent medicines and Coca-Cola—but at a scapegoat minority. In this case, the scapegoat was the southern black population. Cocaine powder was cheap to those who could not afford alcohol. To poor blacks unable to buy liquor, it was readily available as the "5-cent sniff." The use of cocaine was especially

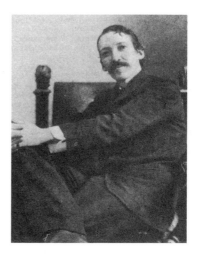

Robert Louis Stevenson used cocaine for inspiration, and is said to have written The Strange Case of Dr. Jekyll and Mr. Hyde in a single six-day and night binge. The story of a talented physician turning into a crazed madman may have been an early glimpse of cocaine psychosis.

NEGRO COCAINE "FIENDS" ARE A NEW SOUTHERN MENACE

Murder and Insanity Increasing Among Lower Class Blacks Because They Have Taken to "Sniffing" Since Deprived
of Whisky by Prohibition.

worrisome in the South because of its euphoric and stimulating properties.
Southern whites feared that Negro cocaine users might become oblivious to
their prescribed bounds and attack white society. According to an editorial
in the *Journal of the American Medical Association*, in June 1900, "the Negroes
in some parts of the South are reported as being addicted to a new form of
vice—that of 'cocaine sniffing' or the 'coke habit'."[17] Col. J.W. Watson of
Georgia urged legal action against the sale "of a soda fountain drink
manufactured in Atlanta and known as Coca-Cola" and claimed that "many
of the horrible crimes committed in the Southern States by the colored people
can be traced directly to the cocaine habit." In Atlanta, the Chief of Police
blamed 70 percent of the crimes on cocaine use.

"It has been authoritatively stated that cocaine is often the direct
incentive to the crime of rape by the Negroes"—*U.S. Government
report, 1910* [18]

Anecdotes were told of cocaine giving superhuman strength, cunning,
and efficiency, spurring the black man to "rise above his place." One of the
more bizarre beliefs about cocaine was that it made blacks invulnerable to .32
caliber bullets. The belief was strong enough to convince Southern police
departments to switch to .38 caliber revolvers.[19]

"A large proportion of the wholesale killings in the South during recent
years have been the direct result of cocaine, and frequently the
perpetrators of these crimes have been hitherto inoffensive, law-
abiding Negroes."—*American Medical Association Report, 1913*

"Most of the attacks upon white women of the South are the direct
result of a cocaine-crazed Negro brain"—*Dr. Koch testifying to U.S.
Congress, 1914*

In 1900, Pemberton removed cocaine from Coca-Cola and replaced it
with caffeine, though he kept the distinctive taste—Coca-Cola continues to
be made with decocainized coca leaf extracts. Cocaine, however, was still
available in other drinks and remedies.

The 1906 Pure Food and Drug Act required accurate labeling of the contents of all patent remedies sold in interstate commerce. The new law did not prevent sales of addictive drugs such as opiates and cocaine, but it did limit their distribution. Eight years later, popular cocaine use was outlawed.

Hallucinogens: Mind, Myth, and Madness

The ancient Vedas of India extolled not only marijuana but also other psychoactive drugs. One of these was a bright red mushroom, *Amanita muscaria*, which the northern tribes called *Soma* and revered as a god. In the Rig-Veda, over 100 holy hymns are devoted to the use of *Soma*.

Ancient meets modern

Aldous Huxley used the name *Soma* to refer to a psychedelic drug in his novel *Brave New World*. *Soma* has now become a trade name for carisoprodol, a modern muscle relaxant.

Hallucinogenic plants and animals have been used throughout the world for religious purposes, most notably in the Americas where perhaps 60 different drugs were employed in various forms of the Indian vision quest. This practice was confined to spiritual adventurers, who often risked severe physical and mental illness in pursuit of enlightenment. It was not until the mid-20th century that taking hallucinogenic drugs became a common form of recreation.

ELEUSIAN MYSTERIES

In ancient Greece, a mysterious cult arose at the Athens temple of Eleusis. Up to 3,000 people each year were initiated into the secret rites, including such notables as Aeschylus, Aristotle, Sophocles, and Plato. They were later followed by the Romans: Cicero, Marcus Aurelius, Hadrian, and other Roman emperors. Little is known of these rites, which were kept secret by the threat of death to those who dared describe it. And yet, this threat could not prevent the poet Pindar from writing, "Happy is he who, having seen these rites, goes below the hollow earth; for he knows the end of life and its god-sent beginning."[20] Cicero agreed, and wrote that Athens had given

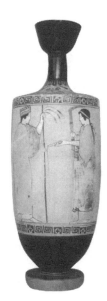

Eleusian vase, 450 BC. Persephone pours a sacred drink, while Triptolemus holds ergot-infected grain, containing LSD.

the world nothing more excellent or divine. Until they were suppressed under Christianity in the 4th century AD, the Eleusian mysteries enthralled the population but their secret remained intact. What could it be?

The answer was suggested by a Swiss chemist, Dr. Albert Hofmann, the discoverer of LSD. He had been studying the toxic effects of a brownish purple mold that grew on improperly stored rye or wheat, and was believed to be responsible for frequent poisonings in Europe. Ergot, from the French word for a rooster spur, is the hard, brown sclerotium of a fungus growing on rye and other grains. As far back as 600 BC, the Assyrians called the growth of ergot a "noxious pustule in the ear of the grain."[21] Epidemics of ergot poisoning took two forms: outbreaks in which the main symptom was epileptic convulsions, or outbreaks with gangrene and ulcers that might cause the loss of the tip of the nose, ear lobes, fingers, toes, and feet. For both of these poisonings, delirium and hallucinations were a common symptom, as was a "Holy Fire" of burning pain in the feet and hands.

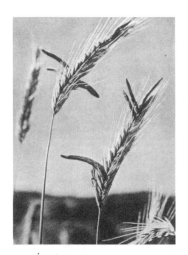

Ergot mold growing on rye

The epidemics came to be called St. Anthony's Fire, after the protecting saint against fire, epilepsy, and infection. St. Anthony lived as a religious hermit in Egypt and died in the year 356. During the Crusades, French knights brought back his remains to Dauphiné for burial, the same location where the earliest recognized outbreak of Holy Fire occurred.

At the time of Dr. Hofmann's research, St. Anthony's Fire continued to plague European villages, with the most recent attacks in France and Belgium in 1953. Hofmann discovered that ergot has at least 30 alkaloids. The most toxic of these are not water-soluble. Therefore, a water infusion might avoid the physically harmful effects while preserving those alkaloids that caused the hallucinogenic effects. Ergot grew readily on *Claviceps purpurea* and other grains native to Greece, and was clearly shown in Eleusian art. The secret of the Eleusian Mysteries had been discovered: the ancients drank a potion containing a substance now known as LSD.

FEAR OF WITCHES

While St. Anthony's Fire caused a great deal of suffering for Europeans, not all exposures to the ergot mold were unintentional. Ergot and Datura were secretly used by occult practitioners to explore psychic realms.[22] Some women did this by mixing the substances with oil to form an unguent which they applied to a broomstick. They then rubbed the stick along the vagina in an efficient method of absorbing the hallucinogenic agent. Woe to those who were caught! The image of a woman—laughing hysterically, naked and riding a broomstick to a psychic realm—was terrifying to the less adventurous public. A woman found in this state was usually declared to be a witch and promptly burned at the stake.

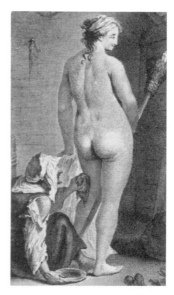

Engraving showing a medieval witch preparing for the sabbat.

An accusation of witchcraft became a ready excuse to punish unruly sectors of society. The period of European history from the 15th to the 17th centuries was a liberating time—the Renaissance, or "age of enlightenment"—when people questioned the traditional dominance of the church and the monarchy. The men in power reacted harshly. The official manual of the inquisitors, the 1489 publication of *Malleus Maleficorum*, the "Hammer of Witches," singled out midwives and their knowledge of herbs. Ergot, which could induce life-saving uterine contractions, was a tool of midwives.

Authorities whipped up hysteria among the public by parading suspected witches and accusing them of causing every natural disaster from fires and illnesses to droughts and crop failures. During this period, an estimated 500,000 people were convicted of witchcraft and burned to death. Eighty-two percent of them were female, typically unmarried women who dared to speak out against their subservient role.

 "In rifleing the closet of the ladie, they found a Pipe of ointment, wherewith she greased a staffe, upon which she ambled and galloped through thick and thin, when and in what manner she listed."
—*Witchcraft investigation, 1324*

With that sort of reaction to their drug adventures, those women who dabbled in the occult understandably became very discrete. Hallucinogens became virtually unknown until their popular rediscovery in the 1950s.

 "I suggest that the best way to understand the cause of the witch mania is to examine its earthly results rather than its heavenly intentions. The principal result of the witch-hunt system (aside from charred bodies) was that the poor came to believe that they were being victimized by witches and devils instead of princes and popes."
—*Marvin Harris, anthropologist* [23]

Do hallucinogens cause hallucinations?

The modern era of hallucinogens began with interest in peyote, followed by the synthesis of mescaline and LSD, and then the rediscovery of the rich history of psychoactive mushrooms. Much of this work was done by Gordon Wasson, a wealthy banker with a fascination for mushrooms and history. Wasson was able to finance expeditions around the world as he developed theories of ancient religions inspired by use of the "sacred mushroom"— showing references in everything from the Bible to the origin of the Christmas tree, in which the presents represent the *Amanita* mushrooms growing at its base. Wasson was joined by the Harvard botanist Richard Evan Schultes, who helped discover and catalog the many varieties of mind-altering mushrooms.

 There are about 5,000 species of mushrooms. About 80 are considered hallucinogenic.

But are these plants really hallucinogenic? The term hallucinogen to describe these substances caused a great deal of debate among drug researchers. Most agree that it is a misnomer. Psychologists in the 1950s thought these drugs would cause effects similar to schizophrenia, and therefore schizophrenic hallucinations. In fact hallucinogenic drugs do not, in general, bring hallucinations. With rare exceptions, such as Datura (see *Chapter 7: Datura*), these drugs do not cause the experience of something that does not exist. A true hallucination is a perception occurring in the absence of environmental stimulation, as might occur in a dream or in psychotic states such as delirium or schizophrenia. So-called hallucinogenic drugs do not cause this. Instead, these drugs simply bring about an alteration in perception or a sense of increased insight or awareness.

Hallucinogen comes from the Latin word *alucinare*, which means "to wander in mind."

If these drugs are not really hallucinogens, what should they be called? A number of suggestions were made. Psychologists proposed "psychotomimetic" and "psycholytic," but these terms were felt to imply too much of a diseased state. Gordon Wasson wanted to call them "entheogens," from the Greek for "a god within," and this term is often used today by those who promote the use of drugs for mystical explorations.[24] "Phantasticant" was preferred by both Richard Evan Schultes and Albert Hofmann. Aldous Huxley was enthusiastic about these mind-altering substances and invented the word "phanerothyme" to describe them. His friend Humphry Osmond disagreed, with a couplet:

> *To fathom hell or soar angelic,*
> *Just take a pinch of psychedelic*

From the Greek for "mind-manifesting," psychedelic became the choice term in the 1960s. Perhaps because it seemed to be too much a part of the counterculture, it never really caught on in government and academic literature. At this time, "psychoactive" is most often used—a correct and neutral term, but overly inclusive since it also includes the opiates, stimulants and depressants. Otherwise, this special class of drugs that cause a peculiar awareness continues to be known as hallucinogens.

SET AND SETTING

After the Second World War, there was a surge in interest in drugs that altered mental functioning. Psychologists found hallucinogens to be unusual and unpredictable drugs, causing experiences that vary widely depending on the characteristics of the user. The same person using the same drug could, on a different occasion, have a very different experience. This unpredictability was considered to be a function of what is called the set and the setting of the drug experience.

The *set* of a drug event refers to the prior expectations of the drug user and the frame of mind in which the drug is taken. An anxious or fearful person expecting a powerful drug will probably have a dramatically different experience from a confident, relaxed user expecting a mild intoxication.

The *setting* refers to the physical and social environment. A drug taken at home among friends will likely produce a different experience from the same drug taken among strange or hostile people or in an uncomfortable environment.

Many hallucinogens generate a sense of dissociation—a disconnection between mind and body—similar to that reported by some religious practitioners. People often describe a sensation of dissolving boundaries, whereby a user might feel that the boundary between the ground and his body no longer exists. To some people, this might be a wonderful feeling of connection with the universe, while to others it could be a horrifying sensation of being sucked into the earth. To one person, the hallucinogenic experience can be an incredible enlightenment, and to another, the most terrifying hell. Set and setting helped explain not only why such different outcomes took place, but also the psychological effects of religious rites and other experiences.

The new hallucinogens, particularly LSD, intrigued not only

psychologists but others as well. The founder of *TIME* magazine, Henry Luce, and his wife Claire Booth Luce were fascinated by LSD and took it many times. They also introduced a number of their friends to it, including the actor Cary Grant who claimed "it has completely changed me," over the course of at least 100 acid trips.

MILITARY TAKES NOTICE

Hallucinogens also attracted the attention of another, less spiritually oriented, group. By the early 1950s, the arms race between the United States and the Soviet Union had created a roughly equal number of atomic and hydrogen bombs and both were experimenting with more novel weapon systems. The first chemical weapons had been developed by Germany, but were never used in the Second World War (some believe that Hitler had an intense dislike of

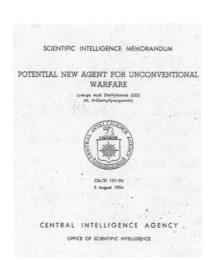

these weapons because he had been gassed as a soldier in the First World War). After the Second World War, both the U.S. and the U.S.S.R. developed enormous stockpiles of chemical weapons: the U.S. produced about 40,000 tons of nerve and blister agents while the U.S.S.R. eventually created about 65,000 tons, much of which is still stored in crumbling concrete bunkers.

By causing a temporary mental instability, LSD was a possible new type of chemical weapon. The CIA took notice when military intelligence reported, erroneously, that the Swiss pharmaceutical firm Sandoz had sent 50 million doses to the Soviets. The CIA rapidly began a program to explore the use of LSD and other hallucinogens as a military agent. Sandoz had synthesized LSD by a laborious process from ergot, and could only produce very small quantities at a time. For this reason, and because of concern about depending on a foreign supplier (its discoverer, Dr. Hofmann, had refused the CIA's request for supplies), the CIA commissioned the American drug company Eli Lilly to synthesize LSD and produce it in large quantities. The Chemical Warfare Service at the Edgewood Arsenal in Maryland went on to stockpile enormous quantities of LSD, testing it on unwitting soldiers and distributing it to investigators around the country. Most of this research was highly classified and the data never released, but rumors soon spread about the powerful effects of LSD in mimicking schizophrenia.

In 1959, the San Francisco columnist Herb Caen ran an announcement that the military would pay anyone $150 to take a new experimental drug called LSD-25. Among those who took the military supplies were the poet Allen Ginsburg and the novelist Ken Kesey, who used his experiences as the basis for his *One Flew Over the Cuckoo's Nest.*

 Many early users of LSD—and its most enthusiastic proponents—were given the drug from supplies created by the military.

PSYCHEDELIC THERAPY

While the military explored the use of hallucinogens to destabilize individuals, psychiatrists were interested in their use for the opposite purpose. Schizophrenia is a mental illness characterized by hallucinations and a detachment from reality. It is found in about one percent of the population throughout the world. The cause of schizophrenia is not well understood, and treatments are far from satisfactory. When news reached psychiatric researchers that a drug had been found that might simulate, or perhaps cure, schizophrenia, there was tremendous interest.

 "There have been numerous reports of how dying individuals, free from pain in LSD ecstasy, have come to perceive the meaning of life and death, and have died in peace, reconciled to their fate, and free from fear."[25]

All psychiatric medications in the 1950s were essentially tranquilizers—they all improved mental illness simply by suppressing the patient's problems and conflicts. By enhancing awareness, rather than suppressing it, hallucinogens held the possibility that they could resolve these problems instead. Mescaline and LSD used during psychoanalysis proved to be remarkably effective in recovering repressed memories. The French psychiatrist Jean Delay claimed that hallucinogens enabled one to go beyond the simple act of remembering, to actually reliving the experience: it is not *reminiscence*, as he put it, but *réviviscence*.

By 1965, between 30,000 and 40,000 psychiatric patients had received LSD therapeutically, and over 2,000 scientific papers were published on the subject. Most of these studies were highly favorable. A 1960 survey of 5,000 patients, covering 25,000 LSD or mescaline sessions, found it was very well tolerated. Another survey in 1966 of 2,742 drug sessions found no resulting psychoses, suicide attempts, or uncontrollable behavior.[26]

LSD was used not only for psychotherapy, but also for terminally ill patients. Doctors in American hospitals observed that the very severe pain suffered by cancer patients, which no longer responded to conventional pain killers, could often be completely relieved by LSD. Patients also slept better afterward, an improvement which lasted as long as ten days. In one formal study, LSD was given to 128 cancer patients in their last months of life. On average, pain disappeared for 12 hours and was subsequently reduced for two to three weeks. There were no adverse medical reactions to the LSD therapy.[27] It was believed that LSD was not acting as a painkiller in the usual sense, but that the perception of pain was altered. Patients were able to turn their thoughts toward religion and face their death with equanimity. When they no longer feared death, they appeared to have less pain.

COUNTERCULTURE CRACKDOWN

Until 1963, LSD, psilocybin, mescaline, and other hallucinogens were entirely legal in the United States. While psychologists, psychiatrists, and pain-management physicians were intrigued by their possible medical uses, writers, artists, and musicians were also attracted by the drugs. A struggling novelist, Jack Kerouac, had been introduced to heroin by William Burroughs, and went on to take the other new drugs. In 1957, he published *On the Road*, a free-wheeling romp through the country in search of nothing more than an interesting experience—no goals, no responsibilities, not much philosophy, and little more than a reaction to the mainstream American quest of post-war stability and prosperity. The book became one of the most influential American novels of the 20th century. In 1965 half of the American population was under 30. Every idea was open to question and every new experience was worth investigating.

 "What had turned the Plains Indians to peyote in the 1870s turned some college-educated whites to LSD in the 1960s; their old cultural forms seemed meaningless, and they needed new symbols and rituals to shape beliefs and guide action."[28]

A few of the most vocal users of hallucinogens went beyond defending them—they turned drugs into a religious crusade. Aldous Huxley was one of the first. In *The Doors of Perception*, published in 1954, he argued that all religions owed their basic beliefs to the visions inspired by hallucinogenic experiences. He went on to take LSD and mescaline hundreds of times, and inspired other writers, artists, and musicians to do the same—including a 1960s rock band that used his title for their name, *The Doors*.

None of the psychedelic proselytizers was as enthusiastic as a Harvard psychologist named Timothy Leary. Described as a very intelligent, charming, and somewhat conniving young man, Leary grew up in a privileged household. His father was President Eisenhower's dentist, and Leary went to West Point but was expelled for being too rebellious. After obtaining a Ph.D. from Berkeley in clinical psychology, the 35-year-old got a job at the Harvard Center for Personality Research. In 1960, at age 40, he was vacationing in Mexico when he first took psilocybin. According to his colleagues, Leary was always looking for an opportunity to step beyond the mainstream, a chance for notoriety. Now he had found it. From psilocybin, he moved to LSD and shared his supplies with students, staff, faculty, and anyone interested. Leary and another Harvard psychologist, Richard Alpert, obtained Government grants to study the effects of the drug on perception. They also used it in prisons for a rehabilitation program that showed some signs of success.

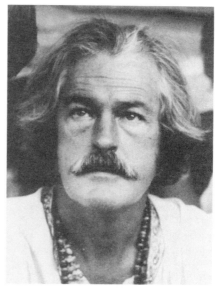

"The only hope is dope."—Timothy Leary (1920-1996)

"Leary is the most dangerous man in America."—President Richard Nixon

By 1963, their enthusiasm had gone beyond academic research. When others complained that LSD was being used indiscriminately and for kicks, Leary replied by saying it *should* be used indiscriminately and for kicks. Leary and Alpert took LSD and gave it to students while gradually drifting away from structured academic research into a recreational party where everyone was encouraged to take it. "Turn on, tune in, drop out," they urged the students. Leary and Alpert, however, did not drop out from the university. They were fired.

Once out of the university, Leary and Alpert had free rein to popularize LSD. It became the drug of the 60s and the hippie movement. Leary played a cat-and-mouse game with the FBI as he made himself the Johnny Appleseed of LSD, encouraging everyone to use it and threatening to have his followers put it into municipal water supplies. He was eventually caught, imprisoned, and escaped with the help of the Weather Underground, a militant group of the most extreme anti-Government activists. Leary found asylum in Algeria in a bizarre alliance with Eldridge Cleaver and the Black Panthers, where the

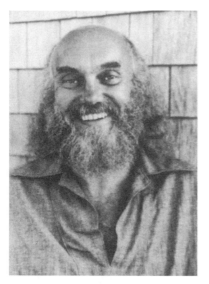

Richard Alpert, aka Baba Ram Dass

black revolutionaries were forced to share quarters with the white acid-head, to their mutual discomfort. Along with his wife and a retinue of hippies and rock stars, Leary had smuggled in 20,000 hits of LSD and was planning to turn on all of Africa.[29] Leary was recaptured in 1973, spent three years in prison, and was then released under an arrangement in which he informed on his former associates. Later on, he toured the country as a stand-up comedian poking fun at his own religious fervor, and giving joint lectures with G. Gordon Liddy, the FBI agent who had arrested him and later achieved his own dubious fame as a Watergate criminal. Although, right up to his death, Leary always denied that LSD had any detrimental effects, he was considered by many to have permanent mental illness from too many acid trips.

After Leary's imprisonment, Dr. Richard Alpert did indeed drop out. He went to India and resurfaced as Baba Ram Dass—the quintessential and often caricaturized new age guru.

 "Psychedelic drugs cause panic and temporary insanity in people who have not taken them."—Timothy Leary and Richard Alpert

The medical community was not quite sure what to do with a substance that appeared non-toxic but was clearly being abused, and the bizarre behavior of Leary and other enthusiasts did not help. The American Medical Association consulted the Harvard campus physician, Dr. Farnsworth. He urged stringent

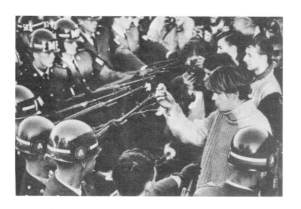

controls. President Kennedy was on the Board of Regents of Harvard University when Leary and Alpert were kicked out. Kennedy himself was not dramatically opposed to drugs. He was said to have smoked marijuana on at least one occasion in the White House and had experimented with cocaine. His brother Robert Kennedy, the Attorney General, was also known to have taken either LSD or psilocybin in the spring of 1963. Jack Kennedy casually side-stepped the issue, preferring to avoid further confrontation with the growing anti-war protests, at which recreational drugs were rampant. The anti-war and drug movements—one political, the other anti-political—had become almost indistinguishable.

On October 16, 1966, the first "Human Be-in" was held in New York and San Francisco. The same day, California outlawed LSD. Shortly after, the Federal Government followed suit, and Sandoz, the only legitimate source of LSD, turned over the supply in its New Jersey facility.

President Johnson was intensely against LSD, and singled it out for denunciation in his State of the Union address. In 1967, a complete Federal ban on hallucinogens was the first bill he proposed. The National Institute of Mental Health was forced to end its research programs on hallucinogenic drugs.

Making hallucinogens illegal only intensified the anti-war protestors' hatred of the President. The press spread rumors that 100,000 people would be coming to San Francisco in the summer of 1967 to take drugs. It was a self-fulfilling prophecy that brought countless young people to the dubiously named Summer of Love. Many of the writers who had extolled the use of hallucinogens for religious or mystical insight were appalled at the reckless and crime-ridden drug scene that resulted.

The antics of Ken Kesey and his "merry pranksters," who drove across the country in an old school bus dispensing LSD, probably helped turn public opinion against all hallucinogens.

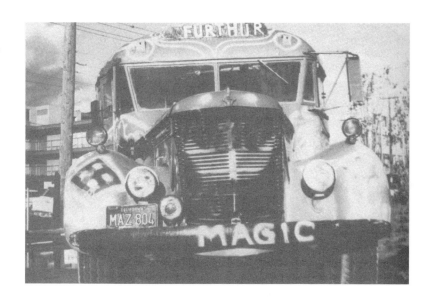

Some put the blame on Leary and Alpert, for urging powerful drugs on unprepared adolescents. Aldous Huxley complained that Leary's behavior was "the reaction of a mischievous Irish boy to the headmaster of his school … why, oh why, does he have to be such an ass?"[30] In an irony of history, the bizarre antics of people such as Timothy Leary, who had pushed most vigorously for the liberal use of hallucinogens, were probably a major reason that these drugs became illegal.

"By January of 1968 most of the flower children had abandoned the scene and it was dominated by speed freaks, addicts, alcoholics, motor-cycle hoodlums, and the teenage runaways and schizoid or inadequate personalities they preyed on."[31]

By 1970, it was estimated that between one and two million Americans had taken LSD. The chairman of the New York County Medical Society's Subcommittee on Narcotics Addiction stated that LSD was "more dangerous than heroin." That year, a new Federal law included hallucinogens among the most dangerous drugs and declared illegal as Schedule I substances, the most stringent level.

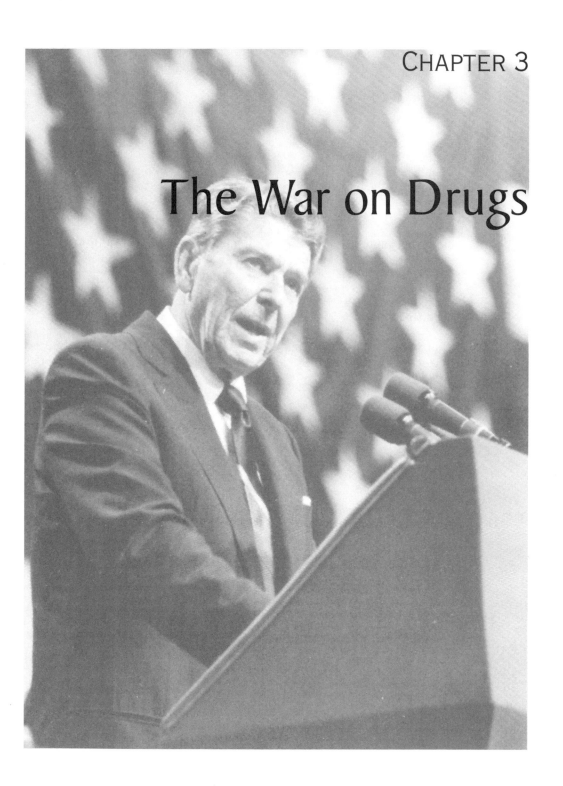

CHAPTER 3

The War on Drugs

On June 1, 1998, a letter was sent to the Secretary General of
the United Nations with the following statement:[1]

Every decade the United Nations adopts new international conventions,
focused largely on criminalization and punishment, that restrict the ability
of individual nations to devise effective solutions to local drug problems.
Every year governments enact more punitive and costly drug control
measures. Every day politicians endorse harsher new drug war strategies.

What is the result? U.N. agencies estimate the annual revenue generated
by the illegal drug industry at $400 billion, or the equivalent of roughly
eight per cent of total international trade. This industry has empowered
organized criminals, corrupted governments at all levels, eroded internal
security, stimulated violence, and distorted both economic markets and
moral values. These are the consequences not of drug use per se, but of
decades of failed and futile drug war policies.

In many parts of the world, drug war politics impede public health efforts
to stem the spread of HIV, hepatitis and other infectious diseases. Human
rights are violated, environmental assaults perpetrated and prisons
inundated with hundreds of thousands of drug law violators. Scarce
resources better expended on health, education and economic
development are squandered on ever more expensive interdiction efforts.
Realistic proposals to reduce drug-related crime, disease and death are
abandoned in favor of rhetorical proposals to create drug-free societies.

Persisting in our current policies will only result in more drug abuse, more
empowerment of drug markets and criminals, and more disease and
suffering. Too often those who call for open debate, rigorous analysis of
current policies, and serious consideration of alternatives are accused of
"surrendering." But the true surrender is when fear and inertia combine to
shut off debate, suppress critical analysis, and dismiss all alternatives to
current policies.

Attached to this letter were 47 pages of signatures from people in 44 countries.
The signatures included 11 Nobel Prize winners, 7 heads of state,
and the United Nations' own former Secretary General.
No legislators signed from the United States, the country that controls the global drug war.

A Century of Increasing Drug Control

"We are the drug-habit nation."—H.W. Wiley, 1911

At the beginning of the 20th century, the United States had few laws controlling drugs. Medications were unregulated and could be formulated by anyone. They were sold without prescription and often with little or no indication of their contents. Drugs, in general, were poorly understood and their use considered a matter of personal choice and responsibility.

> In 1900, an estimated 2% of all physicians and 1% of all nurses were addicted to patent medicine opiates.

Alcohol, on the other hand, was very well understood. It had been a matter of intense controversy from the beginning of European colonization of the United States, with some immigrant groups highly in favor of their beloved beer and spirits, while others were adamantly opposed to the "devil's drink." By the mid-19th century, alcohol was prohibited by law in a number of states. The reasons were complex: some people shunned alcohol because of religious belief, others because of the injury they saw liquor cause to individuals and their families, and yet others for economic reasons as they found drunken workers less productive (for example, Henry Ford immediately fired any worker who drank alcohol, even when the worker drank only while off-duty). When concern eventually did develop over the unregulated use of patent medicines, it was not about the opium, heroin, or cocaine they contained, but their high percentage of alcohol.

The first state drug laws were passed in the West, in response to the large numbers of immigrants from China. Oriental workers had been brought in to help build mines and railroads, but then feared as surplus labor during the economic depression of the 1890s. California passed a law forbidding further immigration from China, and the new drug laws were part of a thinly disguised program of discrimination against the resident Chinese. San Francisco passed the first law against opium use in 1875. However, it applied only to raw opium and did not address other patent medicine opiates such as opium tinctures, morphine, or codeine. The law was specifically targeted against the opium dens frequented by Orientals: whereas the Chinese habit of smoking opium seemed foreign and menacing, opium-based patent medicines were considered American remedies.

By the end of the 19th century, addiction to narcotic patent medicines had become a significant public health problem. Many pharmacists and physicians sold drugs indiscriminately for immense profit. "If the illicit sales of the drugs were stopped," according to a Government report at the time, "quite ten percent of the retail drug stores of the United States would be put out of business."[2]

Public health officials later estimated that in 1900, about 250,000 Americans out of a population of 75 million—about 1 in 300—were opium addicts. Another 200,000 were cocaine addicts. The majority of these were genteel middle-class women.[3]

1906: Pure Food and Drug Act

The Federal Pure Food and Drug Act forced the patent medicine industry to list on the bottle labels the presence of ingredients such as alcohol, opiates, cocaine, and cannabis. The Act did not prohibit any drugs. It was passed only because of concern about hidden ingredients. Children's medicine, for example, often contained morphine or heroin, and deaths from overdose were commonplace. The law was passed simply to warn the buyer of the contents.

 "Until labeling requirements were mandated in 1906, not only did manufacturers not list the narcotic or alcohol contents, they often positively denied its presence when it was plentiful in the substance." [4]

1909: Smoking Opium Exclusion Act

The rampant use of opiate medications was not just an American problem. Concern about opiate abuse around the world, particularly in China, led to a series of international conferences—the first attempt to stem the global drug trade. The United States took a lead role in controlling the production and distribution of narcotics, specifically opiates at first, followed by cocaine, and then other substances that became prominent drugs of abuse.

The Smoking Opium Exclusion Act was a response to an outcry against the "filthy Oriental habit" and made imports of opium illegal for any purpose except legitimate pharmaceutical use. Notably, it addressed only smoking opium—favored by the Chinese—and not tinctures and other medicinal forms that were in widespread use by other Americans.

1915: HARRISON NARCOTIC ACT

Led by Congressman Francis Barton Harrison, the first major national anti-narcotic law was passed in 1914 and came into force the following year. The Harrison Narcotic Act was originally passed as a record-keeping law, intended to curb the excessive prescription of narcotics and prevent addiction. The law, as it was initially drawn up, prohibited opium (and its derivatives), cocaine, and cannabis. The inclusion of cannabis was protested by the National Wholesale Druggists' Association because it did not appear to be habit-forming. The medical community was divided on the subject. Some favored the continued legal status of cannabis as a relatively non-addictive drug with evident medicinal value. Others were alarmed at the widespread abuse of cannabis for clearly recreational purposes, especially among the Syrian community in New York. To avoid stalling the Act, marijuana was left out of the final bill. It was not regulated under Federal law until 1937.

The Harrison Narcotic Act became effective on March 1, 1915. Almost immediately, the cost of heroin on the streets rose from $6.50 an ounce to about $100 dollars an ounce.[5]

It is largely because of this Act that the word narcotic has come to mean any illegal drug, and later gave rise to the Bureau of Narcotics, and other laws and institutions using that term. Legally, the definition of narcotic is any substance included in the Harrison Narcotic Act: opiates and cocaine.

"The problem of narcotic drug addiction has passed all the bounds of reasonable comprehension ... and has become the greatest evil with which the Commonwealth has to contend."
—New York Legislature, 1917

1917: THE FIRST WAR ON DRUGS

While passage of the Harrison Act made heroin and cocaine more expensive, it did little to diminish their popularity. By the start of the First World War, drug use was considered an epidemic. Addicts were seen as a social menace, a threat to the war effort, and a corruption of American society. The result was a much touted national "War on Drugs" with heavier prison sentences for users. Heroin production was outlawed in 1924 but the drug continued to be legally imported for restricted use. In 1956, it was completely outlawed and all remaining stocks were surrendered to the Federal Government.

Veterans who had become addicted during the war were tolerated, in part out of sympathy for their suffering and patriotism, and in part because not much could be done to help them.

 War veteran addicts scrounged for money to buy drugs, often picking up scrap metal. They became known as "junk men" and then simply as "junkies".

Non-veteran addicts were treated less sympathetically. By 1930, 35 percent of all new convicts in the U.S. were being indicted under the Harrison Narcotic Act.

1920: Prohibition

In 1917, Congress passed the Volstead Act, a constitutional amendment prohibiting the production and sale of alcohol. After a lengthy process of state-by-state ratification, the notorious Eighteenth Amendment came into effect on January 16, 1920.

There had been frequent movements for the prohibition of alcohol almost since the first settlement of the United States, but they had never gained quite enough support. The First World War finally tipped the balance, when anti-German sentiment was mobilized against the beer-serving German taverns. The U.S. had been at war since April 1917. The prohibition campaign convinced the public that the production of liquor was part of a German plot to sap America's strength and willpower, and deplete the cereal grains that were needed for bread for soldiers and starving Europeans.

 The lesson of Prohibition was clear: if a desired substance is not provided legally, it will be provided illegally.

Within a year of its imposition, it became obvious that Prohibition was not working. People were drinking as much as before. Indeed, the consumption of alcohol *increased* among women and adolescents, who saw it as a forbidden luxury. Overall, the consumption of beer decreased, but that of distilled spirits dramatically rose to compensate. Some, like the Jamaican ginger extract (the notorious "Jake") were 75 to 80 percent alcohol—far more potent than legal drinks before Prohibition.

 "What we prohibit, we cannot control."—J.P. Morgan

Where previously the manufacture and distribution of alcohol had been controlled by the Government and enriched the tax base, it was now controlled by criminals and financed corruption. In 1920, it had taken decades of campaigns to mobilize enough support to pass and ratify the Eighteenth Amendment. Thirteen years later, it took just ten months to repeal it.

1937: MARIHUANA TAX ACT

In the booming economy of the 1920s, Mexican immigrants were welcomed into the western states as workers for farms and industries. However, the Great Depression of 1929 brought a backlash against Mexicans as an unwelcome labor surplus. They came to be associated in the popular press with marijuana, and as early as 1919 there were complaints of increased crime and violence due to their use of the drug.

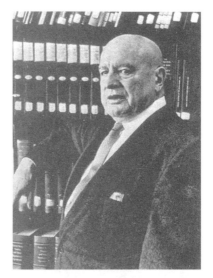

Harry J. Anslinger (1892-1975), hard-line Commissioner of the Federal Bureau of Narcotics, morphine addict

The spread of marijuana was also blamed on immigrants from India: at a national narcotics conference, the delegate from San Francisco railed against the "large influx of Hindoos ... demanding cannabis." A citizen group calling itself the American Coalition was formed to fight new immigration, mainly by whipping up public hysteria about the influx of drugs brought by the newcomers. None was more vehement than Harry Anslinger, Commissioner of the Federal Bureau of Narcotics from 1930 to 1962. Anslinger had first made his reputation during Prohibition, during which he pursued rum-runners with a vigor that embarrassed his superiors. After Prohibition, he turned his attention to the drug trade, making wild claims about the evils of marijuana and narcotics even as he supplied his close friend, Senator Joseph McCarthy, with illicit morphine and later became an addict himself.

 "Marijuana, perhaps now the most insidious of our narcotics, is a direct by-product of unrestricted Mexican immigration. ... Mexican peddlers have been caught distributing sample marijuana cigarets to school children." [6]

Anti-Mexican sentiment in the western states was not enough, however, to convince the Federal Government to make marijuana illegal. The movement needed the help of an influential national figure. It found one in the newspaper publisher William Randolph Hearst. Cannabis was the best and most economical raw material in the manufacture of paper. But Hearst had invested heavily in northwestern forest paper mills. To protect his operations from competitive cannabis paper, he wanted to make cannabis illegal. He commanded his newspapers to use the Mexican word *marijuana* to replace the earlier terms cannabis and marihuana, to "make it sound more foreign and menacing,"[7] and took every opportunity to characterize marijuana as a dangerous drug.

 "Marijuana, while no more habit-forming than ordinary cigarette smoking, offers a shorter cut to complete madness than any other drug."[8]

On October 1, 1937, the United States Congress passed the Marihuana Tax Act. Rather than an outright law against marijuana, the Tax Act merely prohibited the transfer of marijuana without purchase of a transfer tax stamp.

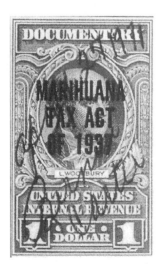

Marihuana Tax stamp, issued to Dr. Alexander Shulgin, 1956 (courtesy of A. Shulgin)

Each time the drug changed hands, the possessor was required to pay a $100 per ounce tax. Failure to do so was a federal offense. Not surprisingly, such stamps were rarely issued and marijuana effectively became illegal. It was prohibited in this way until the Tax Act was superceded by the Controlled Substances Act of 1970.

Not everyone was convinced of the hazards of marijuana. In the 1940s, the Mayor of New York, Fiorello La Guardia, commissioned a study of marijuana which found no evidence of addiction, tolerance or withdrawal, and no association with aggressive or antisocial behavior. The Federal Government ignored the study's findings.

During Prohibition, the Government's warnings on the dangers of alcohol had been widely ridiculed and diminished its credibility as an objective voice of health promotion. Now, with the same vigor, the evils of marijuana were exaggerated in Government and educational publications. The only result was a further loss of credibility in Government pronouncements on drugs.[9]

 "[The marijuana smoker] will suddenly turn with murderous violence upon whomever is nearest to him. He will run amuck with knife, axe, gun, or anything else that is close at hand, and will kill or maim without any reason."—*American Journal of Nursing, 1936*

1965: Drug Abuse Control Amendments

In 1951, amphetamine abuse became a major concern. The Harrison Narcotic Act was amended to demand prison sentences for offenders, followed by the Narcotics Control Act of 1956, which made these sentences mandatory and eliminated probation and parole. It did little to stop the proliferation of amphetamines. On the contrary, new types of amphetamines began to be produced in meth labs on the West Coast. The Government responded with the Narcotics Manufacturing Act of 1960 and the Racketeer Influenced and Corrupt Organizations Act (RICO) of 1962, making it easier to control the racketeering and organized crime that had entered the amphetamine trade.

The 1960s brought another great drug epidemic in the United States. It was caused by a number of factors: the unprecedented prosperity after the Second World War, the disillusionment and rebellion that accompanied the Vietnam War, and the Bohemian and Beatnik quest for mind-altering experiences. Most of all, it was due to one demographic fact—the 76 million adolescents of the post-war baby boom, an enormous, young generation feeling invulnerable and willing to try anything new.

President Lyndon Johnson was vehemently opposed to hallucinogenic drugs, holding them responsible for the social turmoil of the 1960s. The Drug Abuse Control Amendments of 1965 (DACA) amended the Food, Drug and Cosmetic Act of 1938 by prohibiting depressant, stimulant and hallucinogenic substances. Individual hallucinogenic drugs were not specified; DACA simply referred to any substance with a "hallucinogenic effect on the central nervous system." Curiously, DACA made an exemption for the personal use of substances such as psilocybin and psilocin. This loophole was closed by a subsequent law in 1968.

1970: Comprehensive Drug Abuse Prevention & Control Act

Drugs had so far been controlled by a collection of laws regulating individual drugs. For opiates alone, there were separate laws for possession, for importation, and even for the domestic cultivation of the opium poppy (the Opium Poppy Control Act, 1942). This legislative patchwork could not keep up with the novel types of hallucinogens and designer drugs that popped up each year. Rampant use of drugs both old and new prompted the Government to overhaul all drug laws and combine them into a single regulation for controlled substances.

The Comprehensive Drug Abuse Prevention and Control Act of 1970 became the legal foundation of drug regulation in the United States. It was a consolidation of all previous laws regulating the manufacture and distribution of narcotics, stimulants, depressants, hallucinogens, anabolic steroids, and any other chemicals considered to have a potential for abuse.[10]

This law continues to be the controlling authority in the United States. Most other industrialized countries have adopted a similar comprehensive law, and the United Nations has enacted a code that has roughly the same structure and appearance in order to regulate international drug trafficking.

1972: NIXON'S WAR ON DRUGS

By the time of Nixon's presidency, drugs had become a major public issue. Most arguments for or against their use dwelt on issues of civil rights and free speech, and indirectly led to arguments about governmental authority and the Vietnam War.

A national survey in 1971 reported that 40 percent of Americans aged 18 to 21 had used marijuana. While college students were discovering hallucinogens, soldiers in Vietnam were discovering heroin. An estimated 25 percent of American servicemen used both marijuana and heroin, and, just as in the First World War, veterans brought narcotics back into mainstream society (sometimes quite literally: heroin was often smuggled inside the corpses of dead soldiers). In 1971, it was estimated that 10 to 15 percent of all army troops were addicted to heroin, and 20 to 35 percent were using it.

In 1968, Richard Nixon gained the presidency by promising to "restore law and order," with a major focus on drug control. In 1972, he declared a "total war against dangerous drugs." Nixon campaigned effectively to portray the drug epidemic as a foreign threat to Americans and vowed to stop economic aid to countries that allowed drug trafficking. In 1973, he moved drug control from the Food and Drug Administration (FDA), which is under the Department of Commerce, to the newly created Drug Enforcement Administration (DEA), a branch of the Department of Justice. The move was

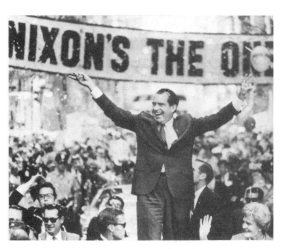

"America has the largest number of heroin addicts of any nation in the world. ... The problem has assumed the dimensions of a national emergency. ... If we cannot destroy the drug menace in America, then it will surely in turn destroy us."
—President Richard Nixon, 1971

more than symbolic. Illicit drug use became punished with a zeal unequaled in the history of the country, and drug convicts began to fill the prisons.

 "No President has equaled Nixon's antagonism to drug abuse."
—David F. Musto, The American Disease [11]

In 1976, wearied of the Vietnam War and endless domestic conflicts, public sentiment turned to the more lenient administration of Jimmy Carter. In 1977, Carter formally recommended legalizing the personal use of marijuana in amounts up to an ounce.

 "Penalties against possession of a drug should not be more damaging to an individual than the use of the drug itself; and where they are, they should be changed. Nowhere is this more clear than in the laws against possession of marihuana in private for personal use."
—President Jimmy Carter

1981: REAGAN'S WAR ON DRUGS

The relaxed attitude toward drugs reached a peak in 1979, when an estimated ten percent of all Americans regularly used illegal drugs. The huge market created powerful international crime syndicates, most notably in coca growing regions of Latin America. The economies of Colombia, Bolivia and Peru became dominated by the drug trade. Almost all of the drugs were destined for the American consumer.

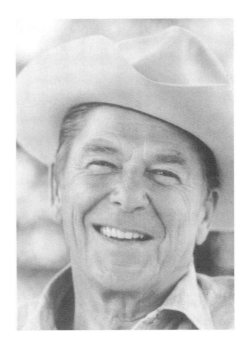

The greatest cause for alarm was not marijuana or cocaine, but crack—a newer, less expensive form of cocaine that proliferated among inner-city neighborhoods. Crack was not seen as a benign or mind-expanding drug like marijuana. It was highly addictive and associated with poverty and crime. Even those who used other recreational drugs were horrified by the spread of crack and a wave of public hysteria about its evils swept the country. Most people thought that it was an entirely new drug that caused instant addiction and violent insanity, particularly among African Americans.

*"Any user of illicit drugs is an
accomplice to murder."
—First Lady Nancy Reagan [12]*

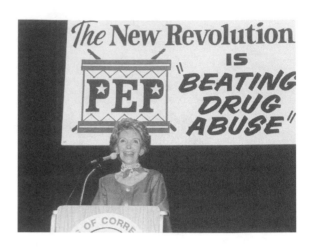

How much of this fear was based on fact, and how much stemmed from a deeper fear of inner-city blacks, is debatable. What is clear, however, is that the fear of crack was remarkably similar to the fear of cocaine at the turn of the century, right down to the image of drugged black men attacking whites.

Popular sentiment once again turned against drugs. A Gallup poll in 1980 had shown that 53 percent favored the legalization of small amounts of drugs. By 1986, this had shrunk to 27 percent.

The newly elected President responded forcefully. The control of drugs had always been a domestic issue. An old statute, the Posse Comitatus, prohibited military forces from involvement in civil law enforcement, unless specifically authorized by Congress. The regulation had been passed after the American Civil War to prevent further military activity in the South. In 1981, Congress passed the Department of Defense Authorization Act, allowing military forces to be used in drug interdiction.

On January 30, 1982, President Reagan formally declared his War on Drugs. First Lady Nancy Reagan weighed in with a campaign to "Just Say No" to drugs. Under his administration, and followed by President Bush, penalties were dramatically increased for drug possession and distribution. Jails were expanded to accommodate the additional prisoners and billions of dollars set aside for new prison construction.

The War on Drugs focused on the supply, not the demand. Of the dramatic increase in the domestic budget to combat drugs, 70 percent was dedicated to stopping drugs at the source and just 30 percent to education, prevention and treatment of the users. Huge increases in foreign aid were given to Bolivia, Colombia, Ecuador, Peru, and Mexico to enlist their support in the effort. Most of the countries that supplied the American drug trade were reluctant to take drastic steps to reduce production, and did so half-heartedly. It was a tough economic choice between the loss of income from cash crops and the loss of foreign aid.[13] American efforts to interdict the foreign drug trade sometimes went beyond economic inducements to outright military intervention. The domestic War on Drugs became an international conflict as accusations of drug production provided the excuse to conduct subversive military campaigns in countries from Nicaragua to Afghanistan. How many of these threats were real and how many imagined has yet to be determined.

1984: COMPREHENSIVE CRIME CONTROL ACT

Normally, a drug is legal until a law is passed by the Government specifically designating it as illegal. By the mid-1980s, new recreational drugs were appearing faster than the legislature could pass laws against them. The Comprehensive Crime Control Act of 1984 was an amendment to the CSA which allowed the Administrator of the DEA to directly place a substance into Schedule I, on a temporary basis, side-stepping the normal political process. The order could take place immediately and make the substance illegal for one year (with an extension of six months) until the legislature had a chance to review it.

The impact of this law was subtle but very profound. For the first time in history, a drug could be made illegal without review by the elected Government.

1986: ANTI-DRUG ABUSE ACT

In 1951 mandatory minimum sentences had been introduced for those convicted of illegal drug possession. These sentences were considered to be unnecessarily severe and were not very effective. They were inconsistently enforced and finally repealed in 1970.

 Average prison sentence for drugs[14]
Before mandatory minimums = 1.9 years
After mandatory minimums   = 6.9 years

Under Reagan's administration, the Federal Sentencing Reform Act of 1984 reintroduced mandatory minimums and made them broader and more stringent than the earlier laws. By then, however, 49 states had already taken action to provide minimum sentences for drug infractions.

In 1986, the Anti-Drug Abuse Act provided mandatory minimum sentences specifically for the possession of cocaine. The new law imposed a prison sentence of 5 to 40 years for cocaine possession—and this sentence could not

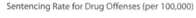

Sentencing Rate for Drug Offenses (per 100,000)

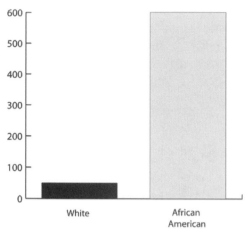

African Americans use illegal drugs less than whites, but they are sentenced at a much higher rate[15]

be suspended, nor could the convict be paroled or placed on probation. The mandatory minimum applied to 500 grams (about one pound) of powder cocaine, but just 5 grams of crack cocaine. Since blacks and those on lower incomes were much more likely to use crack than powdered cocaine, they were also more likely to find themselves in prison. The majority of crack offenders (86 percent) were black, but most powder cocaine users (70 percent) were white. In 1991, mandatory minimums were applied to 59 percent of Federal seizures of crack, but just 3 percent of seizures of powder cocaine. Notably, the mandatory minimum law did not apply to convictions for methamphetamine, of which 66 percent were white, or LSD, of which 97 percent were white.

Five grams of crack was chosen because it is a common unit on the street; in one 12-month period, only 13 percent of Federal crack seizures were for less than that amount. For example, a wholesale dealer possessing 495 grams of powder cocaine would not face a mandatory minimum sentence, but he could supply each of 99 street-level dealers with 5 grams of powder converted to crack—and all of them would be liable for mandatory minimums. If sentencing for powder cocaine had been the same as for crack, mandatory minimums would have tripled from 27 percent to 76 percent of total cocaine convictions.

1986: CONTROLLED SUBSTANCES ANALOGUE ENFORCEMENT ACT

Despite the sweeping regulations of the Controlled Substances Act, new "designer drugs" continued to pop up, and were legal until the DEA took action to restrict them. On October 27, 1986, just days before the national elections, an Amendment to the CSA was passed to remedy this situation. Under this amendment, any analog of a controlled substance—any drug that is chemically similar or has a similar stimulant, depressant, or hallucinogenic effect as a Schedule I or Schedule II controlled substance—would also automatically be illegal.

The amendment allowed new drugs to be declared illegal without the need to demonstrate their abuse. Many new synthetic amphetamines and hallucinogens were controlled in this way. For example, the new synthetic drugs CY-19 (4-phosphoryloxy-N,N-diethyltryptamine), and CZ-74 (4-hydroxy-N,N diethyl-tryptamine), had been legal substitutes for psilocybin. After this Amendment, these substances automatically became illegal as analogs of psilocybin, even though they are not mentioned in the law.

1993: CLINTON'S WAR ON DRUGS

President William Jefferson Clinton entered office with a widely publicized admission of having smoked (but not inhaled) marijuana as a young man. It was assumed that he would follow the policies of President Carter and take steps to decriminalize drugs. This seemed to be the case during his first term, when his attitude toward the White House Office of National Drug Control Policy was considered to be "benign neglect." Running hard for his second term, Clinton declared his own War on Drugs and appointed a retired four-star military general, Barry McCaffrey, to direct the effort.

Clinton's drug war was no more successful than earlier campaigns to stem drug use. Despite a massive increase in Federal spending on drug control, from about $1.5 billion in 1989 to $18.5 billion in 2000, the average price of a gram of pure cocaine steadily dropped from a peak of about $300 in 1981 to less than $100, with a similar decrease in the price of heroin.[16] Meanwhile, the number of heroin users in 2000—975,000—was twice that of 1993.

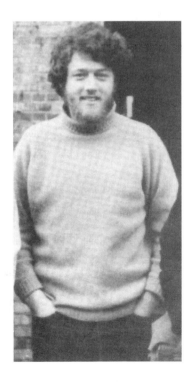

In the Central and South America, and the Caribbean, the United States increased pressure on governments to fall in line behind drug interdiction efforts, often creating anger in these countries at the heavy-handed tactics to solve what is generally perceived as an American domestic problem. For example, the current Operation Libertador involves 36 Latin American and Caribbean countries and territories. The program costs $500 million per year, but only $5 million to $6 million of this is used to reduce demand.[17]

Like the earlier wars on drugs, Clinton's effort generated a lot of publicity but a variable, and probably negligible, change in American use of recreational drugs. As Prohibition showed: if demand exists, someone will find a way to supply it.

Clinton was expected to have a lenient approach to drugs. Instead, during his time in office the annual number of Americans arrested for marijuana rose by 43 percent.

The United States has far more prisoners than any other industrialized country, most of them for drug offenses. Yet the use of drugs remains about the same.[18]

Comparative Rates of Imprisonment (per 100,000 population)

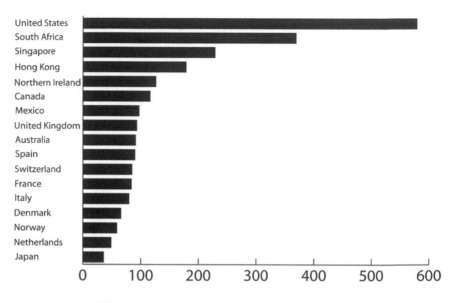

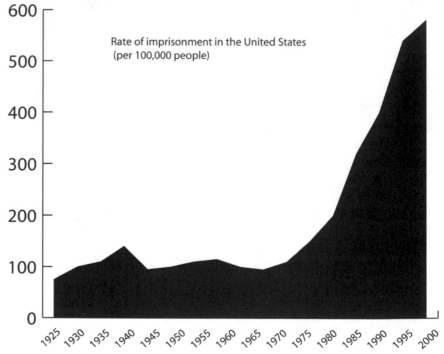

Rate of imprisonment in the United States (per 100,000 people)

2001: BUSH'S WAR ON DRUGS

President George W. Bush won a closely fought campaign by promising a return to conservative values—a policy which historically has included increased punishment for drug users and sellers. It is difficult to imagine how this could happen. During the past two administrations, the money allocated for drug interdiction has risen 1,200 percent. Punishment for drug sellers has become, on average, greater than that for murder. Mandatory imprisonment for drug users has created a huge increase in the prison population, of which 65 percent are there for drug convictions. And yet, the overall use of illegal drugs is about the same.

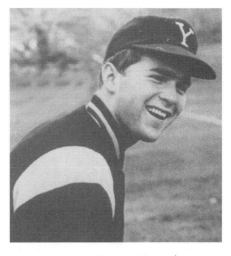

As a young man George W. Bush reportedly used illegal drugs such as cocaine. He faces a greater challenge than any previous president in controlling drugs.

Government officials justify these efforts by pointing to a slight decrease in the use of cocaine, while ignoring the increase in MDMA; they point to a decrease in heroin use in New York, while ignoring the increase in other cities; they point to statistics that show that children have increased awareness of the dangers of illegal drugs, while ignoring studies that show that these same children think the dangers are exaggerated and drugs are just one more forbidden pleasure.

 "What the drug war has done is to drive the price of drugs up, so the more the price of drugs go up, the more money there is to corrupt people."—*Jamaican police Col. Trevor McMillan*

 "We now have guns, ammunition, gang warfare that we didn't have before."—*Trinidad government official* [19]

The War on Drugs, by any objective measure, has been a failure. Other countries—notably Canada, Great Britain, and other European nations—are beginning to question the drug war and are considering methods of controlling drugs that do not involve imprisonment for users. The United States has resisted this approach, but may not be able to do so for much longer.

How Is A Drug Made Illegal?

The Comprehensive Drug Abuse Prevention and Control Act of 1970 continues to be the current law controlling drugs in the United States. Under Title II of this Act, known as the Controlled Substances Act (CSA), the main criteria used to declare a drug illegal is not the physical or mental danger from using the drug, but its potential for abuse.

HOW DOES A SUBSTANCE BECOME A "DRUG OF ABUSE"?

According to law, abuse means that a drug is used in a manner that is not approved by the Government. For example, an approved use might be a doctor's prescription of morphine to relieve pain, or even self-medication of dextromethorphan to relieve a cough. Abuse would be taking morphine or dextromethorphan without the doctor's recommendation or without the medical condition. Drugs are made illegal when their potential for abuse becomes high enough to produce a threat to individual or public safety.

Neither the term "drug" nor "potential for abuse" is specifically defined in the CSA. Because "drug" can be interpreted in various ways, the Government typically uses the phrase "drug or other substance." According to congressional discussion, the indicators that a drug or other substance has a potential for abuse are:

1. There is evidence that individuals are taking the substance in amounts sufficient to create a hazard to their health or to the safety of other individuals or to the community.

2. There is significant diversion of the substance from legitimate drug channels.

3. Individuals are taking the drug or other substance on their own initiative rather than on the basis of medical advice from a practitioner licensed by law to administer such drugs.

4. A new drug is similar to a substance already known to have a high potential for abuse, making it reasonable to assume that it will also be abused.

FIVE SCHEDULES OF CONTROLLED SUBSTANCES

Under the CSA, controlled substances are divided into five levels of control, depending on their potential for abuse.

Schedule I   These drugs are considered to have a very high abuse potential and no accepted medical use. Physicians do not have the authority to prescribe them, with rare exceptions. Examples include heroin, marijuana, and LSD.

Schedule II   These drugs are considered to have a very high abuse potential but also an accepted medical use. Physicians may prescribe them, but only within quite stringent regulations. Examples include morphine, cocaine, amphetamines, and barbiturates.

Schedule III   These drugs are considered to have a high abuse potential but also accepted medical use. Physicians routinely prescribe them. Examples include lesser concentrations of the opiates and barbiturates.

Schedule IV   These drugs are considered to have a moderate abuse potential but also accepted medical use. Physicians routinely prescribe them. Examples include the benzodiazepines such as Valium and many antidepressant medications.

Schedule V   These drugs are considered to have a low but significant abuse potential, and accepted medical use. They may be purchased without a prescription. Examples include cough and cold remedies such as dextromethorphan.

The decision as to whether a drug should be scheduled under the CSA is made by the Secretary of the Department of Health and Human Services (HHS), in consultation with the Food and Drug Administration (FDA), the National Institute of Drug Abuse (NIDA), and other agencies which may provide scientific information about the drug.

Two decisions are made. The first is whether a drug has abuse potential, and therefore should be controlled under the CSA. This decision is made by the Secretary of the HHS. The second is under what Schedule the drug should be listed. This is made by the Administrator of the Drug Enforcement Administration (DEA).

As outlined in Section 201 (c), [21 U.S.C. 811 (c)], the Administrator of the DEA determines the scheduling of a substance by considering the following:

1.   The drug's actual or relative potential for abuse.

2.   The drug's pharmacological effects: whether the drug is a narcotic, depressant, stimulant, or hallucinogen.

3.   Current scientific knowledge regarding the substance: all data of the physical and mental effects of the drug.

4. Its history and current pattern of abuse: where, when, and by whom the drug is abused.

5. The scope, duration, and significance of abuse: what is the economic and social impact of regulating the use of the drug?

6. What, if any, danger does the drug pose to the public health?

7. The drug's psychological or physiological dependence liability: is it addictive?

8. Is the substance an immediate precursor of a substance already controlled (allowing its manufacture)?

After considering all of these factors, the DEA Administrator makes a recommendation to the HHS under which Schedule to place the controlled substance. Although the DEA has the power to make the final classification, the evaluations of the HHS are binding on the DEA with respect to scientific and medical matters. Therefore, the DEA may elect to control a substance at a lower level than recommended by the HHS, or not to control it at all, but if the HHS recommends that a substance *not* be controlled, the DEA may not control that substance. (The DEA may, however, issue a temporary emergency order to control a drug.)

Once the recommendations have been made, the HHS Secretary forwards them to the Attorney General, who generally approves all such recommendations, and delegates the action back to the DEA for implementation.

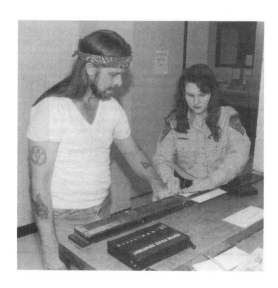

The process of adding, deleting, or changing the control Schedule of a drug can be started by any interested party. It is usually initiated by the HHS, but it can also be started directly by the DEA, or by a petition from any interested group: for example, the drug manufacturer, a medical society or association, a pharmacy association, a public interest group concerned with drug abuse, a state or local government agency, or even an individual citizen. All of these petitions eventually end up with the DEA, which may undertake an investigation before issuing the final determination. The DEA may begin an investigation of a drug at any time, based upon information received from law enforcement laboratories, state and local law enforcement and regulatory agencies, or other sources of information.

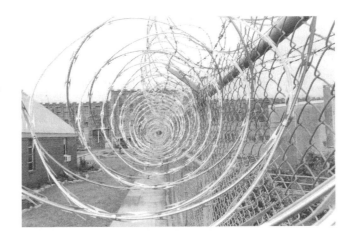

When the DEA Administrator has determined that a drug or other substance should be controlled, decontrolled, or rescheduled, a proposal to take action is published in the Federal Register. This proposal invites all interested parties to file comments with the DEA, or to request a hearing with the DEA. If no hearing is requested, the DEA will evaluate all of the comments received and publish a final order in the Federal Register based on these comments. This order will set the effective dates for controlling the drug.

If a hearing is requested, the DEA will enter discussions with the interested group and attempt a satisfactory compromise to any disagreement. If a compromise cannot be reached, a hearing will be held before an Administrative Law Judge, who will take evidence on factual issues and hear arguments on legal questions regarding the control of the drug. At the close of this hearing, the Administrative Law Judge prepares a report of findings of fact and conclusions of law, and submits a recommendation to the DEA Administrator. The Administrator will review these documents, as well as the underlying material, and prepare yet another report of findings of fact and conclusions of law (which usually just repeats that of the Administrative Law Judge), and publishes a final order in the Federal Register.

Once the final order is published, anyone has 30 days to appeal to a U.S. Court of Appeals to challenge it. Unless stayed by this Court, the final order then becomes law.[20]

 Keeping up with drug regulations can be complicated. The easiest way is to check the Federal Register online: www.access.gpo.gov/su_docs/aces/aces140.html

Drugs Illegal in the United States

SCHEDULE I CONTROLLED SUBSTANCES

Schedule I substances are considered to have a very high abuse potential, no acceptable medical use, and to be unsafe for use under medical supervision. The following list is taken from the Controlled Substances Act (*21 Code of Federal Regulations, Part 1308—Schedules of Controlled Substances*). Alternate and chemical names are given in parentheses.

Opiates
1. Acetyl-alpha-methylfentanyl (N-[1-(1-methyl-2-phenethyl)-4-piperidinyl]-N-phenylacetamide)
2. Acetylmethadol
3. Allylprodine
4. Alphacetylmethadol
5. Alphameprodine
6. Alphamethadol
7. Alpha-methylfentanyl
8. Alpha-methylthiofentanyl
9. Benzethidine
10. Betacetylmethadol
11. Beta-hydroxyfentanyl
12. Beta-hydroxy-3-methylfentanyl
13. Betameprodine
14. Betamethadol
15. Betaprodine
16. Clonitazene
17. Dextromoramide
18. Diampromide
19. Diethylthiambutene
20. Difenoxin
21. Dimenoxadol
22. Dimepheptanol
23. Dimethylthiambutene
24. Dioxaphetyl butyrate
25. Dipipanone
26. Ethylmethylthiambutene
27. Etonitazene
28. Etoxeridine
29. Furethidine
30. Hydroxypethidine
31. Ketobemidone
32. Levomoramide
33. Levophenacylmorphan
34. 3-Methylfentanyl
35. 3-Methylthiofentanyl
36. Morpheridine
37. MPPP (1-methyl-4-phenyl-4-propionoxypiperidine)
38. Noracymethadol
39. Norlevophanol
40. Normethadone
41. Norpipanone
42. Para-fluorofentanyl
43. PEPAP (1-(2-phenethyl)-4-phenyl-4-acetoxypiperidine)

44. Phenadoxone
45. Phenampromide
46. Phenomorphan
47. Phenoperidine
48. Piritramide
49. Proheptazine
50. Properidine
51. Propiram
52. Racemoramide
53. Thiofentanyl (N-phenyl-N-[1-(2-thienyl)ethyl-4-piperidinyl]-propamide)
54. Tilidine
55. Trimeperidine

Opium derivatives
1.   Acetorphine
2.   Acetyldihydrocodeine
3.   Benzylmorphine
4.   Codeine methylbromide
5.   Codeine-N-Oxide
6.   Cyprenorphine
7.   Desomorphine
8.   Dihydromorphine
9.   Drotebanol
10. Etorphine
11. Heroin
12. Hydromorphinol
13. Methyldesorphine
14. Methyldihydromorphine
15. Morphine methylbromide
16. Morphine methylsulfonate
17. Morphine-N-Oxide
18. Myrophine
19. Nicocodeine
20. Nicomorphine
21. Normophine
22. Pholcodine
23. Thebacon

Hallucinogenic substances
1.   Alpha-ethyltryptamine (etryptamine, Monase, AET,α–AT)
2.   4-Bromo-2,5-dimethoxy-amphetamine (4-bromo-2,5-DMA; 4-bromo-2,5-dimethoxy-α-methylphenethylamine)
3.   4-Bromo-2,5-dimethoxy-phenethylamine (alpha-desmethyl DOB; 2C-B, Nexus)
4.   2,5-Demethoxy-amphetamine (2,5-dimethoxy-α-methylphenylamine; 2,5-DMA)
5.   2,5-Dimethoxy-4-ethyl-amphetamine (DOET)
6.   4-Methoxyamphetamine (4-methoxy-α-methyl-phenethylamine; PMA)
7.   5-Methoxy-3,4-methylenedioxy-amphetamine
8.   4-Methyl-2,5-dimethoxy-amphetamine (4-methyl-2,5-dimethoxy-methylphenethylamine; DOM, STP)
9.   3,4-Methylenedioxy-amphetamine (MDA)
10. 3,4-Methylenedioxy-methamphetamine (MDMA)
11. 3,4-Methylenedioxy-N-ethylamphetamine (N-ethyl MDA, MDE, MDEA)
12. N-hydroxy-3,4-methylenedioxy-amphetamine (N-hydroxy MDA)
13. 3,4,5-Trimethoxy-amphetamine
14. Bufotenine (3-(β-Dimethylaminoethyl)-5-hydroxyindole; 3-(2-dimethylaminoethyl) 5-indolol; N,N-dimethylserotonin; 5-hydroxy-N,N-dimethyltryptamine; mappine)
15. Diethyltryptamine (DET)
16. Dimethyltryptamine (DMT)

17.   Ibogaine (Tabermanthe iboga; 7-Ethyl-6,6-β,7,8,9,10,12,13-octahydro-2-methoxy-6,9-methano-5H-pyrido [1′,2′:1,2] azepino [5,4-b] indole)
18.   Lysergic acid diethylamide (LSD)
19.   Marihuana
20.   Mescaline
21.   Parahexyl (Synhexyl; 3-Hexyl-1-hydroxy-7,8,9,10-tetrahydro-6,6,9-trimethyl-6H-dibenzo[b,d]pyran)
22.   Peyote (all parts of the plant Lophophora williamsii Lemaire)
23.   N-ethyl-3-piperidyl benzilate
24.   N-methyl-3-piperidyl benzilate
25.   Psilocybin
26.   Psilocyn
27.   Tetrahydrocannabinols
28.   Ethylamine analog of phencyclidine (PCE; cyclohexamine; N-ethyl-1-phenylcyclohexylamine)
29.   Pyrrolidine analog of phencyclidine (PCPy; PHP; 1-(1-phenylcyclohexyl)-pyrrolidine)
30.   Thiophene analog of phencyclidine (TPCP; TCP; 1-[1-(2-thienyl)-cyclohexyl]-piperidine)
31.   1-[1-(2-Thienyl)cyclohexyl]pyrrolidine (TCPy)

Depressants
1.   Mecloqualone
2.   Methaqualone
3.   Gamma-hydroxybutyrate (GHB)
4.   Flunitrazepam

Stimulants
1.   Aminorex (aminoxaphen; 2-amino-5-phenyl-2-oxazoline; 4,5-dihydro-5-phenyl-2-oxazolamine)
2.   Cathinone (norephedrone; 2-amino-1-phenyl-1-propanone; alpha-aminopropiophenone; 2-aminopropiophenone)
3.   Fenethylline
4.   Methcathinone (ephedrine; methylcathinone; 2-(methylamino)-propiophenone; alpha-(methylamino)-propiophenone; monomethylpropion)
5.   (±)cis-4-methylaminorex
6.   N-ethylamphetamine
7.   N,N-dimethylamphetamine (N,N-alpha-trimethyl-benzeneethanamine; N,N-alpha-trimethylphenethylamine)

Temporary listing of substances subject to emergency scheduling
1.   N-[1-benzyl-4-piperidyl]-N-phenylpropanamide (benzylfentanyl)
2.   N-[1-(2-thienyl)methyl-4-piperidyl]-N-phenylpropanamide (thenylfentanyl)

Schedule II Controlled Substances

Schedule II substances have a very high abuse potential, but also have some legitimate medical uses, and may lead to severe psychological or physical dependence. They may be prescribed by a medical doctor with a permit from the Drug Enforcement Administration. Some of these drugs may be at a lesser schedule of control in lower potencies.

Opium and opiates
1.   Raw opium
2.   Opium extracts
3.   Opium fluid
4.   Powdered opium
5.   Granulated opium
6.   Tincture of opium
7.   Codeine
8.   Ethylmorphine
9.   Etorphine hydrochloride
10.   Hydrocodone

11.   Hydromorphone
12.   Metopon
13.   Morphine
14.   Oxycodone
15.   Oxymorphone
16.   Thebaine

Opiate derivatives

1.   Alfentanyl
2.   Alphaprodine
3.   Anileridine
4.   Bezitramide
5.   Bulk dextropropoxyphene
6.   Carfentanil
7.   Dihydrocodeine
8.   Diphenoxylate
9.   Fentanyl
10.   Isomethadone
11.   Levo-alphacetylmethadol (LAAM)
12.   Levomethorphan
13.   Levorphanol
14.   Metazocine
15.   Methadone
16.   Methadone-intermediate (4-cyano-2-demethylamino-4,4-diphenyl butane)
17.   Moramide-intermediate (2-methyl-3-morpholino-1,1-diphenylpropane-carboxylic acid)
18.   Pethidine (meperidine)
19.   Pethidine-intermediate-A (4-cyano-1-methyl-4-phenylpiperidine)
20.   Pethidine-intermediate-B (ethyl-4-phenylpiperidine-4-carboxylate)
21.   Pethidine-intermediate-C (1-methyl-4-phenylpiperidine-4-carboxylic acid)
22.   Phenazocine
23.   Piminodine
24.   Racemethorphan
25.   Racemorphan
26.   Remifentanil
27.   Sufentanil

Stimulants

1.   Amphetamine
2.   Methamphetamine
3.   Phenmetrazine
4.   Methylphenidate

Depressants

1.   Amobarbital
2.   Glutethimide
3.   Pentobarbital
4.   Phencyclidine (PCP)
5.   Secobarbital

Hallucinogenic substances

1.   Nabilone

Immediate precursors

1.   Phenylacetone (P2P, phenyl-2-propanone, benzylmethyl ketone)
2.   1-Phenylcyclohexylamine
3.   1-Piperidinocyclohexanecarbonitrile (PCC)

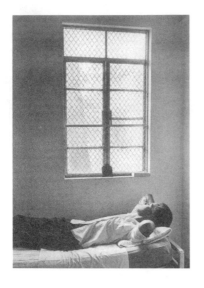

Federal and State Drug Laws

Federal and state laws against drugs are complex, change from year to year, and are often enforced erratically, depending on the judge, the circumstances, and characteristics of the defendant. Because of the highly publicized on-going war on drugs, penalties have become increasingly severe. Some of the state regulations border on absurdity. For example, in two recent incidents, a child was thrown out of school for giving Advil to another child,[21] and a seventh-grader was suspended for giving a zinc cough lozenge to a friend.[22] Some states have tried to liberalize drug laws, particularly with respect to marijuana. Even in these states, however, Federal laws remain in effect.

TYPES OF DRUG CRIME

Crimes are classified as misdemeanor or felony offenses. A misdemeanor is a minor crime that might result in a fine, some public service, or maybe a short jail sentence. A felony is more serious. Individuals convicted of a felony may lose their profession and the future right to hold many types of job.

Many states, and the Federal system, have adopted mandatory sentencing laws, according to which the judge has no discretion to pass a lenient sentence based on the circumstances. The simple facts determine the prison sentence, which also may not allow parole. For example, there have been several cases of women who unknowingly carried drugs for their husbands or boyfriends. When caught, they were given mandatory ten-year prison terms.

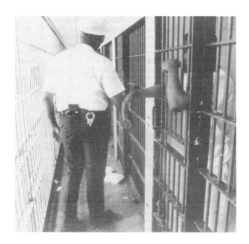

Many states, and the Federal Government, have forfeiture laws, whereby property used in a crime is confiscated. The Federal Government has parking lots and hangars filled with motorcycles, cars, boats, and aircraft seized from people selling drugs. Seized property also includes real estate. Consider the following situation: a teenage boy does a little small-time dealing from his parents' house and car. They find out about it and tell him to stop. If the boy is caught, and the prosecutor can prove that his parents knew about it, they could lose both their home and their car under drug forfeiture laws.

Possession

Laws regulating the control of drugs most commonly refer to possession of the substance. This is often mistakenly believed to mean only physical possession of the drug. In fact, the legal definition of possession is extended to include *control* of the drug, whether or not it is in direct possession, and *physical proximity*, when the drug is nearby but not necessarily on the person. If a drug is found in someone's car, for example, a charge of possession can be made even if it is argued that the drug belongs to someone else.

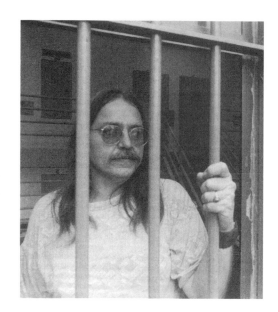

Intent to distribute

Drug crimes are not only a matter of possessing or selling the drug. Many casual drug users do not realize that possessing even a relatively small amount of a drug may automatically be considered "intent to distribute," regardless of whether the drug is for use or for sale. With crack cocaine, this can be as little as five grams, about a teaspoon.

Conspiracy

A person associated with people who possess or sell drugs may be convicted of conspiracy, even if they never touch the drugs themselves. Seemingly innocent acts—lending a friend a car, cashing a check, or allowing a dealer to use a telephone—can be construed as complicity in a drug deal, and bring a prison sentence for conspiring to sell drugs.

Federal drug penalties: marijuana, as of January 1, 1996 [23]

Amount	First Offense	Second Offense
Marijuana: Less than 50 kg Hashish: 10 kg or more Hash oil: 1 kg or more	*Prison:* Maximum 5 years *Fine:* Maximum $250,000 individual $1 million other	*Prison:* Maximum 10 years *Fine:* Maximum $500,000 individual $2 million other
Marijuana: 50 to 99 kg or 50 to 99 plants	*Prison:* Maximum 20 years If death or serious injury: mininum 20 years maximum life *Fine:* Maximum $1 million individual $5 million other	*Prison:* Maximum 30 years If death or serious injury: maximum life *Fine:* Maximum $2 million individual $10 million other
Marijuana: 100 to 999 kg or 100 to 999 plants	*Prison:* Minimum 5 years Maximum 40 years If death or serious injury: mininum 20 years maximum life *Fine:* Maximum $2 million individual $5 million other	*Prison:* Minimum 10 years Maximum life If death or serious injury: maximum life *Fine:* Maximum $4 million individual $10 million other
Marijuana: more than 1000 kg or 1000 plants	*Prison:* Minimum 10 years Maximum life If death or serious injury: mininum 20 years maximum life *Fine:* Maximum $4 million individual $10 million other	*Prison:* Minimum 20 years Maximum life If death or serious injury: maximum life *Fine:* Maximum $8 million individual $20 million other

Federal drug penalties: other drugs, as of January 1, 1996 [24]

Drug & Amount	First Offense	Second Offense
Any illegal drug (except marijuana, hashish, hash oil) Any amount	*Prison:* Maximum 20 years If death or serious injury: mininum 20 years maximum life *Fine:* Maximum $1 million individual $5 million other	*Prison:* Maximum 30 years If death or serious injury: maximum life *Fine:* Maximum $2 million individual $10 million other
Methamphetamine 10-99 gm pure 100-999 gm mixture **Heroin** 100-999 gm mixture **Cocaine** 500-4999 gm mixture **Cocaine base** 5-49 gm mixture **PCP** 10-99 gm pure 100-999 gm mixture **LSD** 1-9 gm mixture **Fentanyl** 40-399 gm mixture **Fentanyl analogue** 10-99 gm mixture	*Prison:* Minimum 5 years Maximum 40 years If death or serious injury: mininum 20 years maximum life *Fine:* Maximum $2 million individual $5 million other	*Prison:* Minimum 10 years Maximum life If death or serious injury: maximum life *Fine:* Maximum $4 million individual $10 million other
Methamphetamine 100 gm or more pure 1 kg or more mixture **Heroin** 1 kg or more mixture **Cocaine** 5 kg or more mixture **Cocaine base** 50 gm or more mixture **PCP** 100 gm or more pure 1 kg or more mixture **LSD** 10 gm or more mixture **Fentanyl** 400 gm or more mixture **Fentanyl analogue** 100 gm or more mixture	*Prison:* Minimum 10 years Maximum life If death or serious injury: mininum 20 years maximum life *Fine:* Maximum $4 million individual $10 million other	*Prison:* Minimum 20 years Maximum life If death or serious injury: minimum life *Fine:* Maximum $8 million individual $20 million other

"BUT OFFICER …!"

"My friend gave me a ride downtown and the cops pulled him over. They found a couple of rocks of crack in the open ashtray. That was not my stuff, but they charged me too. Can they do that?"

Yes they can. Possession of a drug does not mean that you have to control it or have it in your hand or pocket.

In this case, the police can't tell who put the rocks in the ashtray, since it was right between the two of you. Unless your friend claims it, he can say that it was yours. The police can arrest anyone they think might have the drugs.

"I use drugs, but I never sold them. The cops busted me with some heroin and I got charged with possession for sale. How can they do that?"

The police do not have to prove you were selling drugs, only that you had an intention to sell drugs. They can decide this on the basis of the situation and their opinion. For example, if the drug was in many small packages, or found with weighing scales, this will be enough to prove that you wanted to sell the drugs.

"I got some new stuff. It's supposed to be just like Demerol, but it is a different chemical. So it is legal. There is no law against it. Check it out!"

Not true. Until 1986, a drug was legal unless the Government made it illegal. Now, any substance that resembles an illegal drug—or has the same effects and might be used in the same way—may be considered illegal as if it was the actual drug.

"There were six of us in a car and the others were smoking up. It got really thick in there. I didn't smoke myself, but the next day I tested positive for marijuana. Can I get off?"

Probably not. The law does not allow "passive inhalation" as an excuse for testing positive for marijuana at the Federal cutoff levels (see *Chapter 5*).

*"My buddy FedEx'd me an ounce of weed. They must have opened and
searched the package because right after it was delivered, I got busted. I
thought that was illegal! They can't search a package without a warrant,
can they?"*

Packages sent through the U.S. Postal Service may not be searched
without a warrant if they are sent at a post office. If dropped into a mailbox,
however, they may be opened freely.

FedEx and UPS are private services and not part of the U.S. Postal
Service. Packages sent by these services do not come under the Postal regulation,
and may be opened freely.

*"How is it that I can't buy morphine here, but I can go to Mexico and get
some to bring back—and it's legal?"*

Under current law, U.S. citizens are allowed to import into the U.S. a
"personal use" supply of pharmaceuticals. These include Schedule II controlled
substances, such as morphine and cocaine (but not Schedule I substances).

In Mexico and many other countries, it is possible to get a prescription,
or buy these substances, from unscrupulous doctors or pharmacies. This
loophole has been exploited by many drug dealers who resell the drugs illegally
in the U.S. Under the Controlled Substances Trafficking Prohibition Act of
1998, the "personal use" amount was reduced to no more than fifty pills or
"generally a two-week supply."

For this personal use exemption, the traveler must have a valid
prescription for the drug, the imported drug must be in the original container
in which it was dispensed, with a clear label of contents, and a declaration
must be made to an appropriate official of the U.S. Customs Service.

*"An undercover police officer was trying to buy some Ecstasy from me. I
knew he was a cop, so I just sold him some aspirin with the lettering
rubbed off. I was pretty happy with my scam, but I got busted anyway!
How can they do that?"*

Under the "imitation controlled substance law," it doesn't matter if the
substance sold was actually a drug. The point is that it was represented as an
illegal drug, which carries the same penalty as selling the actual illegal drug.

"I got arrested with a few hits of LSD. It was my first time in court and the prosecutor let me plead to the possession for one day in jail and probation. No big deal, right?"

Any drug conviction will affect your life permanently. You will have a difficult time ever getting Government employment, a professional license, or a job in which you must be bonded. In some states, you could lose your eligibility to receive public assistance or even to drive a car. If you are an immigrant, you may be deported. A conviction for drugs is a terrible thing to carry for the rest of your life.

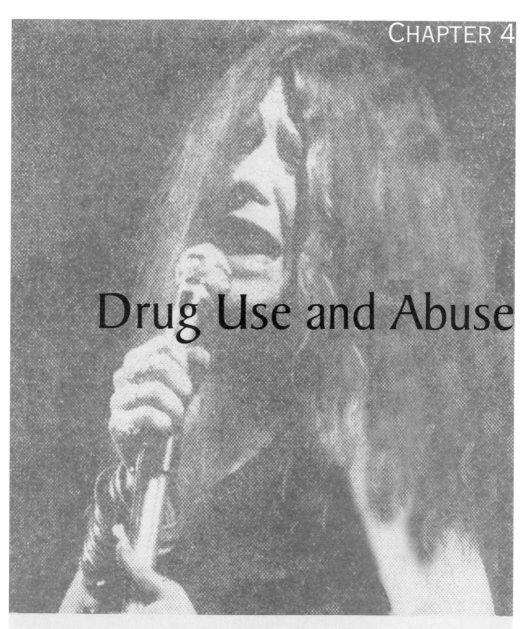

CHAPTER 4

Drug Use and Abuse

Death of Janis Joplin Attributed To Accidental Heroin Overdose

"I'm almost sorry for people who haven't been alcoholic,
because I know things a person who's never been sick doesn't know."
—*First Lady Betty Ford*

The Notion of Substance Abuse

Substance abuse has a different meaning in the legal sense from the psychiatric sense. Legally, abuse refers to substances that are used for non-medical or non-legitimate purposes. Using a drug just for fun is therefore considered abuse of a drug.

The psychiatric meaning of abuse considers the outcome rather than the purpose of use. According to the standard definition, given by the American Psychiatric Association in their Diagnostic and Statistical Manual of Mental Disorders,[1] substance abuse is:

A maladaptive pattern of substance use leading to clinically significant impairment or distress, as manifested by one (or more) of the following, occurring within a 12-month period:

1.   Recurrent substance use resulting in a failure to fulfill major role obligations at work, school, or home

2.   Recurrent substance use in situations in which it is physically hazardous

3.   Recurrent substance-related legal problems

4.   Continued substance use despite having persistent or recurrent social or interpersonal problems caused or exacerbated by the effects of the substance

In short, abuse is defined as "the continued use of a drug despite negative consequences."[2]

 Who got them started on illegal drugs?
20% used drugs with their parents
19% used drugs with another relative
1% were introduced to drugs by a dealer

TYPES OF ILLEGAL DRUG USE

When does drug use become abuse? Typically, people do not start to use drugs with the intention of disrupting their lives or becoming addicted. Drug use usually begins with curiosity, encouragement by friends, or a desire to find relief from boredom, pain, anxiety or depression. Use shades into abuse when drug activity starts to cause problems in the person's life.

Illegal drug use can be considered to fall into one of the following categories, where any level of use may progress to the next:

Experimental use
This is short-term, random use of one or more drugs. It usually occurs out of curiosity, encouragement by friends, or a desire to reach an altered state of mind.

↳ **Recreational use**
This occurs most often with friends who get together occasionally to take the drug, either out of interest or pleasure.

↳ **Circumstantial use**
By this point, the drug is used for a specific purpose: to cope with a problem or achieve a certain mood. The user may take the drug with friends, with acquaintances, with strangers, or alone. They may take it in binges, backing off when they need less or when problems from using the drug overcome the benefit.

↳ **Compulsive use**
This is drug addiction. The user's life is dominated by getting and using the drug. Everything else is less important. Addicts may be able to function quite well as long as they have access to the drug and use it in a regulated way, but their use can easily become uncontrollable and lead to physical, social, and legal problems.

Drug Use Illnesses

SINGLE-DOSE PROBLEMS
People using illegal drugs rarely know how much of the drug they are taking and what else is in the substance. They rely on the word of the person who sold it to them—not a very dependable source of information. No matter how long or often a drug has been taken, each time a drug is used there is a danger of a bad reaction resulting from impurities in the drug, from infection, from overdose, or other physical conditions.

A bad reaction to the single use of a drug can occur after minutes, hours, days, or even years. For example, in the 1960s, injecting amphetamines and opiates became popular, with users often sharing needles. Thirty years later, thousands of these people developed irreversible liver damage from the newly discovered Hepatitis C virus, which had been dormant in the liver, slowly destroying it ever since that initial infection from sharing dirty needles. Just a single use may have resulted in lifelong infection with Hepatitis C or HIV.

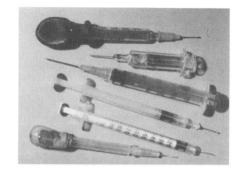

INTRAVENOUS DRUG USE

When a drug is taken by smoking, snorting, chewing, or ingesting, the body has an opportunity to protect itself by immune cells on the surface of the lungs and mucosal membranes. If a drug is injected, it bypasses these defenses.

Injectable medications are sterile and designed to dissolve easily in the bloodstream. Most injected illegal drugs consist of non-sterile powders or crushed pills dissolved in water. The fine particles irritate the blood vessels, setting off a chain of reactions that lead to vascular inflammation and permanent damage. Undissolved fragments can lodge in tiny blood vessels of the lungs, heart, brain, and eyes, causing hemorrhage, strokes, and blindness.

Non-infectious lung disease from intravenous drug use[3]

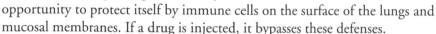

Atelectasis
Bronchopleural fistula
Pneumomediastinum
Pneumothorax
Pulmonary edema
Pulmonary embolism of needle fragments
Pulmonary fibrosis
Pulmonary talcosis

Injecting drugs also poses a high risk of infection from contaminated drugs and needles. Skin injury is the most obvious sign of intravenous drug use, with scars from needle punctures along the veins of the arms, back of the hands, top of the feet, and the neck. Even the veins of the abdomen and penis have been used. Veins irritated by drugs will quickly collapse or harden and can no longer be injected. Drugs may then be shot directly into skin or muscle, causing infectious abscesses and further scarring.

To protect the veins from small pill fragments, many intravenous users filter the drug through a pinch of cotton. This practice might screen out some of the larger fragments, but results in the injection of even tinier fragments of the cotton itself, which can cause a strong immune reaction from the body.

"Cotton fever" begins about 10 to 20 minutes after injection, with headache, chills, breathlessness, nausea, vomiting, and pain in the muscles, joints, abdomen, and low back. These symptoms tend to disappear without treatment within 12 to 24 hours.[4]

Infections due to intravenous drug use[5]

Bone and joint infection
Brain abscess
Candidal meningitis
Cellulitis (skin infection)
Cerebral mucormycosis
Endocarditis
Endophthalmitis
Epidural abscess
Fungal cerebritis
Fungal meningitis
Gas gangrene
Gonorrhea
HTLV-1, HTLV-2
HIV
Malaria
Penile gangrene
Phlebitis (vein infection)
Spinal abscess
Syphilis
Systemic candidiasis
Tetanus
Tick-borne relapsing fever
Tubercular meningitis
Tuberculosis
Viral hepatitis (types A, B, C, and D)
Wound botulism

Using sterile needles can prevent the most likely cause of infection—sharing dirty needles. Many public health specialists have recommended the legal, non-prescription purchase of syringes, or free needle-exchange programs. Statistics show that access to clean needles can prevent infectious disease: in states where syringes are given out in needle-exchange programs, HIV infection rates for IV drug users hover around 35 percent, compared with 80 percent in states without needle-exchange programs.[6]

How do intravenous drug users die?
Autopsies done on people who died from intravenous drug use show that only 11 percent died from overdose. About half died from infections, especially the HIV virus causing AIDS.

OVERDOSE

To avoid serious or permanent injury, anyone who has overdosed on drugs should be taken to the Emergency Department. It is very important to notify the ED of the drugs the person might have taken (including prescription drugs). Without knowing this, it is difficult for the ED to administer the proper treatment.

"Get a tox screen!"
Many people believe that an Emergency Department can quickly discover which drugs someone has taken. This may be true on television, but in reality the ED toxicology screen only looks for a few, most common drugs, and the results can take a long time.

　　　　For proper treatment, it is very important that you tell the ED exactly what drugs the patient might have taken.[7]

Treatments of overdose generally follow one of three principles:

Get the drug out of the body
This can be done by pumping the stomach, giving medications that cause vomiting or diarrhea, or giving medications that bind to the drug (such as activated charcoal) or neutralize it.

Counter the effects of the drug
The action of the drug can be balanced by giving medications that do the opposite. For example, sedatives may be given to a person who has overdosed on amphetamines, or a stimulant given for an overdose of depressants.

Block the action of the drug in the brain
By blocking the neurotransmitter receptors, the action of the drug will be prevented until it is flushed out of the system. For example, naloxone is used to block the opiate receptor in the treatment of opiate overdose.

LONG-TERM PROBLEMS

Long-term repeated use of a drug can cause a variety of problems. Some of these are due to the development of tolerance, resulting in a withdrawal syndrome if the drug is stopped. Others arise from the cumulative impact of the drug on the body: for example, repeated use of MDMA and amphetamines causes a gradual erosion of brain nerve cells, which may not be noticed until old age.

Other long-term effects include nasal ulceration or perforation from heavy cocaine use, collapsed veins from repeated injection, and burned fingers from smoking crack.

The most common long-term effect is a loss of interest and motivation in life. Drugs are a passive type of experience. With chronic use a person can become more passive in general, relying on an external source of mental experiences.

90% of strokes in people 20 to 40 years old are due to drugs,[8] usually cocaine, stimulants or opiates.

A stroke can occur any time: with the first, the tenth, or the hundredth use of the drug.

WITHDRAWAL

Not all drugs cause a withdrawal syndrome when the user stops taking them. Those that do, generally produce withdrawal effects that are opposite from the effects of the drug. For example, the use of opiates causes numbness, euphoria, dry skin and mouth, constipation, slow pulse, low blood pressure, and pinpoint pupils. The opposite occurs when opiate use is stopped: pain, anxiety, sweating and runny nose, diarrhea, rapid pulse, high blood pressure, and dilated pupils (see *Opiates*).

For most drugs, withdrawal is usually just uncomfortable, but for some drugs it can be hazardous or even fatal.

The treatment of withdrawal takes two approaches:

👍 **Suppress withdrawal by giving a chemically similar medication**
This is usually done by giving a medication that is longer lasting and less psychoactive than the drug being withdrawn. For example, methadone (an opiate) is given for opiate withdrawal.

👍 **Treat the symptoms of withdrawal**
The specific symptoms of withdrawal may be treated to make the process less miserable. For example, clonidine may be given to relieve the flu-like feelings of opiate withdrawal.[9]

PREGNANCY

The fetus is exposed to almost every drug taken by a woman, and is very sensitive to its effects. Unfortunately, many women are not even aware that they are pregnant during the first eight weeks, the time of the greatest risk to the unborn child.

 Drugs of any kind can be very toxic to the fetus. Unless specifically approved by a physician, pregnant women should stop the use of all drugs, including tobacco, alcohol, and herbal medications.

Pregnancy, especially in women who take heroin, may not be obvious because many women stop menstruating when they become heavy drug users.[10]

Surveys show that about one in ten infants have been exposed to illegal drugs during pregnancy. The result is a great increase in the risk of miscarriage and infant deformity. Even with an apparently healthy baby, the risk of sudden infant death syndrome (SIDS) is much higher if the mother has used recreational drugs.[11]

If mom uses ...	the risk of SIDS is
PCP	4 times higher
Cocaine	8 times higher
Opiates	18 times higher

Addiction

Besides the danger of overdose, the greatest risk of drugs is addiction. While overdose is a physical problem, addiction is a matter of behavior. In itself, addiction may not cause serious illness or injury, but its effect on the life of the drug user can be devastating.

 "I'll die young, but it's like kissing God."—*Lenny Bruce, talking about his drug addiction.*

SUBSTANCE DEPENDENCE

In medical studies, "substance dependence" is the term used for addiction. There are two types of substance dependence: psychological dependence and physical dependence. Psychological dependence is a craving for the drug, so that the user is desperate to get more.[12] Physical dependence means that there are physical symptoms of withdrawal when the person stops using the drug, such as hangover, body aches, or a flu-like feeling.[13] Addiction is generally considered to be a condition of psychological dependence with or without accompanying physical dependence. A drug user can be addicted even though there are no withdrawal symptoms.

 Addiction is the repetitive, compulsive use of a substance despite negative consequences to the user.

According to the American Psychiatric Association,[14] substance dependence is defined as a maladaptive pattern of substance use leading to impairment or distress, with at least three of the following:

☹ **Tolerance**
A need for increasing amounts of the substance to achieve the desired effect, or a diminished effect with the same amount.

☹ **Withdrawal**
A syndrome of impairment or distress that occurs when use of the substance is stopped, and relieved when it is taken again.

☹ **Increasing amounts**
The substance is taken in larger amounts or over a longer period than was intended.

☹ **Attempts to stop use**
There is a persistent desire or unsuccessful efforts to cut down or control the use of the substance.

☹ **Drug-seeking behavior**
A great deal of time is spent in activities necessary to obtain the substance, or recover from its effects.

☹ **Neglecting other activities**
Important social, occupational, or recreational activities are given up or reduced because of the substance use.

☹ **Drug problems**
The person continues to use the substance even though he or she knows that it is causing physical or psychological problems.

 "Wouldn't you? Yes you would. You would lie, cheat, inform on your friends, steal, do anything to satisfy total need. Because you would be in a state of total sickness, total possession, and not in a position to act any other way."—*William Burroughs, Naked Lunch.*

Animal studies

In experiments with animals that are habituated to a drug—given the drug long enough to establish addiction—the animals will start to dose themselves in ways remarkably similar to humans. If monkeys and rats are trained to press a lever to deliver an intravenous dose of cocaine, they will do so up to 300 times for a single injection. If they are given free access to cocaine, they will continue to take it even after they have seizures. While most animals will not take dangerous amounts of alcohol, nicotine, or heroin, they will take cocaine until they kill themselves. They will go on long binges and, after a few days, many of them will give themselves a lethal dose.[15]

I Iumans show the same behavior: usually the only thing that stops a serious cocaine addict is running out of cocaine.

Addiction and the brain

It is believed that the part of the brain most responsible for the rewarding—and probably addictive—effects of some drugs is the nucleus accumbens (see *Chapter 6*). These cells use the neurotransmitter dopamine, which is increased by drugs such as nicotine, cocaine, and amphetamines.

All addictive drugs appear to set up a pleasure-reward-withdrawal cycle in the brain that creates craving for more of the drug.

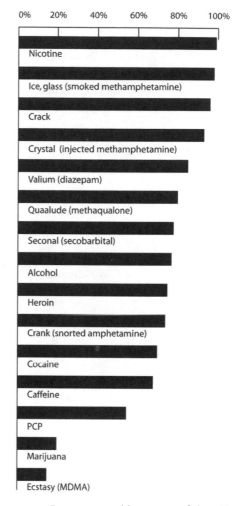

| 0% | 20% | 40% | 60% | 80% | 100% |

Nicotine

Ice, glass (smoked methamphetamine)

Crack

Crystal (injected methamphetamine)

Valium (diazepam)

Quaalude (methaqualone)

Seconal (secobarbital)

Alcohol

Heroin

Crank (snorted amphetamine)

Cocaine

Caffeine

PCP

Marijuana

Ecstasy (MDMA)

Experts rate addictiveness of drugs[16]

"… sudden leaving off the uses of opium after a long and lavish use [caused] great and even intolerable distresses, anxieties and depressions of the spirit, which commonly end in a most miserable death, attended with strange agonies, unless men return to the use of opium; which soon raises them again, and certainly restores them."—*John Jones, The Mysteries of Opium Revealed, 1700* [17]

Is addiction genetic?

Not all individuals respond the same way to addictive substances. Some quickly become dependent while others never do. Most people become addicted only after using the drug for a long time. For example, only about three percent of those who use cocaine, and less than one percent who use medically prescribed opiates, develop any form of addiction.

It is likely that there are many factors determining whether an individual will become substance dependent, including a genetic component. Studies of adopted children show that their risk of addiction is more similar to that of their biological parents than that of their adoptive parents. People who have become dependent on one substance are also more likely to become dependent on other substances, leading to the concept of an "addictive personality."

STAGES OF ADDICTION

Addiction does not occur immediately, but usually follows from a gradual process in which the drug becomes increasingly important to the person's life.

Experimental stage

Taking drugs usually starts with experimental use. This may be simple curiosity, a rite of passage into a social group, or the result of peer pressure.

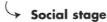

Social stage

At this stage, the person still feels normal, but the use of the drug is a big part of social acceptance and identity.

Instrumental stage

The user now takes the drug for a specific purpose: for pleasure, or to cope with anger, shame, guilt, boredom, stress, or loneliness. Signs of dependency begin to appear. The user drifts away from old friends and spends much more time with others, who also use the drug heavily. At this point, the main form of socializing and recreation is getting high. There is tolerance, leading to more drug use, and extreme mood swings. The person no longer feels normal—either high with the drug, or irritable, anxious, depressed, and craving the drug.

Compulsive stage

In the final stage of addiction, the user is preoccupied with the drug and will do anything to get it, including theft and prostitution. The addict will hide drugs, even from friends. Most addicts do not recognize their dependence, but become lost in arrogance and illusions of grandiosity.[18]

Despite the popular notion that most drug users are addicts, in fact only a small percentage of users fall into this category. About 80 percent of heroin users, for example, are "chippers"—using occasionally and non-addictively. Drug use may lead to addiction, but usually falls somewhere short of that. Most people stop before they ever become addicted.

STAGES OF RECOVERY

A tremendous amount of research has been devoted to helping addicts recover from addiction. It is now believed that this recovery takes place in six stages, from thinking to acting:[19]

Precontemplation
Before change can take place, a person needs to recognize the problem. Addicts typically deny that a problem exists, or blame their genetic makeup, family—anything or anybody but themselves.

Contemplation
Once the person recognizes the problem, a plan is made to change, usually within the next six months. True change, however, may be years away. At this point, most addicts are focused on the past, on the problem—when they should be thinking about the future, and the solution.

Preparation
This involves the addict setting a date for action and publicly announcing they intend to change their behavior. A plan of action is important, including coping strategies.

Action
An enormous commitment of time and energy may be required. The addict will benefit from strong encouragement and support.

Maintenance
Once the goal is achieved, the addict has to remain focused to avoid lapses and relapses. This stage can last from six months to a lifetime.

Termination
When temptation no longer exists, the former addict may consider the problem resolved. Some experts argue, however, that addiction is a life-long issue that never entirely disappears.

TWELVE-STEP PROGRAMS

In 1934, two recovering alcoholics, Bill Wilson and Dr. Bob Smith, met while looking for mutual support to stay sober. A year later, in Akron, Ohio, they founded Alcoholics Anonymous. The goal of this self-help group was simple: by gathering in a social group (where, ironically, most drink coffee and smoke tobacco—two other highly addictive drugs), they could share their stories and provide mutual support for recovery from alcohol addiction. The principle of AA, as it came to be known, is "once an alcoholic, always an alcoholic." Alcoholism is considered a chronic disease that can flare up any time, and the former alcoholic must be aware of this for the rest of his life. Recovery takes place by following 12 steps:[20]

Step 1   Admitted we were powerless over alcohol—that our lives had become unmanageable.

Step 2   Came to believe that a Power greater than ourselves could restore us to sanity.

Step 3   Made a decision to turn our will and our lives over to the care of God as we understood Him.

Step 4   Made a searching and fearless moral inventory of ourselves.

Step 5   Admitted to God, to ourselves, and to another human being the exact nature of our wrongs.

Step 6   Were entirely ready to have God remove all these defects of character.

Step 7   Humbly asked Him to remove our shortcomings.

Step 8   Made a list of all persons we had harmed, and became willing to make amends to them all.

Step 9   Made direct amends to such people wherever possible, except when to do so would injure them or others.

Step 10   Continued to take personal inventory and when we were wrong promptly admitted it.

Step 11   Sought through prayer and meditation to improve our conscious contact with God as we understood Him, praying only for knowledge of His will for us and the power to carry that out.

Step 12   Having had a spiritual awakening as the result of these steps, we tried to carry this message to alcoholics, and to practice these principles in all our affairs.

Although many people objected to the heavy emphasis on religion (7 of the 12 steps refer to God or a spiritual power), AA is considered to be one of the most effective means of resolving alcoholism.

The success of AA led to its adaptation for other substance addictions. Narcotics Anonymous groups are organized the same way. Fewer people are involved in NA groups but they appear to be effective in helping addicts recover from their addiction.

Drug Resistance Educational Programs

FADS AND FASHIONS

Like other fashions, the popularity of any drug goes through cycles. Marijuana use declines, but is followed by an increase in crack. Crack gives way to MDMA and GHB. Then the trend swings back to marijuana. These cycles make it difficult to evaluate the effectiveness of programs to discourage drug use. Is the decline in cocaine use due to massive Government intervention? Or is it due to shifting trends—cocaine becoming less popular and being replaced by the increased use of MDMA? Enormous efforts have been made by the Government to stop illegal drug use, with some statistical success. But the fact remains that the use of mind-altering drugs is still widespread.

The most extensive anti-drug educational program is Drug Abuse Resistance Education. The DARE program sends police officers to middle and junior highschools to meet with students in the classroom and work through a programmed syllabus in 17 weekly sessions. DARE was founded in 1981 by former Los Angeles Police Chief Daryl Gates. It now operates in about 80 percent of American school districts, serving some 36 million students in 10,000 communities, with an annual cost of about $700 million. DARE is also used in 49 other countries, with strong U.S. encouragement and economic support.

Is it effective in decreasing illegal drug use? The results of DARE evaluations are contradictory. While most appear to show a decrease in selected drug use, a detailed study by Richard Clayton of the University of Kentucky for the years 1987-1992 could find little effect by DARE on later drug use among Kentucky schoolchildren who participated in the program. Similar studies in North Carolina and Minnesota reached the same conclusion.[21]

Other anti-drug educational programs, including Students Taught Awareness and Resistance (STAR), Life Skills Training (LST), and Prevention Dimension take a different approach. These programs give less emphasis to the criminal aspects of drug use and focus instead on helping students identify, understand, and resist the daily pressures they encounter to use tobacco, alcohol, and other drugs. This type of "social influences" approach may be more effective than that of DARE.

In the United States, Government-supported educational programs are coordinated by the Office of National Drug Control Policy (ONDCP) headed by the president-appointed "drug czar." The position is currently held by John Walters, a previous assistant to William Bennett, who is expected to advocate similar policies of increased punishment for drug offenders. The ONDCP develops strategies to wage the war on drugs, and works with community organizations, especially the Partnership for a Drug Free America.[22] Their programs focus mainly on describing the hazards of drug use, and discouraging use by warnings of illness and threats of punishment. The efficacy of this approach is questionable since it does little to educate the public about the drugs involved. Americans pride themselves on resistance to authority and prefer to make an individual decision about what is good for them. Drug "education" that does not describe drugs, but simply tells students not to use them, may do little to discourage potential users.

TOP TEN REASONS WHY PEOPLE USE ILLEGAL DRUGS

1. To numb the body

The opiates, barbiturates, methaqualone, and other drugs have historically been taken to help the user escape pain, dissociate from the body, and achieve a sort of mental vacation. Prostitutes have always favored drugs for this reason. Today, an increasing number of people suffer from "body dysphoria," a feeling of simply not liking your physical appearance. Mind-altering drugs allow a respite from these feelings, a "time-out" in which the user can enjoy an interlude in which the body is no longer a source of embarrassment and suffering.

2. Recreation

Throughout history, drugs have been taken simply for pleasure. The earliest recreational drugs were the opiates and marijuana, later joined by alcohol, caffeine, and tobacco. Recreation is probably the most common reason for illegal drug use today.

3. To join a social group

Many people use illegal drugs to participate in a social group. This can occur through peer pressure, through a desire to join a group that uses a drug, or simply as a part of group activity and an excuse to get together. Sharing a drug, whether alcohol or marijuana, can be a vital part of a social group. It can be uncomfortable to be the only one at the party who doesn't join in.

4. Social functioning

MDMA gained popularity as a way to help shy, inhibited people to open up socially. The same was true for amphetamines (which were even prescribed for this purpose). Cocaine is used by many people in the belief that it gives them an alertness, ebullience, and gregariousness that helps their business dealings.

5.   Mind expansion

For thousands of years, the hallucinogens have been taken to explore other realms of consciousness. History is replete with descriptions such as the *Soma* of ancient India, the Eleusian rites of ancient Greece, and the many drug rituals of the ancient civilizations of the Americas.

In the 1950s, a renewed interest in drug-induced altered states of consciousness spurred the rediscovery of old drugs and the invention of countless new ones. This practice continues unabated and is not likely to stop.

6.   Religion

Closely related to altered consciousness is the use of a drug specifically to contact God, to ask for personal direction, to obtain an answer to a question, or simply to deepen religious faith. The most prominent example of this is the use of peyote by the Native American Church (see *Peyote and Mescaline*), but it is also used less formally by people coping with terminal illness and other spiritual issues. Drugs for this purpose are known as entheogens ("contacting the God within"), and have a growing number of users.

7.   To improve performance

Some illegal drugs are believed to increase strength, endurance, or alertness. Historically, peyote was used by the Tarahumara for their marathon foot races and ibogaine was used by Africans in days-long lion hunts. Today, stimulants such as amphetamines and cocaine are often taken for energy and endurance. MDMA is used at raves to dance all night, and PCP has been favored by urban gangs to increase aggressiveness and tolerance of violent injury.

8.   To change the body

Amphetamines are often taken for weight loss. GHB was first used to increase muscle mass, and was widely sold in gyms and health clubs for this purpose.

9.   Self-medication

Illegal drugs may be taken for a specific illness, without medical supervision. The medicinal use of marijuana is a common example. More commonly, and less reasonably, a drug is used to help cope with anxiety, depression, and other illnesses that would more effectively be managed by a health professional.

10.   Because they are illegal

The surest way to encourage some people to do something is to specifically forbid it. This lesson is as old as humanity; it is told in the Greek myth of Pandora, the story of the forbidden fruit in the Bible's Book of Genesis, and in the creation myths of most of the world's religions. Some people, even those who shun legal drugs, will take illegal drugs just because they are illegal. Adolescents, in particular, tend to question authority and flaunt risk-taking behavior.

TOP TEN REASONS WHY PEOPLE DO NOT USE ILLEGAL DRUGS

1.   Social agreement

Social norms are a strong incentive against using drugs. Even among users of illegal drugs, some drugs are accepted and others shunned. It has often been observed that those who use hallucinogens disdain the opiate users ("junkies"), while opiate users think people are crazy to use hallucinogens ("acid-heads").

On the larger level, social norms are the very reason why some drugs are illegal. People in the United States do not take these drugs because they are not part of the American culture. In other countries alcohol may be illegal while other psychoactive drugs are not.

2.   Lack of purity

Some people might use illegal drugs diverted from medical use, but do not use other illegal drugs because of a reasonable concern about their purity. For example, some prescription narcotic addicts would not consider using street heroin.

One reason MDMA and Rohypnol have become popular among highschool and college students is because they mistakenly think they are taking high-quality pharmaceuticals rather than illegally produced drugs.

3.   Toxicity

Illegal drugs are usually illegal because they have been shown to cause serious injury to the body or mind. Most people respect this hazard and stay away from them.

4.   Lack of knowledge

Many people are justifiably concerned about taking a possibly hazardous substance about which little is known.

Once a drug has been designated a Schedule I Controlled Substance, it becomes very difficult for researchers to obtain permission to study that drug. The result is that most of what is known about substances such as LSD dates from the 1950s and 60s, and very little is known about more recent drugs, such as 2C-B. This lack of knowledge can both help and hinder drug education programs, by replacing research and fact with rumor and propaganda.

5.   Lack of supervision

Many people have a realistic concern about the effects of an illegal drug and will only take it under adequate supervision. Since this type of supervision is seldom available, they do not use these drugs. The lack of safe and controlled settings is a reasonable discouragement for the use of psychoactive drugs.

An increasing number of people are going to Native American Church ceremonies to participate in the structured use of peyote (see *Peyote and Mescaline*), or traveling to South America on guided tours that feature participation in ayahuasca rituals. These are people who would not otherwise take an illegal drug, but feel safe in these settings.

6.   Lack of availability

The popular African drugs ibogaine and cathinone are rarely used in America in part because they are difficult to find. The same is true of many other drugs that are not well distributed. Decreasing availability is the major emphasis of the war on drugs.

7.   Impaired performance

All psychoactive drugs impair intellectual performance, usually by decreasing alertness or concentration. Most also impair physical performance. For this reason, many people avoid both legal and illegal drugs.

Athletes, pilots, professional drivers, parolees, and anyone in occupations with drug-surveillance programs have a special need to avoid illegal drugs since they will lose their jobs or privileges if they are caught using any unauthorized drug.

8.   Fear of addiction

Many people avoid using cocaine, opiates, amphetamines, and other illegal drugs because they are afraid of becoming addicted.

9.   Expense

Illegal drugs are simply too expensive for many people, especially children and adolescents, even if they have no qualms about the other issues.

10.   Because they are illegal

Regardless of other issues, respect for the law and the threat of punishment are enough for most people to decide against the use of illegal drugs.

CHAPTER 5

Drugs at Work: Employee Drug Testing

"Substance abuse is arguably the number one public health problem
in the United States, affecting 18 percent of the population at some time in their lives
and costing $144 billion per year in health care and job loss."
—*Department of Health and Human Services*

Hazards of Drug Use in Industry

For thousands of years, laborers have used drugs for stimulation, for strength, for relaxation, to numb themselves against suffering, or just to avoid boredom and help pass the time at work. The only difference today is the much greater variety of drugs available.

Drugs are commonplace in almost every type of work. The most widespread is caffeine, used by everyone from airline pilots to Zen monks. Alcohol is also a commonly used work drug, although it may not be recognized as such. As anyone who attends conferences knows, the real work is usually done at the "mixers" where alcohol is an important social lubricant. Other drugs may be used less openly, but are pervasive in many jobs. During the Second World War, soldiers as well as factory workers used amphetamines to increase performance. Many continued to do so after the war, to the extent that amphetamines eventually accounted for 20 percent of all prescriptions, most of which were used for increased energy, weight loss, and improved performance.

 A study of long-distance truck drivers found that 62% reported at least occasional illicit drug use while driving.[1]

Each occupation seems to favor certain types of drugs. For example, many writers are notorious alcoholics. Artists and musicians prefer marijuana and hallucinogens for inspiration. Entertainers and businessmen use cocaine for alertness and stamina, while prostitutes use opiates for their numbing effects.

While people's right to use recreational drugs is controversial, most agree that illegal drugs have no business in the workplace. Drug use by workers, however, remains a significant problem in the United States. In 1997, the National Household Survey on Drug Abuse found that there were 6.3 million illicit drug users among the 81.8 million people in U.S. workforce, and a survey by NIDA found that 5 percent of employed people age 20 to 40 had used cocaine in the past month.

There are three major concerns in worksite drug use: employee intoxication, employee reliability, and employee drug-seeking behavior. From the business owner's point of view, drugs result in the following:

- Intoxicated employees are a safety hazard to themselves, to co-workers, and to the public. This is true not only of such obvious professions as truck driver or air traffic controller, but for people working in almost any job where they can injure themselves or miss important information. Accidents and injuries are a huge cost for employers, since they must pay not only for treatment but also the wages of the employee who is off duty in addition to the wages for the replacement worker.

- Health care utilization—not only for injuries, but for *all* health problems—is estimated to be 300 percent higher for drug-using employees. They tend to get sick more often and have more chronic health problems. This can be a very high cost for employers who provide health care for their employees.

In most countries, the highest cost in the manufacture of an automobile is steel. In the United States, it is employee health care. About one third of the cost of a new car is for the automobile workers' health insurance.

- Employees who use drugs have a greater absenteeism. They are frequently away from work because of drug-related symptoms or drug-seeking behavior, and appear to be less committed to their work.

- Job turnover is higher among drug-using employees. There may be a number of reasons for this, but the result is the same: the employer must advertise, interview, hire, and train a new worker.

- Drug-using employees are less productive even while on the job. This is true for any drug, including tobacco. Smokers are 10 to 30 percent less productive than non-smoking employees. An employee going through withdrawal symptoms may not be productive at all. In general, drug-using employees are about one third less productive than those who do not use drugs.

- Because illegal drugs affect the central nervous system, they dull the mind and make learning more difficult. Employee training takes longer and is less effective—another direct cost to the employer.

- A final concern is security issues or theft by drug-using employees. Many operations in which security is a major concern will not only dismiss drug-using employees, but will refuse to hire an applicant who has a record of *ever* using illegal drugs.

Concern about drug use in the workplace reached a peak in the 1980s. It is debatable how much of this was due to a genuine increase in worker drug use, and how much was simply driven by the Federal Government's overall anti-drug program. The emphasis on worksite drug control was considered a useful way to increase drug awareness and decrease use, both in

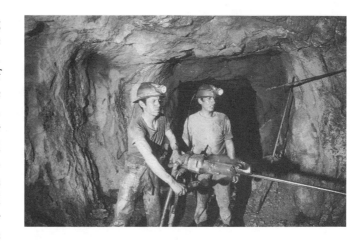

and out of the workplace. For example, there is no evidence that there has ever been a commercial airline accident because of pilot drug use.[2] Strict drug monitoring of pilots was instituted anyway, largely to enhance the public's sense of safety.

On September 15, 1986, President Ronald Reagan signed an Executive Order requiring Federal agencies to establish an employee drug-testing program.[3] A comprehensive program was developed by the Department of Transportation (DOT) and the United States Coast Guard (USCG).[4] Each of the DOT administrations expanded the program in their operations: the Federal Aviation Administration (FAA), which oversees pilots and air traffic controllers; the Federal Highway Administration (FHWA), which oversees professional drivers; the Federal Railroad Administration (FRA); the Federal Transit Administration (FTA); and Research and Special Programs Administration (RSPA), which regulates pipelines. The Nuclear Regulatory Commission (NRC) uses more stringent standards.[5]

Employees subjected to random drug tests

Highway (truck, bus) drivers	7,333,000
Railroad workers	97,000
Aviation (pilots, etc.)	364,000
Transit (bus, subway, etc.) drivers	204,000
Pipeline workers	190,000
Maritime (ships, etc)	132,000
TOTAL	8,320,2000

In 1988, the follow-up Drug Free Workplace Act required all Federal grantees and contractors having a contract for property or services of $25,000 or more to have programs for a drug free workplace. Now, almost all major companies and Federal agencies have drug monitoring programs in place. Drug screening is done not only for truck drivers and airline pilots, but also schoolteachers, athletes, and people preparing to adopt children.

Refusing a drug screen is entirely legal, but will result in the loss of the job or position. And if a worker is fired for refusing to take a drug test, it is virtually impossible for him or her to collect unemployment benefits.

FEDERAL REGULATIONS: THE NIDA 5
Federal drug testing rules authorize testing only for five types of drugs:

1.   Marijuana
2.   Opiates (codeine, morphine, and heroin)
3.   Cocaine
4.   Amphetamine and methamphetamine
5.   PCP (Phencyclidine)

These were recommended by the National Institute of Drug Abuse (NIDA) as the most common and worrisome drugs of abuse,[6] and have come to be known as the NIDA 5.

Under the Federal drug testing programs, the laboratory methods use immunoassay for the initial screening and gas chromatography/mass spectrometry (GC/MS) for confirmation. All cutoff levels are in nanograms per milliliter (ng/mL), which is approximately one part per billion.

Federal drug testing cutoff levels

Initial Test Cutoff Levels	(ng/mL)	Confirmatory Levels	(ng/mL)
Marijuana metabolites	50	Marijuana metabolite*	15
Cocaine metabolites	300	Cocaine metabolite**	150
Opiate metabolites	2000		
		Morphine	2000
		Codeine	2000
		6-AM	10
PCP	25	PCP	25
Amphetamines	1000		
		Amphetamine	500
		Methamphetamine	500

*   Confirmation for marijuana is by testing for the THC metabolite 11-nor-delta-9-THC-9-carboxylic acid.
**   Confirmation for cocaine is by testing for the cocaine metabolite benzoyl-ecgonine.

If a screening test is positive for opiates, the confirmation test will look for the specific type of opiate: morphine, codeine, or 6-AM (indicating heroin). If a screening test is positive for amphetamines, the confirmation test will look specifically for amphetamine and methamphetamine.

Workplace Drug Monitoring

All employees, whether staff or management, fulltime or part-time, are usually included in the drug-testing program. A "mature minor," typically at least age 15, can agree to the test without parental consent.[7]

AMERICANS WITH DISABILITIES ACT

The Americans with Disabilities Act (ADA) was enacted in 1990 to protect people with disabilities from discrimination in the workplace. It applies to Government agencies and all employers with 15 or more employees.

Most people think the disabled are those who are blind, paralyzed, or have other obvious impairments, but disabilities also include psychological conditions, such as depression and schizophrenia, and drug addiction. It is estimated that about 45 million people, or one out of six Americans, are considered disabled.

Under ADA, drug addiction *in the past* is considered a disability and protected, but current illicit drug use is not. Therefore, employers are prohibited from asking about your former drug or alcohol use, but can ask about and test your current use. They can also ask about your criminal record.

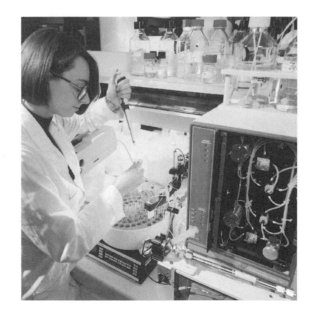

Under ADA, job candidates may not be discriminated against by a medical examination. Urine testing for alcohol is defined as a medical examination, and is therefore not allowed. But the testing of illegal drugs is *not* considered a medical examination, and is allowed.

DRUG TESTING PROGRAMS

Drug testing programs in industry are usually one of six types:

Pre-employment *or* pre-placement

A pre-employment drug test is given after an applicant has been considered for a job, but before the employment offer has been made. This practice has been questioned legally. Most companies now use a pre-placement test, which is given after an offer of employment has been made. The offer of employment is made conditional upon passing the drug screen. This is also called a post-offer test.

Reasonable suspicion, *also known as* reasonable cause *or* for cause

A reasonable suspicion test is given to an employee who is suspected of using a prohibited drug. In DOT-regulated programs, "reasonable suspicion" occurs when a supervisor (some DOT programs require two supervisors) has observed conduct or appearance suggesting drug use. In non-DOT programs, the basis for reasonable suspicion may be defined by state law, company policy, or by company agreements with the employee's union.

Post-accident *or* post-incident

Many companies have a policy in which a drug test is automatically given to any employee involved in an accident or other serious incident.

Questions an employer cannot ask during a job interview [8]

What prescription drugs do you use?
Have you ever abused drugs or alcohol?
Have you ever been in drug or alcohol treatment?
Have you ever had a driving under the influence (DUI) charge?

Questions an employer can ask during a job interview

Do you drink?
Do you currently use illegal drugs?
Have you ever been convicted for a drug offense?
Have you ever had a driving under the influence (DUI) conviction?

Random

A test is given to employees selected at random, without warning.

Return-to-duty

A test given to an employee who has previously had a positive drug test or has previously refused to submit to testing (and was therefore removed from work), before he or she returns to work.

Follow-up

Testing done on a frequent, unannounced schedule after an employee has passed a return-to-duty test. Most DOT programs require a minimum of 6 follow-up tests in the first 12 months, and continue follow-up testing for up to 5 years.

HOW ARE PEOPLE TESTED FOR DRUGS?

Drug use can be determined by testing almost any tissue in the body. For example, fatal accident victims are often tested by analysis of the vitreous humor inside the eyeball. Some bodily tissues can be tested for toxic substances after a period of months or even years—such as the bones or hair of historical figures who died hundreds of years ago.

In current industrial testing programs, the following body materials are used:

- **Urine** testing is by far the most common. It is easy to collect, can be collected on the job site, and is a good indicator of recent drug use. Urine is tested in most workplace programs, as well as treatment and correction programs. Almost all drugs can be detected in urine; an exception is methaqualone.

- **Hair** testing is preferred by the gambling industry for pre-employment screening because it is easy to do without special facilities. It is also used for investigations when other tests are not available, such as criminal cases or deaths. Hair can be tested for most drugs.

  The advantage of testing hair is the long period of detection: the life span of a typical hair ranges from about four months for hairs from the eyelashes or armpit, to four years for hair from the scalp. Hair grows at a rate of about one quarter to one half inch per month. Drugs enter the hair while it is growing and therefore present a record of drug use during the entire period of growth.

  For drug testing, hair samples are usually taken from the back of the head. In a bald person, hair from another part of the body may be used. For people without hair, or who have shaved themselves completely, fingernails may be used.

  Hair testing is less accurate than other methods because of contamination from shampoo residues, hair treatments, smoke, air pollution, and other environmental effects. Another disadvantage is that people have different types of hair, which may affect the readings in the analysis. Dark-haired people such as Hispanics, Asians, and African Americans have a higher concentration of melanin, which incorporates and retains drugs to a higher degree. The result is that a dark-haired person can be ten to fifty times more likely to test positive than a lighter-haired person who used the same amount of drugs.[9] Because of these concerns, most Federal programs do not engage in hair testing.[10]

- **Blood** testing is most commonly done for clinical, diagnostic, and drug overdose purposes. It is routine in hospital emergency rooms. Blood testing can be done even with a severely intoxicated, injured, or dead person, and is therefore favored for post-accident investigation. Almost all drugs can be tested in blood, although THC (marijuana) is particularly difficult to measure.

☞   **Sweat** testing is commonly used in the criminal justice system for monitoring parolees and prisoners. The PharmChek patch is a waterproof adhesive pad about the size of a playing card. It is worn like a bandage for about one week. It is then removed and sent for analysis to PharmChem Laboratories in Menlo Park, California.[11] Sweat testing can be done for cocaine, morphine, 6-AM (heroin), codeine, amphetamine, methamphetamine, THC, PCP, and methadone.

☞   **Oral fluid** (saliva) testing is done only for private insurance evaluations, since the technique is not considered reliable enough under Federal guidelines. A swab is rubbed on the inside of the cheek and then placed in a sealed container and sent off for testing. Saliva will show amphetamines, barbiturates, cocaine, marijuana, opiates, and PCP. Oral fluid testing is more efficient than urine at detecting recent use but is less effective after three days. Advantages include the ease of collection and difficulty of adulteration or substitution, and this form of testing may soon become standard.[12]

CHAIN OF CUSTODY

Since a positive drug test can have a devastating effect on a person's livelihood, and their future prospects for a job, it is critically important that great care is taken to ensure that the testing process is secure and confidential. To do this, the testing specimen is handled in a very precise way, called the "chain of custody."

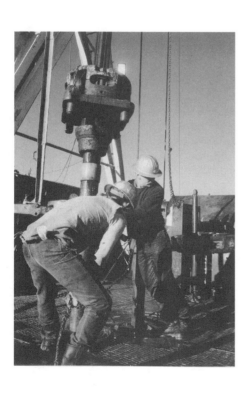

Most drug testing is carried out by collecting a small amount of urine from the employee—about one ounce, or 30 mL. The chain of custody is the process of documenting the transfer of the urine specimen from the donor to the collector, from the collector to the courier, from the courier to the laboratory, and within the laboratory from one person or department to another. Each collection procedure is documented on a custody and control form (CCF), also known as a chain-of-custody form (COC). Most programs use a standard seven-copy Federal CCF, also known as the NIDA Form.[13]

TAMPERED SPECIMENS

Urine specimens are collected in a controlled setting, such as a designated collection booth or bathroom. If it is suspected that the specimen has been tampered with, a special collection may be authorized in which the donor is actually observed urinating into the cup. Tampering is suspected when:

⊘   The urine specimen is outside the allowable temperature range, which is within 1 degree C (1.8 degrees F) of the donor's body temperature.[14] Since the urine supposedly just came out of the body, it should be the same temperature as the donor. If it is not in the allowable temperature range, the urine sample will be suspected as falsified.

⊘   The donor is observed attempting to submit a substituted or adulterated specimen.[15] Most drug testing bathrooms will have a blue die in the toilet water to prevent the donor from adding water to the urine.

⊘   The urine specimen is too diluted (see below, *Diluted Urine*).

⊘   If the laboratory cannot analyze a specimen because of contamination, a "Specimen unsuitable" report will come back to the collecting site, and the donor will be suspected of tampering with the specimen.

The "shy bladder" excuse

Some employees try to avoid a urine test by simply saying they have no urge to urinate, or cannot urinate because they are shy. When "shy bladder" occurs, the donor will be expected to drink up to 40 ounces of fluids and wait for up to three hours. If he or she still cannot urinate, it will be considered a refusal to be tested unless a physician provides a documented medical reason for this condition.

THE URINATOR™

IT'S NOT A DRINK OR AN ADDITIVE !

IT'S A REUSABLE ELECTRONIC DEVICE !

CAN BE USED BY MEN AND WOMEN

IT DOES THE PEEING - SO YOU DON'T HAVE TO!

Attempts to avoid urine drug testing can be quite creative. This product might work—unless a special collection is authorized. If caught, the donor could face severe penalties for trying to falsify a drug test.

LABORATORY ANALYSIS

Drug-testing laboratories must be extremely reliable and legally precise to avoid falsely accusing someone of taking drugs. A negative test may be wrong, but a

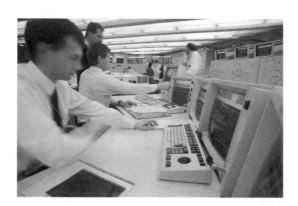

positive test must be one hundred percent accurate. To ensure that a drug detected in a sample is not from accidental exposure, a certain amount of the drug must be present for the sample to be considered positive. This amount is termed the "cutoff value" and is established for each type of drug assay. If the specimen's drug concentration is at or above the cutoff, the result is positive; if the specimen's drug concentration is below the cutoff, the result is negative. "Negative," in this case, does not mean that no drug was det-

ected, but simply that the amount of the drug (if any) was not high enough to meet the established cutoff concentration for that assay.

After a laboratory receives the specimen, it checks the Custody and Control Form for completeness and accuracy. The specimen is then examined for evidence of tampering. If everything is in order, the drug testing takes place.

Screening tests

There are two steps to laboratory testing: screening and confirmation. A screening test is used to "rule out" drug use. It should be quick, cheap, and easy to perform on large groups of people. It is not necessarily very accurate. A typical screening test might use immunoassay.

Immunoassay tests give a simple "yes" or "no" answer. They are sensitive to very minute quantities of a drug but not very specific for it, so that a positive result could be to due to the presence of a related substance. For example, it is very easy to do a screening test for amphetamines, but a great many substances will give a falsely positive test.

If the screening test is negative, nothing more is done. If it is positive, a second, confirmatory test is done.

Confirmation tests

Confirmation tests are extremely accurate, but they also tend to be time-consuming, expensive, and not very practical for large groups of people. Their purpose is to "rule in" drug use. Confirmation cutoff levels are set for each drug that indicate the direct use of that drug. It is almost impossible to fool a confirmation test; however, many small companies or organizations do not bother with this expensive additional procedure.

For a confirmation test, the laboratory takes a further sample from the specimen and starts a new internal chain-of-custody form for that sample. Confirmation testing uses two analytical techniques: gas chromatography and mass spectrometry (GC/MS). Gas chromatography is used to physically separate the different substances present in the specimen. Mass spectrometry can then be used to identify these individual substances. With GC/MS, the specific molecule that corresponds with a drug or drug metabolite can be identified.

Specimens that test negative for drugs are discarded. Specimens that test positive are frozen and stored for at least 12 months in case they need to be used as legal evidence or tested again.

Can Drug Tests Be Fooled?

Not surprisingly, many people try to fool the drug tests. Some of their methods interfere only with immunoassays and not with GC/MS, which may be effective because the sample can clear the screening process and never reach the confirmatory level. If the laboratory has any reason to suspect adulteration, however, the confirmation test will usually show the true amount of the drug.

ADULTERATION PRODUCTS

There are many products advertised in magazines or on the Internet that claim to fool drug tests. In general, these substances are easily available by mail order and specialty shops. However, currently four states (Texas, Pennsylvania, Nebraska, South Carolina) have laws prohibiting possession or sale of drug-test adulterants. The more popular products include:

Klear *or* Whizzies

These products contain nitrite, which interferes with the GC/MS assay for THC. The specimen may screen positive for marijuana, but the marijuana metabolite used for confirmation cannot be detected by GC/MS. Unfortunately, nitrite also removes the substance used by the laboratory as an internal standard for detection of the marijuana metabolite. If the laboratory fails to recover this substance, it will test for nitrite by GC/MS.

Naturally high urine nitrite levels can be caused by urinary tract infections and by eating foods such as beef jerky, which can cause urinary nitrite concentrations as high as 300 ng/mL. However, using Klear (potassium nitrite) or Whizzies (sodium nitrite) will produce a urine nitrite concentration greater than 500 ng/mL, and the laboratory will report the sample as adulterated.

Mary Jane's Super Clean

This product contains alkylphoxysulfonate, which is also present (and much cheaper) in Joy and other dishwashing detergents. If this is added to urine, it may cause an apparent decrease of marijuana metabolites when tested by immunoassay. The results of GC/MS analysis will not be changed.

In theory, the product works as a surfactant, by forming tiny droplets which trap drug molecules and make them "invisible" to the antibodies used in immunoassay tests. Adding Visine eye drops to urine has the same effect. Current laboratories have a number of methods to detect this type of adulteration, making it less effective than in previous years.

Salt

Sodium and chloride are normally found in urine but occur in especially high concentrations when salt has been added as an adulterant. High concentrations of salt can cause a decrease in the apparent concentrations of many drugs when tested by immunoassay.

UrinAid, Clear Choice, or Glutaraldehyde

These products contain glutaraldehyde, which interferes with immunoassays of all NIDA-5 drugs. When glutaraldehyde is added to a urine specimen, it makes the immunoassay uninterpretable. It does not interfere with GC/MS results. Gluteraldehyde is not found in normal urine. If the laboratory finds glutaraldehyde in the specimen, it will be reported as adulterated.

Urine Luck

Besides a clever name, Urine Luck uses a clever process to fool marijuana tests. It contains the salt pyridinium chlorochromate, which dissolves in urine to form pyridine. The effect of pyridine is similar to nitrite by interfering with the detection of marijuana. If the laboratory cannot recover the marijuana metabolite standard, it may test the specimen for pyridine by GC/MS and report it as adulterated.

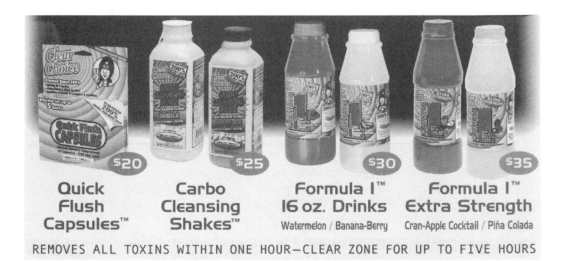

Quick Flush Capsules™	Carbo Cleansing Shakes™	Formula 1™ 16 oz. Drinks	Formula 1™ Extra Strength
$20	$25	$30	$35
		Watermelon / Banana-Berry	Cran-Apple Cocktail / Piña Colada

REMOVES ALL TOXINS WITHIN ONE HOUR—CLEAR ZONE FOR UP TO FIVE HOURS

DILUTED URINE

The easiest and simplest way to fool a drug test is by diluting urine. Some people try to add water to the urine sample, but this may be difficult in a proper testing place. The most common way is to drink a lot of fluids beforehand, and avoid early-morning urine (which has the highest drug concentration).

Because urine contains dissolved substances, it is more dense than water. Normal urine has a specific gravity of about 1.025 (the specific gravity of water is 1.000). If the urine sample has a specific gravity of less than 1.003, representing an eight-fold dilution, the laboratory will reject the sample.

Urine also contains a certain amount of creatinine, which is produced by the muscles of the body. Normal urine has a creatinine level of about 150 mg/dL. If the sample urine is less than 20 mg/dL, again suggesting an eight-fold dilution, the sample will be rejected.[16] Creatine, the popular body-building supplement, is not the same as creatinine, and taking large amounts of creatine will produce only an insignificant increase in urinary creatinine.

Testing urine for specific gravity and for creatinine prevents donors from fooling the drug tests by pouring water into the sample, or drinking enormous quantities of water to dilute their urine and therefore also dilute any drugs that might be present.

 The solution to pollution is dilution.

To a certain extent, diluting urine does increase the chance of beating a drug test. Some drug-using employees will take furosemide (Lasix), a prescription diuretic which causes a very dilute urine. To avoid the problem of having their urine rejected because of an insufficient creatinine concentration, they will eat a lot of red meat beforehand. It is questionable whether this strategy works. Drinking large quantities of water, or taking Lasix, can dilute urine as much as tenfold and therefore lower drug concentrations. But this can also reduce the specific gravity below 1.003, in which case the laboratory reports it as a dilute specimen, and it is rejected. If the specimen is at or below 1.001, this is very close to water and the laboratory report will state "Specimen substituted: Not consistent with normal human urine." This suggests that the drug test has been falsified.

There are many products that claim to cleanse the system of drugs, or at least help the user escape detection. Most of these products are supposed to be taken with large amounts of water, and they work by simply diluting the urine. In general, they do not actually interfere with the drug test. Some also contain vitamin B complex to make the urine more yellow, so that it doesn't look so diluted.

Some "beat the drug test" products that act by diluting urine

Clear Choice Herbal Detox Tea
Detoxify Carbo Clean
Eliminator
HealthTech Pre-Cleanse Formula
Naturally Klean Herbal Tea
Quick Tabs

Quick Flush Capsules and Tea
Ready-Clean
Test Free
Test Pure
THC Terminator Drink
The Stuff

In general, products that claim to beat the drug tests are a waste of money and give the user a false sense of confidence. In some states, these products are illegal. The manufacture, sale, or use of adulterants is a misdemeanor crime in Nebraska,[17] Pennsylvania, and Texas.[18]

LEGAL MEDICATIONS THAT CAN CAUSE POSITIVE DRUG TESTS

A positive drug test may be caused by many prescription medicines:

This drug test ...	may be positive with this legal medication
Amphetamines	Adderall tablets
	Atapryl tablets
	Biphetamine capsules
	Carbex tablets
	Desoxyn Gradumet tablets
	Dexedrine tablets and capsules
	Dextrostat tablets
	Didrex tablets
	Eldepryl tablets
	Selegiline tablets
	Vicks Inhaler
Barbiturates	Anolor 300 capsules
	Arco-Lase Plus tablets
	Axocet capsules
	Bellatal tablets
	Bupap tablets
	Donnatal tablets, capsules, and elixir
	Esgic and Esgic-Plus tablets and capsules
	Fioricet tablets and capsules
	Medigesic capsules
	Nembutal capsules, solution, and suppositories
	Pacaps capsules
	Phrenilin tablets and capsules
	Quadrinal tablets
	Repan and Repan-CF tablets and capsules
	Seconal sodium capsules
	Sedapap tablets
	Tenake capsules
	Tuinal pulvules

Cocaine	cocaine hydrochloride (used in ear, nose, throat, or dental surgery) TAC (Tetracaine, Adrenaline, and Cocaine preparation used in emergency rooms to numb the skin) Brompton's Cocktail (contains cocaine and morphine or heroin, for extreme pain in dying patients).
Marijuana	Marinol Capsules Marijuana approved for medical condition
Methaqualone	none
Opiates	Acetaminophen with codeine Amogel PG Brompton's Cocktail (see above) Brontex Butalbital, aspirin, caffeine, and codeine capsules Capital and codeine suspension Codimal PH syrup Deconsal C expectorant and syrup Diabismul Dimetane-DC and Dimetane DX cough syrup Duramorph injection Fioricet with codeine capsules Fiorinal with codeine capsules Fiortal with codeine Infantol Pink Infumorph solution Kadian capsules MS Contin tablets MSIR capsules, solution, and tablets MS/L and MS/S Nucofed expectorant, syrup, and capsules OMS concentrate Oramorph SR tablets Paragoric Parepectolin suspension Pediacof cough syrup Phenaphen with codeine capsules Phenergan VC with codeine Poly-Histine CS syrup Promethazine hydrochloride and codeine phosphate syrup RNS suppositories Robitussin A-C and Robitussin-DAC syrup Roxanol and Roxanol 100 solution Ryna-C liquid Ryna-CX liquid Soma compound with codeine Triaminic expectorant with codeine Tussar-2 and Tussar SF and syrup Tussi-Organidin NR and SNR liquid Tylenol with codeine (#1,2,3, or 4)

What Happens When a Drug Test is Positive?

A Medical Review Officer (MRO) is a specially certified medical doctor with training in the interpretation of positive drug tests. Under Federal guidelines, a worker testing positive must have an opportunity to talk about the results with an MRO or appropriate physician to see if there might be another explanation besides drug use. In fact, the MRO may not declare the test positive unless there has been an attempt to contact the specimen donor.

Most MROs try to call the employee by telephone. If a "reasonable attempt" to contact the employee is not successful, the MRO may declare the drug test a verified positive. In other words, it is up to the employee to convince the MRO that there might have been another reason why he or she tested positive.

The MRO interview

"Hello Mr. Smith, this is Dr. Murphy at Bay City Medical Center. I'm calling because your drug test came back positive for amphetamines. Your company doesn't know this yet. I wanted to call you first, to see why this happened. Are you taking any medicines, or do you know of any reason why your test might be positive?"

"Stand-down" is a common employer practice of temporarily removing an employee from a safety-sensitive job if the individual has a confirmed laboratory test but before the MRO has completed the verification process. This practice is prohibited by law—in fact, the MRO is not even allowed to inform the employer of the positive test until it has been verified.

The most common excuse for a positive drug test is that the employee did not personally take drugs but was at a party where others were using drugs.

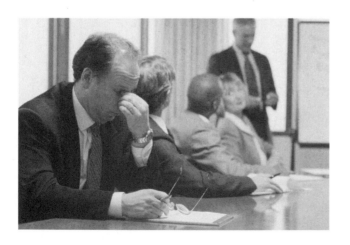

This rationalization is often used for marijuana: "I was in a bar where people were smoking up ... I couldn't help inhaling it." More than a dozen experimental studies on passive inhalation have been published.[19] Some of these researchers were able to cause a positive drug test among people passively inhaling the smoke, but only when the exposure was extremely intense and unrealistic.[20] They concluded that it was almost impossible for someone to test positive because others nearby smoked marijuana.[21] The Government decided that this excuse would not be allowed.

In the early 1980s, some health food stores sold a tea made from coca leaves called *Health Inca Tea*. The tea was supposedly made from "decocainized coca leaves." A study in 1986 showed that this tea contained detectable amounts of cocaine and could cause a benzoyl-ecgonine positive urine test result.[22] The tea is no longer available.

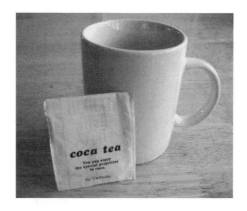

Positive drug test?

A woman denied using cocaine. She claimed that her positive test was due to her body absorbing cocaine from the semen of her boyfriend. The Government did not accept the excuse.

Other excuses have included inhaling cocaine powder when sitting beside someone cutting cocaine, and other seemingly innocent exposures. The Government has determined that these types of exposures are not enough to cause a positive drug test, and has not accepted such excuses.

CHAPTER 6

Chemicals and the Brain

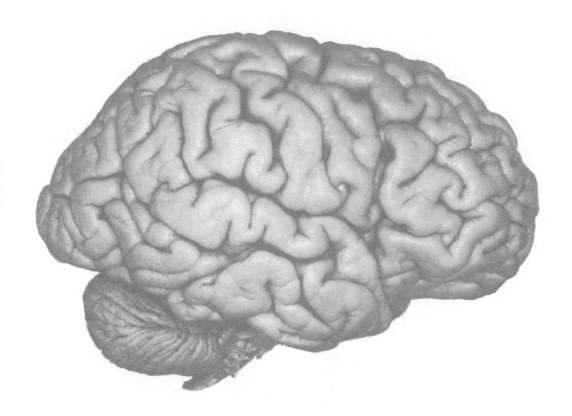

"It started off in chemistry, and went into art and mysticism."
—*Albert Hofmann, discoverer of LSD*

The Quickest Way to the Brain

For psychoactive drugs to be effective, they must enter the bloodstream and get to the brain. Drugs that reach the brain more quickly have a more dramatic effect. Therefore, smoking cocaine (crack) is more intense than snorting powder cocaine, which in turn is more intense than drinking the cocaine wines and elixirs of past centuries.

HOW ARE DRUGS TAKEN?

For practical purposes, there are only five common methods of drug use. These are arranged here in order of the speed with which the drug will reach the brain and begin to have an effect.

Smoking

Smoked or inhaled drugs enter the lungs and are quickly absorbed into the bloodstream through tiny vessels lining the air sacs. Smoke is created when a material is vaporized under heat to form a gas. As the gas spreads into the cooler surrounding air, it condenses into microscopic liquid droplets (which is why smoke feels moist). These droplets catch the light and appear as visible smoke. Because of the very small size of the droplets, much smaller than dust particles, inhaled smoke continues all the way to the lung air sacs, where it comes into contact with the bloodstream and is quickly absorbed. Blood from the lungs continues to the heart and some of it is pumped directly to the brain.

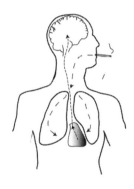

⊕   Time to brain: 7 to 10 seconds

Injecting

This is the most direct way to take a drug, but surprisingly not as fast as smoking. There are several methods of using a needle to inject a drug. It may be injected into a vein ("slamming"), into a muscle ("muscling"), or deep into the skin ("skin popping").

  If the drug is injected into a vein, the blood first returns to the right side of the heart. It then is pumped to the lungs (which is why injected particles can cause injury to the lungs), returned to the left side of the heart, and then pumped to the brain. The other types of injection spread the drug into other tissues. Blood bathing these tissues will eventually pick up the drug, return it to the heart, lungs, and heart again, and then carry it to the brain.

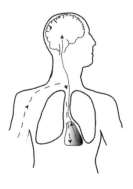

⊕   Time to brain: 15 to 30 seconds if injected into a vein
               3 to 5 minutes if injected into muscle or skin

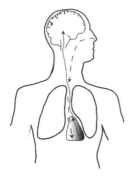

Snorting

Snorting is an expression used in the illegal drug trade meaning to sniff a drug. It comes from the sound made with a quick, loud sniff, like a snorting horse.

Drugs sniffed into the nose are absorbed by blood vessels in the mucous membranes of the nasal passages. Although these blood vessels are very close to the brain, the drug-laden blood first returns to the heart, after which some of it is pumped back to reach the brain.

⏱   Time to brain: 3 to 5 minutes

Contact

Some drugs can be absorbed directly through the skin, or mucous membranes in the eyes, mouth, vagina, or anus (suppositories). Historically, some drugs were taken after first cutting or burning the skin and then applying a drug paste. Today, prisoners occasionally use this method, but it is painful and inefficient.

Fentanyl is marketed in an adhesive patch that can provide a steady release of the drug for several days. Some illicit users of cocaine rub it on a mucous membrane, especially in the vagina or penis. Tiny LSD blotters are sometimes dropped into the space behind the lower eyelid, where the drug is rapidly absorbed. Liquid LSD can also be dropped into the eye, but this is seldom done, perhaps because LSD is rarely sold in liquid form.

⏱   Time to brain: 3 to 5 minutes for the eye
                    15 to 30 minutes for skin and other areas

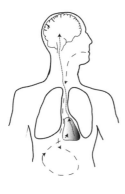

Ingesting

A drug that is eaten, drunk, or taken as a pill first passes down the esophagus to the stomach, where it is mixed with gastric fluids. It then moves on to the small intestine where it is absorbed in the tiny blood vessels lining the walls. Intestinal blood goes to the liver, where the drug may be filtered out or altered. Blood from the liver then reaches the heart and is pumped to the brain.[1] At any step along the way, the drug may be metabolized or degraded, making this method both the safest but also the slowest and least efficient way to take a drug.

⏱   Time to brain: 20 to 30 minutes

Chewing a drug is like a mixture of sniffing and ingesting, with some of the drug absorbed by the mucous membranes of the mouth and the rest of it absorbed by the gastrointestinal tract.

The pupil on drugs

It is a popular belief that dilated pupils show intoxication. Or is it pinpoint pupils?
Here is how the pupils of the eye react to various drugs:

Constricted (miosis)	Dilated (mydriasis)	Jerky (nystagmus)

   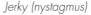

Constricted (miosis)	Dilated (mydriasis)	Jerky (nystagmus)
Barbiturates	Amphetamines	Barbiturates
Codeine	Bufotenine	GHB
Heroin	Cathinone	PCP
Morphine	Cocaine	
Other opiates	DMT	
Glutethimide	Ibogaine	
	LSD	
	MDMA	
	Mescaline	
	Peyote	
	Psilocybin	

BLOOD-BRAIN BARRIER

After the drug molecules arrive at the brain, they diffuse from the blood into the gray matter of the brain itself. To do so, the molecules must pass out of the blood vessels and cross a number of membranes to get into the fluid bathing the nerve cells. This obstacle is referred to as the blood-brain barrier, and not all drugs are able to cross it.

In order for a molecule to slip out of the blood and into the brain, it must be quite small and be able to dissolve in the brain's fatty tissue. This is why psychoactive drug molecules tend to be relatively small and simple, lipophilic ("fat liking"). Bufotenine, for example, does not cross the blood-brain barrier and therefore does not have any psychoactive effect—a feature apparently not realized by the Government when this drug was made illegal. On the other hand, a close relative of bufotenine, 5-methoxy-DMT (see *DMT*), *does* cross into the brain, where it is one of the most powerful hallucinogens known—yet it is legal.

Some drugs are altered in the body into a form that can cross the blood-brain barrier. For example, psilocybin does not actually enter the brain. When psilocybin mushrooms are eaten (or if synthetic psilocybin is taken), the drug is absorbed and passes to the liver. There, it is changed into psilocin, which does have the ability to pass into the brain.

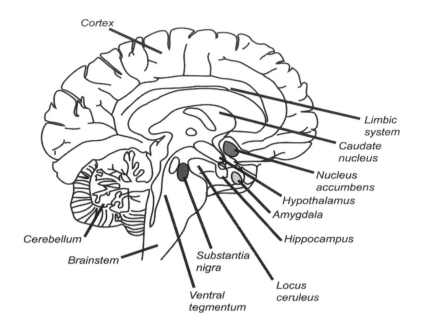

The ability to cross the blood-brain barrier is one of the features that determine the potency of a drug. Heroin, for example, is really just morphine with a couple of molecular groups added on. The add-ons allow it to cross into the brain more readily. Once in the brain, heroin has the same effects as morphine, but because it can get there more quickly, it is overall a more active (and more addictive) drug than morphine.

Mental road map

Once in the brain, drugs have their most pronounced action in certain areas. Each of these areas shows the typical effects of the drug, to the point where an expert can guess the drug's action on the brain just by looking at the signs and symptoms of the drug user.

The brain functions on three main levels: the brainstem, the midbrain, and the cortex. They progress from the most primitive part to the most advanced, and are conveniently arranged in the head from lowest to highest.

The first level of the brain is the brainstem, at the bottom and extending into the spinal cord. This is the most primitive part of the brain. It is present in fish and lower animals, and serves mainly to regulate basic bodily functions such as breathing and sleep. Drugs that affect this level, such as the opiates, GHB, and methaqualone, can result in stupor or coma.

If an overdose is taken, the interference with breathing can cause death.

Behind the brainstem is the cerebellum. It is also considered a primitive part of the brain and is present in primordial animals. This part of the brain coordinates muscle activity, balance, and vision. The stumbling behavior and jerky eyes seen after use of many drugs are typical of their effects on the cerebellum. Ibogaine, for example, may be toxic to the cerebellum and cause the shaking tremor seen in its users (see *Ibogaine*).

Above the brainstem is the next evolutionary extension of the brain, present in reptiles (and sometimes called the "reptilian brain"). Because it is a small, hidden region located midway between the brainstem and the large brain cortex, it is referred to as the midbrain. It has areas which deal with emotions (the limbic system), temperature and pain regulation (the thalamus), hormones (hypothalamus), memory (hippo-

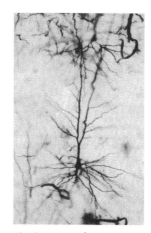

The location of conscious thought? A pyramidal cell from the cerebral cortex

campus), and the sense of reward (nucleus accumbens). Most of all, the midbrain controls the basic functions of survival: instinct, emotions, and the drives for food and sex.

Almost all psychoactive drugs affect the midbrain, and it is here where addiction takes place. The human brain is engineered to seek out and hunt down foods that give pleasure. Cocaine, amphetamines, and other drugs stimulate the pleasure center and provide a feeling of euphoria. But that is not enough to cause addiction. These drugs also target the nucleus accumbens, the reward center. The result is a cycle of pleasure and reward followed by craving, in which the person instinctively goes back for more.

The highest, most developed, part of the brain is the cortex—the folds of gray matter making up the bulk of the volume and clearly distinguishing the human brain from that of other animals. The cortex contributes the functioning of the intellect: language, reasoning, planning, and judgment. All psychoactive drugs have some influence on the cortex, although these actions are poorly understood. The visual cortex (which is located, oddly, at the very back of the brain) may be the site of action of the visually hallucinogenic drugs such as LSD. The frontal cortex is considered to be the site of higher consciousness and insightful judgment, and disturbed by addictive drugs. The result is a craving for pleasure and reward coupled

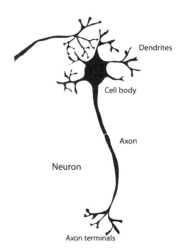

Dendrites

Cell body

Axon

Neuron

Axon terminals

with poor judgment and irrational behavior—precisely the effects seen in addicted people.

The Anatomy of a Neuron

MIND AND MATTER

Perhaps the most remarkable and fascinating feature of psychoactive drugs is that a physical substance can be used to change a mental state. How can this come about? Philosophers have struggled for thousands of years to determine what is real and what is imaginary. Is a thought real? Or is it just a chemical process of the brain? Or is there, as many philosophers believe, no such thing as objective reality?

What is mind? –No matter.
What is matter? –Never mind! [3]

The modern view of psychology increasingly tends to a belief that mental processes can be described by brain chemistry. In this view, "mind" is just a convenient fiction, an expression of behavior, and what we take to be mental processes are in fact the workings of the brain and can be studied and predicted like any other part of the body.[2]

To learn more about the function of psychoactive drugs, therefore, it is useful to take a closer look at the chemistry of the brain and of the drugs themselves. The following section is a very simplified account of how psychoactive drugs work.

ELECTRICAL SIGNALS

All thoughts, sensations, and stimulations of the body are brought about by nerve cells, called neurons. Each neuron can be thought of as an electrical wire with plugs at each end. A chemical signal stimulates the plug and starts the electrical current at one end. The current then runs along the wire to the other end where it produces another chemical signal. This signal, in turn, stimulates the next neuron in line.

René Descartes (1596-1650) originated our concept of mind and body. He described nerve signals to be like a man pulling on a rope to ring a church bell. The modern view is not much different.

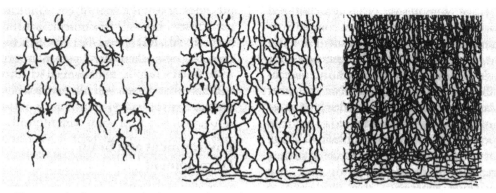

The growth of neurons at birth, 4 months and 16 months respectively

The body has neurons reaching to almost every tissue. These are linked, in chains, to pass signals from one to the other, and particularly to send and receive signals from the brain. The brain itself is mostly made of a massive collection of neurons that primarily pass signals among themselves.

By the time a baby is born, the brain has grown to about one hundred billion neurons. Some neurons die off, or languish, while others continue to grow and make more contacts. The growth and connections between neurons is what we consider to be *learning*. From the moment of birth, the baby begins to learn. All the sights, sounds, smells, touching, and other sensations experienced by the baby help it create new connections among neurons. By age ten, every one of the child's individual neurons will have established, on average, about 1,000 connections with other neurons (with some having up to 200,000 connections), so that the total number of interconnections between neurons amounts to a hundred trillion—or 100,000,000,000,000—possible signals. This unimaginably complex interplay of signals gives rise to what we know as the human mind.

A typical neuron looks like a tree: it has fine roots that come together to form a long trunk which then branches into smaller and smaller twigs. In fact, the root-like receptive parts of a neuron are called dendrites, from the Greek "tree-like." The long trunk is called the axon, ending in a spray of branches called axon terminals.

Neurons are narrow, much thinner than a hair, but their axon extensions can be very long, up to 120 cm (about 4 feet)—long enough to reach many other, even quite distant, neurons in the body or brain. Axons and their terminals grow until they come up against other neurons and then form a snug fit, like a hand in a glove. The tiny space between the surface of one

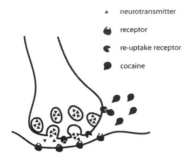

neurotransmitter
receptor
re-uptake receptor
cocaine

Cocaine blocks the re-uptake
of neurotransmitters

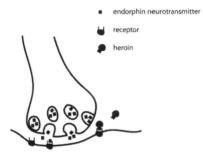

endorphin neurotransmitter
receptor
heroin

Opiates fit the endorphin receptors

In each synapse as many as 10,000 neurotransmitter molecules may be released

neuron terminal and the surface of the next neuron is called a synapse (or synaptic cleft). A synapse is very small, about 1/1000th the width of a human hair.

The trunk of the neuron sends an electrical signal in one direction: it receives a signal from the dendrites and then sends this signal out along the axon to the terminals. When the electrical signal reaches the terminal end, there is a release of chemicals from the terminal into the synapse. These chemicals float across the synapse and stimulate receptors on the dendrites of the next neuron. This triggers a new electrical impulse in that neuron, which sends the signal onwards. In this way, a signal is sent from neuron to neuron throughout the body and brain: electrical-chemical-electrical-chemical.

The chemicals in this electrical-chemical chain that serve to transmit the signal between neurons are called neurotransmitters.

A neuron in a normal resting state has a negative electrical charge, maintained by a high concentration of potassium ions inside the cell. When receptors on its cell surface are stimulated by neurotransmitters, they open a channel in the cell to allow positively charged sodium ions to rush inside. This flood of positive ions causes the interior of the neuron to flip from electrically negative to positive, forming a current that runs all the way to the end of the cell. When it reaches the terminal, the current stimulates neurotransmitters to be released into the next synapse.

After sending a signal, the neuron resets itself. It pumps out sodium ions to restore its normal electrical charge, and replenishes its store of neurotransmitters. The neuron is then ready for the next signal.

Each neuron manufactures its own supply of neurotransmitters, and conserves the supply by reabsorbing the released neurotransmitters from the synapse. This re-absorption also stops the transmission of the signal.

The whole process of neurotransmission takes place very quickly: a neuron can send an electrical signal, reset itself, and send another signal up to 400 times a second.

Sending and Receiving Signals: Neurotransmitters

The electrical circuit model of a neuron is useful way of understanding its function, but as a description it is greatly oversimplified. Neurons are living, growing cells; they are not fixed like an electrical circuit. Almost every neuron is constantly changing its function by adapting to bodily demands, sensations, and environmental influences.

A neuron regulates the production of its neurotransmitters, making more or less of them as needed. It also continually changes the number of receptors on its cell surface according to the amount of stimulation it receives from other cells. If the circuit is over-stimulated, the receptors are downgraded so that fewer and weaker signals get through. If there is too little stimulation, the receptors may be increased and made more sensitive.

The synaptic space itself is also constantly modified. Each neuron's terminals feel and reach out like tentacles. They grow with stimulation and atrophy with disuse. Like muscles, the cells of the brain are "use it or lose it."

A neuron typically produces only one type of neurotransmitter, but some neurons release more than one type, or even different types at different places in the neuron. There may be a cascade effect, in which the release of one neurotransmitter triggers the release of others. In some parts of the brain, for example, a release of serotonin causes a release of enkephalin, which causes the release of dopamine. The combined effect of all of these in the brain's emotional center can be to cause a feeling of well-being.

Locks and keys

A neurotransmitter fits a receptor like a key in a lock. Neurotransmitters released into a synapse bump up against the receptors and bind to them. Once the neurotransmitter binds, the receptor molecule can change its shape and open channels or pores on the neuron's cell membrane, allowing the influx of atoms to result in an electrical current. The receptor then lets go of the neurotransmitter, the neuron pumps the atoms back out of the cell, and electrical stability is restored. Neurotransmitters released into the synapse will continue to bind to the receptors until they are absorbed back into the membrane from which they came. Those that are not absorbed will be deactivated by enzymes or float off into the blood stream.

Excitement and inhibition

Neurons are basically classified into two types: excitatory and inhibitory. In general, excitatory neurons release excitatory types of neurotransmitters that stimulate other neurons, while inhibitory neurons produce inhibitory types of neurotransmitters that have the opposite effect; they stop the transmission of signals. Both are needed, or the system would either shut down from lack of stimulation or be overloaded from too much stimulation.

Psychoactive drugs either act on, or resemble, certain neurotransmitters. Those that involve the excitatory neurotransmitters are called stimulants, and those that involve the inhibitory neurotransmitters are called depressants. (Most hallucinogens involve excitatory neurotransmitters.) Excessive stimulation of excitatory neurons gives a feeling of alertness, increased awareness and concentration, heightened strength and energy. With excessive inhibition, on the other hand, the body and mind is numbed, pain-free, and there is a feeling of deep, dreamy relaxation.

 Overstimulation of either excitatory or inhibitory neurotransmitters can result in pleasurable feelings and euphoria.

For the psychoactive drugs that directly resemble neurotransmitters, the resemblance can vary from a partial similarity to an almost perfect fit. For example, DMT and GHB are chemically very similar to the natural neurotransmitters serotonin and GABA, respectively. Others, such as the opiates, are just similar enough to the endorphins that they are able to bind to the brain's endorphin receptors. The effects of a drug depend on which neurotransmitters it resembles, and its potency is partly determined by how close this resemblance is.

Some psychoactive drugs do not resemble neurotransmitters directly, but produce their effects by increasing the release of natural neurotransmitters. For example, cocaine prevents the re-absorption of norepinephrine, epinephrine, dopamine, and serotonin from the synapse, while amphetamines spur the release of these neurotransmitters. The result of both of these drugs is that the natural neurotransmitters linger in the synapse and therefore have a more intense effect.

At least 80 different neurotransmitters (or neuromodulators) have been described, with more discovered every year. Following are those that are most involved in the effects of psychoactive drugs.

Acetylcholine

Acetylcholine is the neurotransmitter used to stimulate muscles and glands, allowing movement and the discharge of sweat, tears, saliva, and other secretions. Like most other neurotransmitters, its function was discovered by investigating the effects of drugs. Nicotine stimulates one type of acetylcholine receptor, the type found in muscles, and these receptors are therefore called nicotinic receptors. The other type of acetylcholine receptor was discovered by studying the effect of the *Amanita muscaria* mushroom. In addition to causing hallucinations it also causes intense salivation and slowing of the heart. A chemical, muscarine, was isolated and found to be responsible for these physical effects; this type of acetylcholine receptor is now known as the muscarinic receptor.

The side effects of many drugs—dilated pupils, dry mouth, sweating, muscle twitching, irregular heartbeat, etc.—are due to their action on nicotinic and muscarinic receptors.

DOPAMINE

Dopamine neurons help control our appetites for both food and sex. Increased amounts of dopamine produce a feeling of pleasure or reward and encourage people to be more outgoing and exuberant. Too much dopamine is believed to be a feature of schizophrenia.

Psychoactive drugs especially affect dopamine in a deep part of the brain called the ventral tegmentum. Tracts of neurons from this area lead to a very primitive part of the brain called the limbic cortex, which is responsible for the survival instinct and aggressive drive. They also lead to a more recently evolved part of the brain, the frontal cortex, which is responsible for judgment. Too much dopamine, therefore, causes aggressive, reward-seeking behavior as well as disturbed judgment—exactly the compulsive drug-seeking behavior seen with addictive drugs. Cocaine and amphetamines powerfully influence the amount of dopamine present in the synapse.[4]

Dopamine neurons also control purposeful movement. It is the loss of dopamine neurons which causes the shaky, stumbling movements of Parkinson's Disease. Long-term or excessive use of dopamine-affecting drugs has been shown to have the same effects. One such drug, a variant of meperidine, caused a rapid and permanent form of Parkinson's Disease.

EPINEPHRINE

Epinephrine is a neurotransmitter produced by the adrenal gland, located above the kidney. Epinephrine (from the Greek *epi-nephros*, "above kidney") is also called adrenaline (from the Latin *ad-renal*, also meaning "above kidney").

This hormone alerts the entire body, preparing it for fight or flight: the heart rate increases, blood is moved away from the digestive organs to the muscles, and the lungs open up to breathe faster. Body functions that are not necessary for emergencies are inhibited: appetite is suppressed and hunger disappears.

Drugs that mimic epinephrine, such as the amphetamines, are sought out by soldiers, athletes, people who need to stay awake, people trying to lose weight, and people who want to feel more physically and emotionally stimulated.

GABA AND GLUTAMATE

GABA, gamma-aminobutyric acid, has an inhibitory function. Glutamate has an excitatory function. Together, they are by far the most common neurotransmitters in the brain. Both of them are simple amino acids.

New functions for these neurotransmitters are constantly being discovered. GABA serves to relieve pain, by inhibiting the transmission of pain signals, and also affects memory. Many pain relief drugs imitate GABA and are able to bind to GABA receptors. Some extremely powerful examples of these drugs—causing both numbness and memory loss—are the illegal drugs GHB and Rohypnol (see *Flunitrazepam*).

Glutamate has also been found to have many functions, including the formation of memory. PCP is an illegal drug that targets the glutamate receptors, causing both extreme excitement and loss of memory.

NOREPINEPHRINE

Norepinephrine is similar to epinephrine. It is the primary stimulant of the central nervous system. Drugs such as the amphetamines and cocaine increase the amount of norepinephrine, giving a feeling of mental alertness.

OPIOIDS AND ENDORPHINS

After receptors were found for opiate narcotics, it was discovered that the body produced its own opiates to fit these receptors. These morphine-like neurotransmitters were called endorphins (from *endo*genous m*orphine*). They are released during heavy exercise and perhaps other behaviors, such as sex, meditation, or prayer, that provide a feeling of peace and well-being. Endorphins also are released during trauma and help the body deal with extreme pain.

The use of opiate drugs floods the opioid receptors, producing an intense exaggeration of these effects—dulling pain and providing a feeling of euphoria. There are several kinds of opioid receptors, and they create different effects. The main receptor is the mu (also shown in scientific literature as μ) receptor. It stops pain and slows breathing, and provides euphoria. The mu-receptor is most responsible for making opiates addictive. Delta (δ) receptors also give a feeling of euphoria, and sigma (σ) receptors relieve depression, without the reinforcing characteristics of mu-receptor stimulation.

The kappa (κ) receptor stops pain and causes constriction of the pupils, but does not produce a pleasurable feeling. In fact, stimulation of kappa receptors alone produces a very unpleasant feeling of dysphoria, the opposite of euphoria. (The natural neurotransmitters that target kappa receptors are called dynorphins rather than endorphins.) Opiates that stimulate only the kappa receptor can be useful to relieve pain without the worry of addiction.

Opioid receptors and the drugs that target them

Mu	μ	morphine, fentanyl, codeine, naloxone
Delta	δ	none—endogenous opioids primarily
Kappa	κ	dynorphin, nalbuphine, butorphanol
Sigma	σ	PCP, ketamine, pentazocine

SEROTONIN

Also known as 5-hydroxytryptamine (5-HT), serotonin is a widespread neurotransmitter that is necessary for sleep, maintaining body temperature, controlling appetite, preventing seizures, and regulating many other hormones. Serotonin also has a large effect on mood.

At least 14 types of serotonin receptors are known. Excessive stimulation of Type 2 serotonin receptors (5-HT$_2$) causes hallucinations, while the stimulation of Type 3 receptors triggers vomiting. Hallucinogenic drugs characteristically stimulate Type 2 receptors and either stimulate or block the others. Therefore these drugs can also cause vomiting, fever from interfering with temperature regulation, or even seizures. For example, people who take drugs that increase serotonin levels (such as Prozac, Zoloft, Paxil, and others) may have a seizure if they take LSD.[5]

The midbrain controls serotonin in the higher brain regions. Messages from the raphe cells of the midbrain regulate the visual centers in the cerebral cortex and also certain areas of the limbic system, a major center for control of the emotions. The raphe cells work as a kind of brake on this part of the brain. Therefore, if the raphe cells are prevented from working, the visual centers of the brain can become hyperactive and have too much to cope with—resulting in hallucinations.[6]

LSD, psilocybin, DMT, and probably other hallucinogenic drugs mimic the feedback effect of serotonin on the raphe cells and slow their activity, resulting in the psychedelic visual and emotional effects of these drugs.

Stimulating neurotransmitters[7]

Norepinephrine	Increases blood pressure and heart rate
	Relaxes bronchioles
	Activates breakdown of fat
	Stimulates body
	Decreases appetite
Serotonin	Increases body temperature
	Decreases appetite
	Causes hallucinations
Dopamine	Agitates muscles
	Produces euphoria
	Creates addiction
	Increases attention
	Causes nausea and vomiting

DRUGS AND THEIR NEUROTRANSMITTERS

This illegal drug ...	affects primarily these neurotransmitters
Amphetamines	epinephrine, norepinephrine, acetylcholine, dopamine, serotonin
Barbiturates	GABA
Cathinone	epinephrine, norepinephrine, dopamine, serotonin
Cocaine	epinephrine, norepinephrine, dopamine, serotonin
DMT	acetylcholine, serotonin
Flunitrazepam	GABA, glycine
GHB	GABA, dopamine
Ibogaine	dopamine, serotonin, NMDA, norepinephrine
LSD	acetylcholine, dopamine, serotonin
Marijuana	anandamide, acetylcholine, dopamine
MDMA	epinephrine, norepinephrine, dopamine, serotonin
Opiates	endorphins, enkephalins, dopamine
PCP	dopamine, acetylcholine, alpha-endopsychosin

Natural, Synthetic, and Designer Drugs

Psychoactive drugs are often described as one of three types: natural drugs extracted from plants and animals, manufactured synthetic drugs that copy or resemble natural drugs, and "designer drugs" which are variants of manufactured drugs and are accidentally or deliberately created in the laboratory for illegal distribution.

NATURAL DRUGS

Natural drugs come from a wide variety of plants, including flowers, fungi, vines, bushes and trees, and a few come from minerals, insects, and larger animals. Some drugs are found in many different sources. For example, the hallucinogen DMT is present in the seeds, leaves, or bark of a number of unrelated tropical plants, in certain beans, and in the venom of the Colorado River toad.

Natural drugs tend to be more complex than synthetic drugs. For example, peyote has at least 55 pharmacologically active substances, and marijuana has 421 identified substances in 18 different chemical classes. In contrast, the synthetically manufactured versions of these drugs—mescaline and THC—are chemically very simple. There is a good deal of argument among researchers and users about the benefits of natural drugs versus the synthetic variety. Many believe that natural drugs are likely to be less toxic, or are somehow more beneficial, than their synthetic counterpart. The truth is that crude natural and synthetic drugs are not the same, and cannot therefore be compared. Peyote is not identical to mescaline and marijuana is not the same as THC. However, when the natural substance (for example, mescaline derived from peyote) is compared with the synthetic version (mescaline synthesized from chemical precursors), the effect is the same.

SYNTHETIC DRUGS

The synthesis of many psychoactive drugs is not very complex. It can be as simple as cooking basic ingredients on a stove top (see *Ampetamines: Meth labs*). The DEA estimates that there are over 300 ways to manufacture methamphetamine.

Pharmaceutical companies are not permitted to patent a natural drug for exclusive manufacture and sale. Therefore, with less potential profit, there is not much incentive to manufacture these drugs or push for their legal use. The pharmaceutical companies would rather develop, patent, and sell a synthetic drug on which they have exclusive rights. The result is the following:

✘   There is little effort to evaluate the benefits of natural drugs, because these drugs cannot be patented.

✘   Natural drugs that were declared illegal tend to remain illegal, unless there is a politically strong group to lobby for legalization.

✘   New, synthetic drugs are aggressively marketed because there is a high profit potential.

✗   If a synthetic drug has abuse potential, resulting in injury to the user or to
others, it is usually withdrawn from the U.S. market in order to avoid liability
lawsuits. It may continue to be sold in other countries, however. These
drugs may then be illegally imported into the United States (see *MDMA* and
Flunitrazepam).

The home synthesis of psychoactive substances has become increasingly common, and the Internet has made drug recipes readily available. There are even chat groups and forums discussing drug manufacturing methods and problem-solving. The Government has responded by restricting many of the base ingredients to legitimate users, or by allowing purchase in only small quantities. For example, the sale of pseudoephedrine, used to make methamphetamine, is limited to 24 grams to a single buyer. Primary ingredients such as lysergic acid, allylbenzene, and benzaldehyde are more highly restricted and very difficult to obtain by illicit drug manufacturers.

Chemicals likely to be used in the illegal manufacture of drugs are specifically regulated by the Government. List I chemicals include ephedrine and benzaldehyde. List II chemicals are in broader industrial use and include acetone, ethyl ether, toluene and sulfuric acid. Companies that sell listed chemicals are required to keep records of the name and address of purchasers, the method of transfer, and the type of identification used by the purchaser. These records are passed on to the Government.

Home chemists have dealt with these restrictions by looking elsewhere for these base chemicals. One source is essential oils, found in health food and herbal shops.

The DEA, of course, is well aware of these attempts to skirt the law, and routinely subpoenas the customer lists of wholesale distributors of essential oils. A number of illegal drug manufacturers have been convicted on this evidence.[8]

This essential oil yields ...	this illegal drug
Sassafras Oil	MDMA
Calamus Oil	TMA-2
Indian Dill Seed Oil	DMMDA-2
Nutmeg Oil	MMDA
Mace Oil	10% myristicin
Parsley Seed Oil	DMMDA
Oil of Bitter Almonds	benzaldehyde
Oil of Cinnamon	allylbenzene

DESIGNER DRUGS

The term "designer drugs" was coined in the 1980s by Professor Gary Henderson at the University of California, Davis (one of whose former students is the author), after the new signature blue jeans in fashion at the time. Henderson was interested in variants of fentanyl that were being made without fear of prosecution because these new drugs were not specified in the law. One of the most notorious of the clandestine drug manufacturers was Kenneth Baker, who operated a seedy laboratory in California and frustrated DEA agents simply by designing a new variant of fentanyl as soon as his previous output became illegal. After his ninth fentanyl analog, Baker was finally convicted in 1986 under a Federal Food, Drug, and Cosmetic Act violation of failing to register his product.

This loophole was closed in 1986 with the passage of the Controlled Substances Analogue Enforcement Act. Now all present and future variations of illegal drugs are also illegal.

The two common types of designer drugs:
Fentanyl analogs (powerful opioids sold as substitutes for heroin)
Amphetamine analogs (methylated amphetamines and phenethylamines)

Designer drugs are usually stronger and cheaper than the original drug, and are easier to produce in clandestine laboratories. By nature, designer drugs are experimental. Unlike pharmaceutical products, the manufacturers don't carry out research on the drug before sending it out on the streets. In fact, the makers probably don't even know exactly what is in the drug. It is up to the user to find out these effects, and it is not always a pleasant experience.

The first designer drugs were developed by large laboratories but shelved because they did not look promising. In 1962, 4-methyl-aminorex was tested as a weight loss agent, but found to occasionally kill the people who took it. Somehow, the drug was discovered by illicit manufacturers who were less concerned about this side effect. It was sold on the street as Ice and U4Euh. In 1966, it was followed by aminorex, which also caused fatalities but continued to be sold on the street, particularly in Europe.

A designer variant of fentanyl appeared in Philadelphia in the fall of 1988. Dealers called it China White to fool users into thinking they were getting the high-quality heroin known by that name. The new drug, 3-methylfentanyl, was 6,000 times more potent than morphine. Eighteen people died before the word got out about its toxicity.[9]

Designer drugs are not always intentionally created and their effects can be devastating. One of the most remarkable examples of the hazards of designer drugs occurred in San Jose in 1985. An attempt to synthesize meperidine resulted in the accidental production of MPTP (1-*m*ethyl-4-*p*henyl-1,2,3,6-*t*etrahydro*p*yridine). This compound is metabolized in the brain by the monoamine oxidase system to a toxic intermediate (MPP+), which selectively destroys the sustantia nigra. The result was a rapid, severe form of Parkinson's Disease.[10]

The case of the frozen addicts[11]

In 1985, in San Jose, California, a number of men were found paralyzed into a fixed posture. Their brains had been permanently damaged by MPTP, an accidental by-product from an illegal lab trying to make meperidine.

Designer drugs can be considered to be the next step in the natural evolution of mind-altering chemicals.[12] If the pharmaceutical companies do not want to follow the exploration and promotion of these chemicals, for legal or other reasons, non-professionals will take over. Where there is a demand, someone will step in to supply it.

The story of amphetamines shows this progression. Amphetamines were first developed and marketed by the pharmaceutical industry (see *Amphetamines*). The next step involved the development of amphetamine-like agents that were *not* marketed, but taken over by illicit suppliers. These drugs include MDA and MDMA. The final step is designer variants of such drugs, which are produced entirely in illegal laboratories. The new variants include MDEA, DOM, and a whole alphabet soup of other drugs.

Some common designer drugs

BDB	DMA
DMA	DOET
DOM	MDA
MDEA	MDMA
Mecloqualone	5-Methoxy-MDA
Methylaminorex	3-Methylfentanyl
MPPP	NEA
NEXUS	PMA

TESTING DRUG PURITY

A commercially produced pharmaceutical is almost pure. In contrast, the purity of illegal drugs is unspecified: the user may get the supposed drug, a diluted version of the drug, or an entirely different substance.

Every illegal drug has been sold in bogus forms. Almost all street cocaine, for example, is heavily diluted with other substances. In a study of purported mescaline, every sample proved to be something else (usually LSD or PCP). It is very easy to pass off cheap pills and powders as a similar-looking drug.

Because synthetic drugs diverted from pharmaceutical sources have the greatest purity, many illegally made synthetics are made to look like them, with fake labels and packaging. Even natural drugs such as psilocybin may be store-bought mushrooms dusted with amphetamine or another cheap stimulant.

The low purity of illegal drugs also results from sloppy manufacturing. Illicit labs have little regard for precision, proper storage, or avoiding contamination. The result is the production of chemicals of which drug makers have little knowledge.

 "These guys are not gifted when it comes to organic chemistry"—Meth lab investigator

A user is very lucky if a synthetic illegal drug is 90 percent pure—and its purity is more likely to be anywhere from 60 percent down to as little as 10 percent, or it may contain none of the supposed drug at all. What are the other ingredients? They can be anything from fillers such as cornstarch and talcum powder, to cheaper substances that mimic the drug's effects, such as local anesthetics, caffeine, and strychnine (rat poison).

Drugs are "cut" to increase volume by mixing the pure drug with other, cheaper substances. This is usually done with a sharp knife or razor blade, finely chopping and mixing the powders so that it looks like a uniform substance. It is easy to dilute powders in this way, but drugs in hard chunks are more difficult to combine with other substances without the result being quite obviously a mixture—the chunks have to be broken up to mix them, and even then the final product looks clearly diluted. For this reason, rock-like cocaine is often preferred, and even heavily cut cocaine will be sold with a few rocks to make it look more authentic.

There are many tests of drug purity, ranging from sophisticated laboratory methods to relatively crude appraisals. Some commercial laboratories will provide an accurate and confidential analysis of a drug for a small fee (see *Self-Help Resources: Drug Identification*).

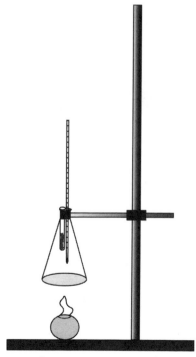

Hot box apparatus to identify drugs

Melting points in degrees Celsius[13]

Cocaine freebase	98	Cocaine hydrochloride (powder)	187
Lidocaine	127	Lactose	203
MDMA (Ecstasy)	148	Vitamine B powder	224
Mannitol	165	Caffeine	237
Methamphetamine	170	PCP	243
Heroin	173	Ephedrine	247
Quinine	177	Baking soda	270

A very effective home method is to check the melting point of a drug. Using an apparatus called a hot box, a flask of mineral oil is placed over a flame. A thermometer is placed in the oil to measure its temperature. Suspended in the oil is a test-tube containing a small amount of the drug. When the drug begins to melt, the temperature is noted. Different chemicals melt at very specific temperatures.

This procedure is so precise that even the percentage of adulteration can be determined. For example, if about 25% of a sample melts at 187 degrees and the rest melts at 203 degrees, it can be assumed that the sample is 25% cocaine and 75% lactose.

A Little Chemistry (Just Enough to Make Sense of It All)

SIMPLE MOLECULES

Psychoactive drugs are simple, small molecules. Drugs that are snorted or taken by mouth are easily absorbed by the body. Others are broken down by stomach acids, or less easily absorbed, and must be smoked or injected to enter the bloodstream.

For a drug to be psychoactive, it must reach the brain. The brain is mostly made of fat. Therefore, psychoactive drugs must be either fat-soluble, or else converted in the body to form a substance that is fat-soluble. For example, heroin and morphine are largely the same molecule: heroin is made of the morphine molecule with the addition of two acetyl groups. This addition makes heroin more fat-soluble than morphine and allows it to reach the brain more effectively, with the result that heroin is more psychoactive than morphine.

The molecules of each class of drugs typically have a common core structure, with a variety of added molecular "functional" groups. The extra parts of the molecule usually help the drug remain stable, withstand the heat of combustion (if the drug is smoked), dissolve in fat or fluids, or pass easily from the bloodstream into the brain.

Most psychoactive drugs contain the element nitrogen and therefore belong to the large class of chemical compounds known as alkaloids. For this reason, the scientific literature often refers to psychoactive drugs as alkaloids. Drugs that have similar effects tend also to have a similar chemical appearance. For example, many drugs from different sources—mescaline from the peyote cactus, LSD from rye fungus, psilocybin from a mushroom, and bufotenine from the Bufo toad—all share a characteristic molecular structure known as the indole ring. It can be expected, then, that a new drug with an indole ring would also have effects similar to these hallucinogens. The practice of taking a known drug and altering it, or adding a functional group, is how many new drugs are made.

The power of drugs can seem tremendous. Consider LSD, the most potent psychoactive substance known. Just 25 micrograms (millionths of a gram) are enough to produce effects. An average postage stamp weighs 60,000 micrograms, equal to 2,400 doses of LSD. Yet, only 0.01 percent, or about one part in ten thousand, of this amount actually reaches the brain. This would appear to be an extremely small amount of drug to have such a dramatic effect on consciousness. Even such a small amount, however, can contain a large number of these very simple molecules. Just 0.1 mg of a hallucinogenic drug—an amount that is barely visible to the naked eye—consists of about 200,000,000,000,000,000 (2×10^{17}) molecules! Each one of these molecules is able to bind to neurotransmitter receptors and affect the brain's chemistry.

 Psychoactive drug molecules are very simple and small, which is why a tiny amount of a drug can have such a dramatic effect.

BREAKING DOWN A DRUG NAME

Drugs have three names: a brand name (or street name, in the case of illegal drugs), a common name, and a chemical name.

For example, consider MDMA. It has a number of street names, including the one by which it is most commonly known, Ecstasy.

MDMA stands for *methylenedioxymethamphetamine*. The chemical name of methamphetamine is methylphenylisopropyl-amine. Therefore, the full chemical name of MDMA is N-methyl-3,4-methylenedioxymethyl-phenylisopropylamine. The name seems lengthy but it is simply a string of parts, each of which indicates a group of atoms. Together, these groups make up the MDMA molecule:

N-methyl	a carbon (C) atom with hydrogen (H) atoms (methyl group) attached to a compound containing nitrogen (N)	
3,4-methylene	a bridge attached at the 3rd and 4th carbons	
dioxy	two oxygen atoms are part of this bridge	
methyl-phenyl	the methyl group is attached to a type of benzene ring	
iso	an abbreviation of isomer, indicating that the following propane unit is an isomer. There are left handed and right-handed isomers. The right-handed one is about three times more potent.	
propyl	a propane unit of three carbon atoms and eight hydrogen atoms in a chain	
amine	an amino group (including nitrogen) attached to the isopropyl unit.	

Methylphenylisopropylamine

Because methylphenylisopropylamine is the chemical formula of methamphetamine, MDMA can also be described by the abbreviated chemical formula *methylenedioxymethamphetamine*, to produce the acronym MDMA.

Changing any of these components creates a different drug. For example, removing the methyl group creates methylenedioxyamphetamine, or MDA.

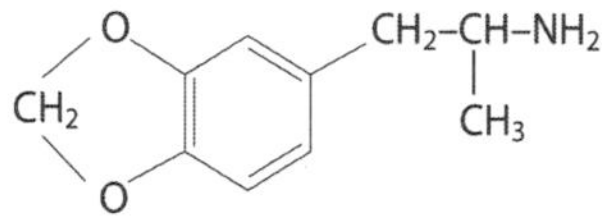

Opiates and opioids

The molecular structure of most opiates (drugs derived from the opium poppy) and opioids (synthetic drugs that resemble the opiates) are composed of a double ring structure. This can be seen in meperidine (Demerol), a popular prescription drug of abuse, and the more powerful opioid, fentanyl.

An attempt by a clandestine lab to make these drugs accidentally resulted in the production of MPTP, a substance that caused rapid and irreversible brain damage. By looking at the molecular structure, it is easy to see the resemblance and why the unprofessional chemists ended up with this simpler, but much more hazardous, product.

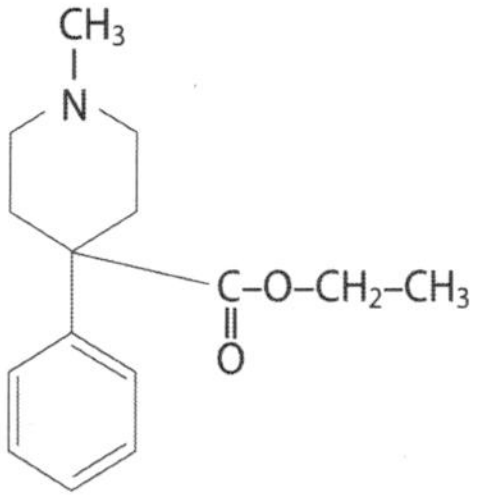

The amphetamine family

Norepinephrine is a major stimulating neurotransmitter in the brain. It can be injected, but will be broken down by stomach acids if taken by mouth. In the late 19th century, it was discovered that norepinephrine was similar to ephedrine, a natural stimulant from the *Ephedra* plant and used in Chinese medicine for thousands of years. Amphetamines were developed partly as a synthetic variant of ephedrine and partly as a form of norepinephrine that could be taken by mouth. Since the discovery of amphetamine, many variants of this molecule have been synthesized, all of which have stimulating properties.

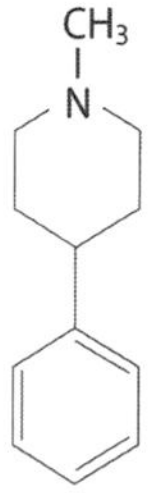

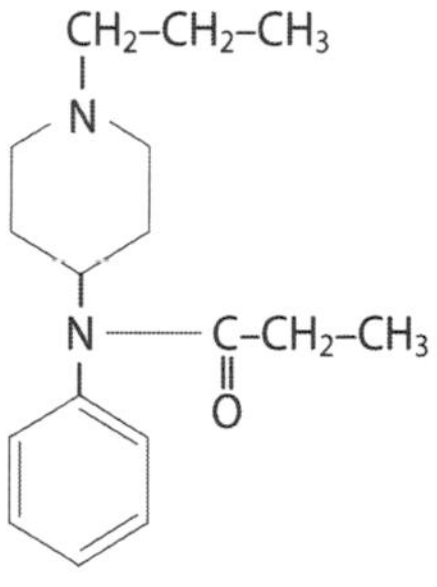

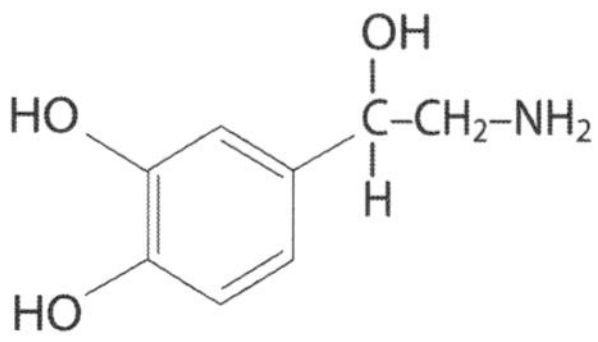

Methylene-dioxy-amphetamine (MDA)

Meperidine

MPTP

Fentanyl

Norepinephrine

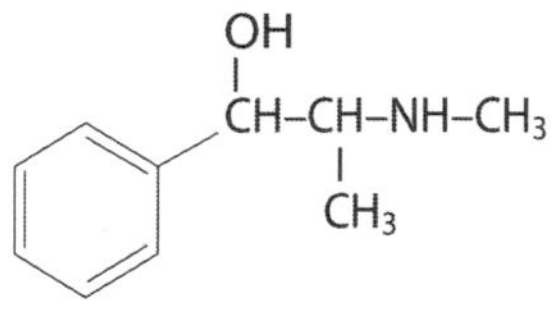

Ephedrine

CH$_2$–CH–NH$_2$
          |
         CH$_3$

Amphetamine

OCH$_3$

CH$_2$–CH–NH$_2$
          |
         CH$_3$

H$_3$C

DOM

Amphetamine increases the amount of dopamine and norepinephrine in the synapse by stepping up their release and interfering with their normal reabsorption. The result is a massive stimulation of the central nervous system, including the pleasure center located in the nucleus accumbens. Amphetamine also increases dopamine in the caudate nucleus and putamen of basal ganglia, which regulate motor control. The over-stimulation of these areas can be seen in the trance-like repetitive actions of heavy amphetamine users.

The amphetamines, together with another group of drugs, the phenethylamines, form a class of substances with only one carbon ring, called the phenylalkylamines. This simple molecular structure can be easily added on to, creating a tremendous variety of new drugs. For example, adding two carboxy (oxygen, carbon, and hydrogen) groups produces DOM. Adding a methyl group gives methamphetamine. Adding two oxygen atoms then gives MDMA. Adding a methyl group to MDMA produces MDEA. Innovative chemists (see *MDMA*) have developed hundreds of new psychoactive drugs, each one slightly different in its effects but all of them sharing the basic stimulating properties of amphetamine.[14]

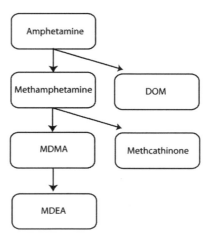

Amphetamine group

ALEPH	4-Methylthio-2,5-dimethoxy-amphetamine
ALEPH-2	4-Ethylthio-2,5-dimethoxy-amphetamine
ALEPH-4	4-Isopropylthio-2,5-dimethoxy-amphetamine
ALEPH-6	4-Phenylthio-2,5-dimethoxy-amphetamine
ALEPH-7	4-Propylthio-2,5-dimethoxy-amphetamine
BEATRICE	2,5-Dimethoxy-4,N-dimethyl-amphetamine
BIS-TOM	2,5-Bismethylthio-4-methyl-amphetamine
4-Br-3,5-DMA	4-Bromo-3,5-dimethoxy-amphetamine
2-Br-4,5-MDA	2-Bromo-4,5-methylenedioxy-amphetamine
3C-BZ	4-Benzyloxy-3,5-dimethoxy-amphetamine
3C-E	4-Ethoxy-3,5-dimethoxy-amphetamine
2,4-DMA	2,4-Dimethoxy-amphetamine
2,5-DMA	2,5-Dimethoxy-amphetamine
3,4-DMA	3,4-Dimethoxy-amphetamine
DMCPA	2-(2,5-Dimethoxy-4-methylphenyl)-cyclopropylamine
DMMDA	2,5-Dimethoxy-3,4-methylenedioxy-amphetamine
DMMDA-2	2,3-Dimethoxy-4,5-methylenedioxy-amphetamine
DOAM	4-Amyl-2,5-dimethoxy-amphetamine
DOB	4-Bromo-2,5-dimethoxy-amphetamine
DOBU	4-Butyl-2,5-dimethoxy-amphetamine
DOC	4-Chloro-2,5-dimethoxy-amphetamine
DOEF	4-(2-Fluoroethyl)-2,5-dimethoxy-amphetamine
DOET	4-Ethyl-2,5-dimethoxy-amphetamine
DOI	4-Iodo-2,5-dimethoxy-amphetamine
DOM (STP)	4-Methyl-2,5-dimethoxy-amphetamine
gamma-DOM	4-Methyl-2,6-dimethoxy-amphetamine
DON	4-Nitro-2,5-dimethoxy-amphetamine
DOPR	4-Propyl-2,5-dimethoxy-amphetamine
EEE	2,4,5-Triethoxy-amphetamine
EEM	2,4-Diethoxy-5-methoxy-amphetamine
EME	2,5-Diethoxy-4-methoxy-amphetamine
EMM	2-Ethoxy-4,5-dimethoxy-amphetamine
F-2	Benzofuran-2-methyl-5-methoxy-6-(2-aminopropane)
F-22	Benzofuran-2,2-dimethyl-5-methoxy-6-(2-aminopropane)
FLEA	N-Hydroxy-N-methyl-3,4-methylenedioxy-amphetamine
G-3	3,4-Trimethylene-2,5-dimethoxy-amphetamine
G-4	3,4-Tetramethylene-2,5-dimethoxy-amphetamine
G-5	3,4-Norbornyl-2,5-dimethoxy-amphetamine
GANESHA	3,4-Dimethyl-2,5-dimethoxy-amphetamine
G-N	1,4-Dimethoxynaphthyl-2-isopropylamine
IDNNA	2,5-Dimethoxy-N,N-dimethyl-4-iodo-amphetamine
IRIS	5-Ethoxy-2-methoxy-4-methyl-amphetamine
4-MA	4-Methoxy-amphetamine
MADAM-6	2,N-Dimethyl-4,5-methylenedioxy-amphetamine
MDA	3,4-Methylenedioxy-amphetamine
MDAL	N-Allyl-3,4-methylenedioxy-amphetamine
MDBU	N-Butyl-3,4-methylenedioxy-amphetamine
MDBZ	N-Benzyl-3,4-methylenedioxy-amphetamine
MDCPM	N-Cyclopropylmethyl-3,4-methylenedioxy-amphetamine
MDDM	N,N-Dimethyl-3,4-methylenedioxy-amphetamine
MDE	N-Ethyl-3,4-methylenedioxy-amphetamine
MDHOET	N-(2-Hydroxyethyl)-3,4-methylenedioxy-amphetamine
MDIP	N-Isopropyl-3,4-methylenedioxy-amphetamine
MDMA	N-Methyl-3,4-methylenedioxy-amphetamine
MDMC	N-Methyl-3,4-ethylenedioxy-amphetamine
MDMEO	N-Methoxy-3,4-methylenedioxy-amphetamine
MDMEOET	N-(2-Methoxyethyl)-3,4-methylenedioxy-amphetamine
MDOH	N-Hydroxy-3,4-methylenedioxy-amphetamine
MDPL	N-Propargyl-3,4-methylenedioxy-amphetamine
MDPR	N-Propyl-3,4 methylenedioxy-amphetamine
MEDA	3,4-Ethylenedioxy-5-methoxy-amphetamine
MEE	2-Methoxy-4,5-diethoxy-amphetamine
MEM	2,5-Dimethoxy-4-ethoxy-amphetamine
META-DOB	5-Bromo-2,4-dimethoxy-amphetamine

META-DOT	5-Methylthio-2,4-dimethoxy-amphetamine
METHYL-DMA	N-Methyl-2,5-dimethoxy-amphetamine
METHYL-DOB	4-Bromo-2,5-dimethoxy-N-methyl-amphetamine
METHYL-MA	N-Methyl-4-methoxy-amphetamine
METHYL-MMDA-2	N-Methyl-2-methoxy-4,5-methylenedioxy-amphetamine
MMDA	3-Methoxy-4,5-methylenedioxy-amphetamine
MMDA-2	2-Methoxy-4,5-methylenedioxy-amphetamine
MMDA-3a	2-Methoxy-3,4-methylenedioxy-amphetamine
MMDA-3b	4-Methoxy-2,3-methylenedioxy-amphetamine
MME	2,4-Dimethoxy-5-ethoxy-amphetamine
MPM	2,5-Dimethoxy-4-propoxy-amphetamine
ORTHO-DOT	2-Methylthio-4,5-dimethoxy-amphetamine
TA	2,3,4,5-Tetramethoxy-amphetamine
TMA	3,4,5-Trimethoxy-amphetamine
TMA-2	2,4,5-Trimethoxy-amphetamine
TMA-3	2,3,4-Trimethoxy-amphetamine
TMA-4	2,3,5-Trimethoxy-amphetamine
TMA-5	2,3,6-Trimethoxy-amphetamine
TMA-6	2,4,6-Trimethoxy-amphetamine
2T-MMDA-3a	2-Methylthio-3,4-methylenedioxy-amphetamine
4T-MMDA-2	4,5-Thiomethyleneoxy-2-methoxy-amphetamine
2-TOET	4-Ethyl-5-methoxy-2-methylthio-amphetamine
5-TOET	4-Ethyl-2-methoxy-5-methylthio-amphetamine
2-TOM	5-Methoxy-4-methyl-2-methylthio-amphetamine
5-TOM	2-Methoxy-4-methyl-5-methylthio-amphetamine
TOMSO	2-Methoxy-4-methyl-5-methylsulfinyl-amphetamine

Phenethylamine group

Mescaline

Phenethylamine is found throughout nature, and is a large component of chocolate. The neurotransmitter dopamine is itself a type of phenethylamine. Like the amphetamines, phenethylamine is a stimulant, but it is rapidly destroyed in the body in its basic form. The following chemical variants allow it to linger longer in the body, and penetrate more easily into the brain. Among psychoactive drugs, mescaline is the only common member of the phenethylamine group. Many other variants of these drugs have been synthesized, the majority of them by Dr. Alexander Shulgin (see *MDMA*).

AEM	alpha-Ethyl-3,4,5-trimethoxy-phenethylamine
AL	4-Allyloxy-3,5-dimethoxy-phenethylamine
ARIADNE	2,5-Dimethoxy-alpha-ethyl-4-methyl-phenethylamine
ASB	3,4-Diethoxy-5-methoxy-phenethylamine
B	4-Butoxy-3,5-dimethoxy-phenethylamine
BOB	4-Bromo-2,5,beta-trimethoxy-phenethylamine
BOD	2,5,beta-Trimethoxy-4-methyl-phenethylamine
BOH	beta-Methoxy-3,4-methylenedioxy-phenethylamine
BOHD	2,5-Dimethoxy-beta-hydroxy-4-methyl-phenethylamine
BOM	3,4,5,beta-Tetramethoxy-phenethylamine
2C-B	4-Bromo-2,5-dimethoxy-phenethylamine
2C-F	4-Fluoro-2,5-dimethoxy-phenethylamine
2C-G	3,4-Dimethyl-2,5-dimethoxy-phenethylamine
2C-G-3	3,4-Trimethylene-2,5-dimethoxy-phenethylamine
2C-G-4	3,4-Tetramethylene-2,5-dimethoxy-phenethylamine
2C-G-5	3,4-Norbornyl-2,5-dimethoxy-phenethylamine
2C-G-N	1,4-Dimethoxynaphthyl-2-ethylamine
2C-H	2,5-Dimethoxy-phenethylamine
2C-I	4-Iodo-2,5-dimethoxy-phenethylamine

2C-N	4-Nitro-2,5-dimethoxy-phenethylamine
2C-O-4	4-Isopropoxy-2,5-dimethoxy-phenethylamine
2C-P	4-Propyl-2,5-dimethoxy-phenethylamine
2C-SE	4-Methylseleno-2,5-dimethoxy-phenethylamine
2C-T	4-Methylthio-2,5-dimethoxy-phenethylamine
2C-T-2	4-Ethylthio-2,5-dimethoxy-phenethylamine
2C-T-4	4-Isopropylthio-2,5-dimethoxy-phenethylamine
gamma-2C-T-4	4-Isopropylthio-2,6-dimethoxy-phenethylamine
2C-T-7	4-Propylthio-2,5-dimethoxy-phenethylamine
2C-T-8	4-Cyclopropylmethylthio-2,5-dimethoxy-phenethylamine
2C-T-9	4-(t)-Butylthio-2,5-dimethoxy-phenethylamine
2C-T-13	4-(2-Methoxyethylthio)-2,5-dimethoxy-phenethylamine
2C-T-15	4-Cyclopropylthio-2,5-dimethoxy-phenethylamine
2C-T-17	4-(s)-Butylthio-2,5-dimethoxy-phenethylamine
2C-T-21	4-(2-Fluoroethylthio)-2,5-dimethoxy-phenethylamine
CPM	4-Cyclopropylmethoxy-3,5-dimethoxy-phenethylamine
4-D	4-Trideuteromethyl-3,5-dimethoxy-phenethylamine
beta-D	beta,beta-Dideutero-3,4,5-trimethoxy-phenethylamine
DESOXY	4-Methyl-3,5-Dimethoxy-phenethylamine
DME	3,4-Dimethoxy-beta-hydroxy-phenethylamine
DMPEA	3,4-Dimethoxy-phenethylamine
E	4-Ethoxy-3,5-dimethoxy-phenethylamine
ETHYL-J	N,alpha-diethyl-3,4-methylenedioxy-phenethylamine
ETHYL-K	N-Ethyl-alpha-propyl-3,4-methylenedioxy-phenethylamine
HOT-2	2,5-Dimethoxy-N-hydroxy-4-ethylthio-phenethylamine
HOT-7	2,5-Dimethoxy-N-hydroxy-4-(n)-propylthio-phenethylamine
HOT-17	2,5-Dimethoxy-N-hydroxy-4-(s)-butylthio-phenethylamine
IM	2,3,4-Trimethoxy-phenethylamine
IP	3,5-Dimethoxy-4-isopropoxy-phenethylamine
J	alpha-Ethyl-3,4-methylenedioxy-phenethylamine
LOPHOPHINE	3-Methoxy-4,5-methylenedioxy-phenethylamine
M	3,4,5-Trimethoxy-phenethylamine
MAL	3,5-Dimethoxy-4-methallyloxy-phenethylamine
MDMP	alpha,alpha,N-Trimethyl-3,4-methylenedioxy-phenethylamine
MDPEA	3,4-Methylenedioxy-phenethylamine
MDPH	alpha,alpha-Dimethyl-3,4-methylenedioxy-phenethylamine
ME	3,4-Dimethoxy-5-ethoxy-phenethylamine
MEPEA	3-Methoxy-4-ethoxy-phenethylamine
METHYL-J	N-Methyl-alpha-ethyl-3,4-methylenedioxy-phenethylamine
METHYL-K	N-Methyl-alpha-propyl-3,4-methylenedioxy-phenethylamine
MP	3,4-Dimethoxy-5-propoxy-phenethylamine
P	3,5-Dimethoxy-4-propoxy-phenethylamine
PE	3,5-Dimethoxy-4-phenethyloxy-phenethylamine
PEA	Phenethylamine
PROPYNYL	4-Propynyloxy-3,5-dimethoxy-phenethylamine
SB	3,5-Diethoxy-4-methoxy-phenethylamine
3-TASB	4-Ethoxy-3-ethylthio-5-methoxy-phenethylamine
4-TASB	3-Ethoxy-4-ethylthio-5-methoxy-phenethylamine
5-TASB	3,4-Diethoxy-5-methylthio-phenethylamine
TB	4-Thiobutoxy-3,5-dimethoxy-phenethylamine
3-TE	4-Ethoxy-5-methoxy-3-methylthio-phenethylamine
4-TE	3,5-Dimethoxy-4-ethylthio-phenethylamine
2-TIM	2-Methylthio-3,4-dimethoxy-phenethylamine
3-TIM	3-Methylthio-2,4-dimethoxy-phenethylamine
4-TIM	4-Methylthio-2,3-dimethoxy-phenethylamine
3-TM	3-Methylthio-4,5-dimethoxy-phenethylamine
4-TM	4-Methylthio-3,5-dimethoxy-phenethylamine
3-TME	4,5-Dimethoxy-3-ethylthio-phenethylamine
4-TME	3-Ethoxy-5-methoxy-4-methylthio-phenethylamine
5-TME	3-Ethoxy-4-methoxy-5-methylthio-phenethylamine
TMPEA	2,4,5-Trimethoxy-phenethylamine
TP	4-Propylthio-3,5-dimethoxy-phenethylamine
TRIS	3,4,5-Triethoxy-phenethylamine
3-TSB	3-Ethoxy-5-ethylthio-4-methoxy-phenethylamine
4-TSB	3,5-Diethoxy-4-methylthio-phenethylamine
3-T-TRIS	4,5-Diethoxy-3-ethylthio-phenethylamine
4-T-TRIS	3,5-Diethoxy-4-ethylthio-phenethylamine

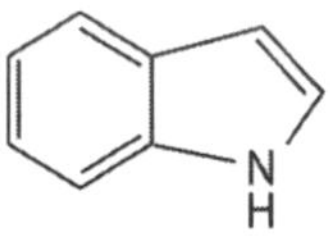

Indole ring

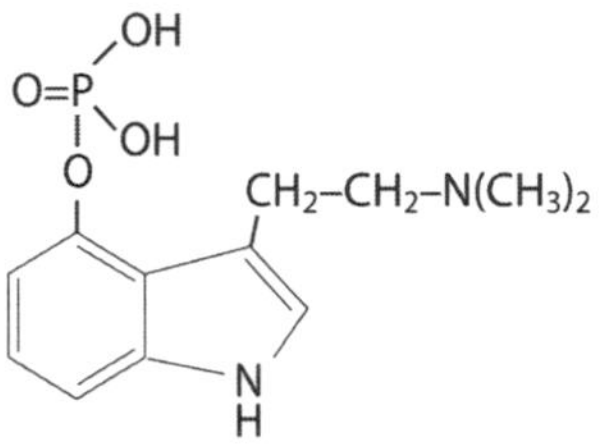

Psilocybin

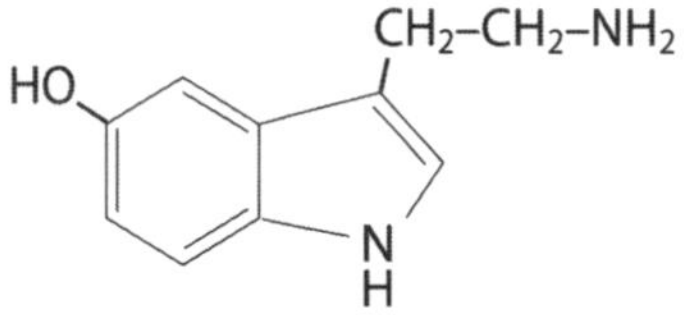

Serotonin

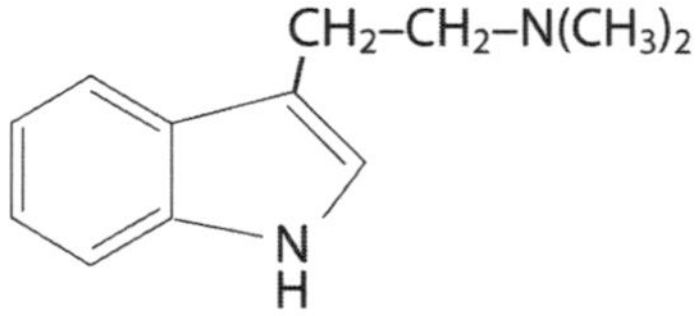

DMT

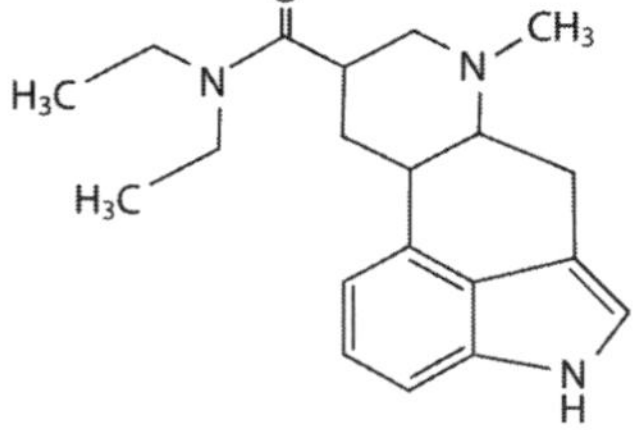

LSD

THE INDOLE HALLUCINOGENS

Hallucinogenic drugs bring out their effects largely by binding to the $5\text{-}HT_2$ type of serotonin receptor. It can be expected, therefore, that the hallucinogens would chemically resemble serotonin. A comparison of their molecules shows that this is indeed the case. Psilocin, the active part of the hallucinogenic psilocybin mushroom, is almost identical to serotonin.

The core of this molecule is the two-ring combination—one six-sided and the other five-sided—known as the indole ring. It is believed to be responsible for the psychoactive effects. Note that many hallucinogens share the indole ring, although they differ in other ways.

The DMT-type hallucinogens are known as tryptamines. DMT itself occurs naturally in the mammalian brain and in the cerebrospinal fluid, although its function there is not well understood. If used as a drug, DMT is not active when taken orally because it is broken down by the enzyme monoamine oxidase (MAO). Some anti-depressant medications contain inhibitors of this enzyme, which if taken would allow DMT to reach the brain. Amazingly, Indians in the Amazon discovered that some plant preparations contain MAO-inhibitors. When they mixed this substance with DMT-containing plants, they were able to develop a hallucinogenic drug (see *Chapter 7: Ayahuasca*).

Metabolism of Drugs

Drugs affect different people differently. It is hard to predict the exact effect of an illegal drug, in part because not enough research has been done to study them. Certain factors, however, are known to influence how well the body can handle a drug.

Age

After age 30, the body produces gradually smaller amounts of the liver enzymes that metabolize drugs. An older person may feel a greater effect from, or cannot tolerate, the same dose as a younger person.

Ethnicity

Different ethnic groups have varying levels of specific enzymes that metabolize drugs. For example, many individuals of Oriental ancestry have lower levels of the enzymes that metabolize alcohol, while Europeans appear to metabolize alcohol more efficiently and are less affected by it. In the same way, it is likely that some ethnic groups metabolize certain drugs less efficiently, and may be more affected by them.

Heredity

Some people have a genetically fast or slow drug-specific metabolism, and it is believed that the tendency to become addicted may be partly a hereditary trait.

About 1 in 12 individuals appears to lack the enzyme cytochrome P450-246, needed to metabolize MDMA. These people may have a fatal reaction to the drug, as noted in many cases of the "sudden death syndrome" (see MDMA).

Sex

Males and females have different rates of metabolizing drugs.

Health

A healthier, well-nourished person may have a better tolerance to a drug, and metabolize it at a faster rate.

Allergy

Some people have allergies to certain drugs.

Psychiatric state

People with mental illness, or extreme moods, may not be able to tolerate some drugs. These people already have a chemical imbalance in the brain. For these people, exposure to even small amounts of hallucinogens could cause severe psychological effects.

Combined drug use

Many drugs cross-react to each other. This may occur because of a combination of effects, or because key metabolic enzymes are tied up so that metabolism is delayed. Combining MDMA with LSD, for example, is done to add the euphoria of MDMA to the hallucinations of LSD. The hazards of MDMA are also affected by other drugs: combining it with drugs such as Prozac may be protective, but combining it with cocaine may be fatal.

Types of Tolerance

Repeated use of a drug usually enables the body to develop tolerance to its effects. Tolerance occurs with all drugs, but it can occur slowly or rapidly, and last for a longer or shorter time, depending on the type of drug. Tolerance to opiates can take weeks or months to evolve and then equally long to resolve, while tolerance to hallucinogens occurs within a day but is resolved within a week.

Tolerance to a drug takes place in several ways:

Dispositional tolerance

The body speeds up the metabolism of the drug in order to eliminate it. This is usually accomplished by an increase in the production of enzymes in the liver that break down the drug. One way of testing the burden of drugs in the body is by measuring these enzymes—if they are high, the body is suffering from the drug effects.

Pharmacologic tolerance

With repeated use, the brain's neurons become less sensitive to the effects of the drug and may even produce an antidote or antagonist to the drug. Most neurons react to the overwhelming presence of a neurotransmitter-like drug by downgrading the receptors for it. With opioids, the brain can actually produce an opioid antagonist, cholecystokinin, to counteract its effects. This type of tolerance is very frustrating to drug users, who require increasingly higher doses to achieve the same effect.

Behavioral tolerance

The brain learns to compensate for the effects of the drug by using parts of the brain that are not affected. This is how chronic alcohol and marijuana users manage to function quite well despite levels of intoxication that would incapacitate people who are less accustomed to the drug.

Reverse tolerance

A drug user may actually become more sensitive to a drug when that drug destroys brain tissue. The excessive sensitivity may alter the overall drug experience to make it less enjoyable. MDMA is an example of a drug that often becomes very disagreeable with extensive use.

Acute tolerance

Also known as tachyphylaxis, this is the almost immediate tolerance to the effect of a drug as the body adapts to it. For example, a single dose of most hallucinogens causes a reduced effect if the drug is taken again, and even if a different type of hallucinogen is taken. For LSD, psilocybin, and other hallucinogens, it may take a week to regain full sensitivity to the drug.

Select tolerance

The body develops tolerance to different aspects of the drug at different rates. For example, mental tolerance may proceed rapidly, so that the user wants a higher dose, but if physical tolerance has not caught up the user may take a fatal overdose. This has often happened with barbiturates.

Inverse tolerance (kindling)
Repeated use of some drugs can suddenly cause an increased sensitivity to it, as the brain anticipates and enhances its effects. For example, long-term marijuana or cocaine users often become *more* sensitive to the drug, and even a fake look-alike drug may give them the drug effect.

A Final Word: The Secret of Psychoactive Drugs

Neurotransmitters are the key to understanding psychoactive drugs. When these drugs enter the brain, they flood the space between neurons and overwhelm the normal communication between cells. The result can be a stepped-up transmission of signals, a block of signals, or a total overload of the brain with dramatic and unpredictable effects.

 The key to understanding drugs is to study neurotransmitters—indeed, most discoveries of neurotransmitters have come from scientific research on the effects of psychoactive drugs.

The simple fact—that psychoactive drugs produce their effects by neurotransmitters—points out their true secret: *All drug sensations, feelings, awareness or hallucinations can also be achieved without drugs.*

Psychoactive drugs work by stimulating the natural function of the brain. All the thoughts, perceptions and behaviors already exist. These drugs do not create anything new. Drugs cannot create sensations or feelings that do not have a natural counterpart.[15]

 "There is no such thing as the drug experience per se—no experience that the drug, as it were, creates." [16]

The most remarkable recent discovery—something that those who practice yoga, meditation, prayer, or other mind-altering techniques have always known—is that *all* effects of psychoactive drugs can be produced naturally and spontaneously. As an associate of Timothy Leary pointed out, "Acid is no better than the traditional methods, it's just faster and sneakier."[17]

Psychoactive drugs are somewhat like an athletic coach. Many athletes believe that they could not perform without someone screaming at them to try harder, to go faster, hang in there, don't give up, take it to the limit, and so on. And perhaps they are right: they would not do as well without the encouragement. But who is actually performing, the athlete or the coach?

Countless studies have shown that the effects of a placebo (a fake drug) can be as strong as the real drug. This is only possible because the experience may be *stimulated* by the drug, but it is not *originated* by the drug. The experience is produced by the brain itself.

 A psychedelic drug is like "an especially active placebo."
—Andrew Weil

CONTACT HIGH

With hallucinogenic drugs, in particular, there is a curious phenomenon that suggests that the drug itself may not be so important in getting high. People who have taken a hallucinogen in the past, especially LSD, often say that they feel the same LSD effects when they are close to someone who is under the influence of a hallucinogen. This feeling, which came to be called a "contact high," can even occur in people who have not taken the drug in 10 or 20 years. But with their memory of the hallucinogenic experience, the mere contact with a person on drugs is enough to trigger a natural psychedelic experience.

The same is true of the phenomenon of post hallucinogenic perceptual disorder, more commonly known as "flashbacks" (see *LSD*). Users of LSD (or other hallucinogens), often report that they have had a brief recurrence of the drug-like state months or even years after taking the drug. By then, any trace of the drug in the body has long vanished. It is likely that something—fatigue, stress, illness, another drug, or perhaps a reminder of the drug trip—triggered a natural re-creation of the drug state.

NON-DRUG ALTERED STATES OF CONSCIOUSNESS

It is not easy to achieve powerful drug-like altered states of consciousness without the aid of these chemical helpers. But it is possible. It has been done for thousands of years using techniques such as intense physical exertion, breathing exercises, prolonged wakefulness, fasting, meditation, and isolation. All of these techniques have been employed by religious adepts specifically for this purpose.

Altered states of consciousness can also occur spontaneously, at a time of crisis, physical injury, or in a moment of discovery, when a new avenue of awareness is opened up.

How do these non-drug states compare with the drug states? Both involve heightened or diminished activity in various parts of the brain. Subjectively, the euphoria, invigoration, or insight reported by practitioners of yoga, for example, are no less intense than those reported by drug users. When studied by EEG, PET, and other methods, the brain states can seem remarkably alike. In the non-drug state, however, the neurotransmitter activity is naturally generated, while in the drug state it is artificially supported—and crashes back to baseline, or below, when the support is taken away.

While the outcome may be similar, at least for a short time, there are two big differences between mental states caused by drugs and those produced in other ways:

Side effects
No drug is perfect. Every drug has some undesirable effects which can become intolerable over the long term.

In contrast, a natural sense of euphoria has no side effect other than an annoyingly unrelenting cheerfulness.

Tolerance
The body will adapt to the artificial stimulation (or depression) provided by a drug, and it will take more and more of the drug to trigger the same experience. In some cases (see MDMA), the intensity of the original experience is never again quite equaled, to the great disappointment of the user.

Conversely, with non-drug stimulation the body actually becomes more proficient at it. The same experience becomes easier, not harder, to achieve and it becomes even more intense. In this way, the brain is like any muscle: if an artificial support is used, the muscle gradually weakens from lack of use. On the other hand, if the muscle is repeatedly exercised, it becomes stronger.

Throughout history, drugs have been used in mystical pursuits to awaken the user to what is possible. They give a glimpse of awareness of another reality. But in most spiritual endeavors, drugs are considered to be ultimately a hindrance to progress. Real achievement, in these beliefs, comes from a personal mastery of the mental state without the need for drugs. Philosopher Alan Watts, who popularized Eastern religious thought, recognized the usefulness of psychoactive drugs to jolt a person out of normal awareness. But he recommended that spiritual aspirants eventually set drugs aside and focus on developing and applying what they learned. "When you get the message," he said, "hang up the phone."

From the beginning of humanity, mind-altering drugs have been used as a sort of mental vacation, or to jump-start a spiritual pursuit. They were used as a temporary "time-out" in which the user could experience a different state of consciousness. In modern times, the same thing is taking place and with a far greater variety of drugs. But like all vacations, experiments, or spiritual retreats, people eventually have to come back to face ordinary life.

"The interesting question is not why people take drugs, but rather why they stop taking them."—*Scientific American* [18]

CHAPTER 7

Just Say Know

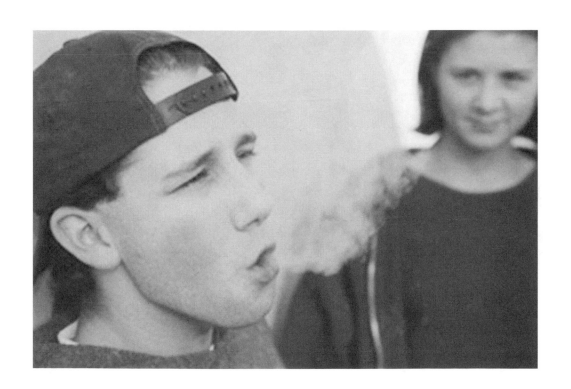

"Recreation is therapy; at least that's what people tell me."
—*Otto Snow, psychoactive drug chemist*

Illegal Drug Use Today

BY THEIR DRUGS SO SHALL YE KNOW THEM

Drugs are a part of cultural identity. From the earliest human societies, drugs that were used by some people but feared by others became a cause of persecution. Drugs are part of the culture of an ethnic group, in the same way that the group's peculiar foods, dress, rituals, and other characteristics give them an identity different from other ethnic groups. And much as a food might be adopted, another group's drug might be adopted as well.

European contact with the Americas introduced new foods to both continents. It also brought knowledge of each other's drugs, probably with equal detriment to both. The Europeans brought alcohol, which has devastated the Native American people. And from the New World, Europeans took back tobacco, which they have probably regretted ever since. The process continues today. Japanese brought *shabu*, smokable methamphetamine, to Hawaii and then California. Russians brought methcathinone. Meanwhile, the United States exported a taste for amphetamines and MDMA to these countries, and to the rest of the world.

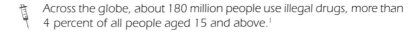

Across the globe, about 180 million people use illegal drugs, more than 4 percent of all people aged 15 and above.[1]

Along with other changes in popular culture—fashions of dress, food, music, and the arts—drug use is trendy. Use of narcotics increases in times of suffering, stimulants in times of industry, depressants during times of stress, and hallucinogens become popular during times of exploration. Today, all of these trends are combined.

The current drug problem could be said to have begun with the American Civil War. During that period, the syringe was invented and thousands of soldiers developed an addiction to morphine. Each successive war has increased the spread of drugs by soldiers into general society. The first great American drug epidemic began in the early years of the 20th century and led to the initial legislation prohibiting heroin and cocaine. Legions of soldiers came back from the First World War either addicted to drugs or drifting into addiction because of social and psychological problems they faced on their return home.

Drug use then declined during the following economic depression, and by the Second World War, it had become so uncommon that it was forgotten as a social problem.

The Second World War, the Korean War, and then the Vietnam War each again brought back veterans addicted to narcotics as a result of both physical and psychological trauma. While soldiers in Vietnam took heroin to numb themselves, back at home the 1960s were a time of exploration. There was a surge of interest in newly discovered psychoactive drugs, along with increased use of the old ones.

By the 1970s, heroin and amphetamines, initially disparaged by the college-educated society, came back in an uneasy mix with marijuana and the hallucinogens. Cocaine became enormously popular and evolved to freebase and crack a decade later.

In every place, in every year, there was concern about the dominant drug of the day. Five years ago it was crack, last year it was heroin, and today, in most American cities, it is MDMA (Ecstasy). In addition to these headline-making drugs, there is now some use of virtually every drug that has ever existed and each year brings a number of new designer drugs. With the Internet and the current globalization of knowledge and commerce, the distribution of any particular drug changes along with other trends in fashion, but it never entirely disappears.

 Drugs today are more varied, more widely known, and most of them more accessible, than ever before.

Every effort of the Government—whether taking military action to stem the flow of foreign drug production, or threatening users and dealers with severe punishment—has had a minimal impact on recreational drug use. The incontrovertible fact is that the United States leads the world in the use of drugs, and this is unlikely to change.

NATIONAL DRUG SURVEYS

At present, 35.6 percent of the population 12 years of age and over has used illegal drugs.[2] Of these, about one in five has used illegal drugs in the past month.[3]

The United States Department of Health and Human Services oversees the National Institute on Drug Abuse (NIDA) and the Substance Abuse and Mental Health Services Administration (SAMHSA). These agencies conduct several major epidemiologic surveys to keep track of drug use.

National Household Survey on Drug Abuse (NHSDA)

An annual survey that began in 1971, the NHSDA is the basic method by which SAMSHA assesses the nature and extent of drug abuse in the general U.S. population. NHSDA data show that the use of illegal drugs tends to begin in teenage years, reaches a high point in young adulthood, and decreases in later life.

National High School Senior Survey

An annual survey conducted by NIDA to measure drug use and attitudes of about 16,000 high school seniors in private and public schools nationwide.

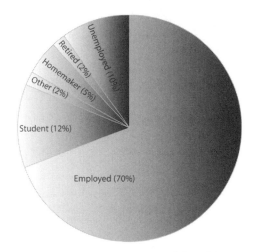

Current users of illegal drugs

Partnership Attitude Tracking Study (PATS)

Funded independently by the Robert Wood Johnston Foundation, this is the largest ongoing study of drug-related attitudes, particularly among children.

The 1996 PATS data of 12,292 interviews showed that 9- to 12-year-olds had become less likely to consider drugs harmful and risky, and more likely to believe that drug use was widespread and acceptable.[4]

Drug Abuse Warning Network (DAWN)

A regular survey conducted by NIDA to track the medical consequences of drug abuse. Data are collected from a sample of more than 700 hospitals and 85 medical examiners located in 26 major metropolitan areas, plus a national panel of hospitals outside these areas. This is the primary way to tally the number of deaths from illegal drugs.

According to DAWN data, the most popular drugs are not the most dangerous. Most deaths are due to prescription drugs, such as Valium, but the greatest *risk* of death, as measured by the likelihood of death per user, is from depressants.[5] Among the popular drugs, only methamphetamine has a very high death rate.

Drug deaths:	Highest number	Highest risk
	codeine	secobarbital (Seconal)
	diazepam (Valium)	methaqualone (Quaalude)
	propoxyphene (Darvon)	glutethimide (Doriden)
	phenobarbital (Luminal)	methamphetamine

No death has ever been attributed to marijuana, and deaths from hallucinogens are extremely rare.

Percent of U.S. household population 12 years of age and older reporting past 30 day illicit drug use by age group, 1997 [6]

Drug	Age Group 12-17	18-25	26-34	35 & older	Total
Any illicit drug	11.4	14.7	7.4	3.6	6.4
Marijuana & hashish	9.4	12.8	6.0	2.6	5.1
Cocaine & crack	1.0	1.2	0.9	0.5	0.7
Hallucinogens	1.9	2.5	0.5	0.3	0.8
Heroin	0.3	0.5	0.2	0.2	0.3
Stimulants (eg amphetamines)	0.6	0.7	0.2	0.2	0.3
Sedatives (eg barbiturates)	0.1	0.2	0.1	0.1	0.1

National Drug Abuse Treatment Unit Survey (NDATUS)

A survey conducted by SAMHSA to collect data on alcohol and drug treatment programs (both public and private).

Drug Services Research Survey (DSRS)

SAMHSA also collects data on provider and patient characteristics in this survey to evaluate the efficacy of drug abuse treatment.

The results of these surveys show that 71 percent of illegal drug users are employed. On the other hand, 6.1 percent of all employed individuals are current users of illegal drugs—5.5 percent of full-time employees and 9 percent of part-time employees. These surveys also show that drugs are used by all sectors of society. Although the "drug problem" may be more visible in some areas, such as the inner cities, this is partly due to poverty and a lack of privacy, and partly due to bias in the popular media.

"The media usually portray cocaine and crack use as a black ghetto phenomenon. This is a racist caricature. There are more drug addicts among middle- and upper-class whites than any other segment of the population, and far more such occasional users. ... Only 13 percent of those using illegal drugs are African American, but they constitute 35 percent of those arrested for simple possession and a staggering 74 percent of those sentenced for drug possession." [7]

STREET TERMS AND SLANG WORDS

Drugs that are legally marketed have a brand name, usually protected by a registered trademark. In the same way, illegal drugs have popular names that are easier to say and remember than their chemical names, and are good for advertising. For example, MDMA sells a lot better as Ecstasy.

The street names may play on the drug name (Rohypnol becomes "Roofies," Benzedrine becomes "Bennies"); hint at the source of the drug ("Thai sticks", "Mexican tar"); its appearance (crack becomes "gravel," LSD is "pink blotters"); and odor (marijuana is "skunk"). Occasionally, the same term is used for different drugs, either purposely to mislead users (see *Chapter 6: Designer drugs*) or arises independently by people who are not familiar with the previous meaning.

There are also popular terms for drug amounts and methods of use: it is easier to say "toke" than "take a deep inhalation and hold it, straining slightly, and then let it out slowly."

New terms appear every year. While most of the older terms eventually fade away, some have been around for centuries (such as "dope"), and a few have entered the common language ("junkie," "cold turkey," "stoned").

For street terms and slang for a specific drug, see the first page of each drug chapter. A list of other terms follows:[8]

Abe	$5 worth of drugs
Acid head	LSD user
Agonies	withdrawal symptoms
Airhead	marijuana user
All lit up	under the influence of drugs
All star	user of multiple drugs
Amped and queer	to be high on cocaine or amphetamines
Amped out	fatigue after using amphetamines
Amping	accelerated heart beat
Anything going on?	Do you have drugs for sale?
Artillary	equipment for injecting drugs
Ate up	someone who's always intoxicated
Babe	drug used for detoxification
Back-to-back	smoking crack after injecting heroin, or using heroin after crack
Backtrack	to allow blood to flow back into a needle during injection
Bad go	bad reaction to a drug
Bad trip	bad experience on an hallucinogen
Bag bride	drug-using prostitute
Bagboy	someone who sells drugs for someone else
Balloon	heroin supplier
Bambs	depressants
Bang	to inject a drug
Barb, Barbies	barbiturate
Base crazies	searching on hands and knees for crack dropped on the floor
Base head	person who bases

Batt	IV needle
Beaners	drugs
Beans	amphetamines, depressants, mescaline
Beat artist	person selling bogus drugs
Beat vials	vials containing sham crack to cheat buyers
Bed bugs	fellow addicts
Beebong	hit
Belt	effects of drugs
Bender	drug party
Big man	drug supplier
Bindle	small envelope or folded paper packet of drug powder
Bing	enough of a drug for one injection
Bingo	to inject a drug
Birdie powder	heroin or cocaine
Biz	bag or portion of drugs
Blanks	low-quality drugs
Blast	to smoke marijuana or crack
Blizzard	white cloud in a pipe used to smoke cocaine
Block busters	depressants
Blow a fix, blow a shot	injection missed the vein and is wasted in the skin
Blow a stick	to smoke marijuana
Blow blue, blow smoke	to inhale cocaine
Blow the vein	rupturing the vein while injecting too quickly
Blue	depressants, crack
Blue angels, birds, dolls, etc.	depressants
Body packer	swallow drug packets for transport
Body stuffer	stuff drugs in the rectum or vagina for transport
Bomb squad	crack-selling crew
Bong	pipe used to smoke marijuana
Boost and shoot	steal to support a habit
Boot the gong	to smoke marijuana
Boxed	in jail
Brick	kilogram of marijuana, crack
Bridge up, bring up	ready a vein for injection
Buck	to shoot someone in the head
Buffe	woman who exchanges oral sex for crack
Bugged	to be covered with sores and abscesses from use of unsterile needles
Bull	narcotics agent or police officer
Burn the main line	to inject a drug
Burned out	collapse of veins from repeated injections
Buzz	under the influence of drugs
Cad, Cadillac	one ounce
Cake	round disks of crack
Cap up	transfer bulk drug to capsules
Carburetor	crack stem attachment
Carpet patrol	crack smokers searching the floor for crack
Chalked up	under the influence of cocaine
Chalking	chemically altering cocaine to make it look more white
Channel	vein into which a drug is injected
Chasing the dragon	to smoke heroin
Chaze	to christen a new bowl or pipe
Check	personal supply of drugs
Chillun	pipe used to smoke hashish
Chinese-eyed	when the eyes become slanted from smoking marijuana
Chipping	using drugs occasionally

Chucks	hunger following withdrawal from heroin
Clips	rows of vials heat-sealed together
Clocking paper	profits from selling drugs
Cluck	crack smoker
Coasting	under the influence of drugs
Cocaine blues	depression after extended cocaine binge
Cod	large amount of money
Cold turkey	sudden withdrawal from drugs
Come home	end a trip from LSD
Cooker	to inject a drug
Cooler	cigarette laced with a drug
Cop	to obtain drugs
Copping zones	areas where drugs can be bought
Cotton	currency
Crack gallery	place where crack is bought and sold
Cranking up	to inject a drug
Crash	to sleep off the effects of drugs
Cushion	vein into which a drug is injected
Deck	packet of heroin
Dime, dime bag	$10 dollars worth of crack
Dipping out	crack runners taking a portion of crack from the vials
Disease	drug of choice
D.L. spot	safe place to buy and use drugs
Do a line	to inhale cocaine
Dog	good friend
Dollar	$100 worth of drugs
Domestic	locally grown marijuana
Doub	$20 worth of crack
Dove	$35 worth of crack
Due	residue of oils trapped in a pipe after smoking crack
Dusting	adding PCP, heroin, or other drug to marijuana
Eight ball	one eighth of an ounce of drugs
Emergency gun	instrument used to inject drugs other than a syringe
Eye opener	crack or amphetamine
Factory	place where drugs are made or packaged
Fall	arrested
Fatty	marijuana cigarette
Fiend	someone who uses drugs alone
Fire, fix	to inject a drug
Five-cent bag	$5 worth of drugs
Flamethrower	cigarette laced with heroin and cocaine
Flag	appearance of blood in the syringe
Flying, fucked up	under the influence of drugs
Gaffus	hypodermic needle
Garbage heads	users who buy crack from dealers instead of cooking it themselves
Geezer, get down	to inject a drug
Gimmick	drug injection equipment
Give wings	to inject someone
Go into a sewer	to inject drugs
Gopher	person paid to pick up drugs
Got it going on	fast sale of drugs
Gravel	crack cocaine
Ground control	caretaker during a hallucinogen experience
Gutter	vein into which a drug is injected
Heeled	having plenty of money

Highbeams	the wide eyes of a person on crack
HO	half ounce of marijuana
Hot box	to fill up a closed area with secondhand marijuana smoke
House fee	money paid to enter a crack house
Hubba pigeon	crack user looking for rocks on the floor after a police raid
Hulling	using others to get drugs
Ice cream habit	occasional use of drugs
Idiot pills	depressants
Jab, job, jack-up, jolt	to inject a drug
Jack	to steal someone else's drugs
Jonesing	need for drugs
Joy pop	to inject a drug
Joy powder	heroin, cocaine
Juggle	to sell drugs to support a habit
Keyed	under the influence of drugs
Kiddie dope	prescription drugs
Klingons	crack addicts
Lace	cocaine and marijuana
Laugh and scratch	to inject a drug
Lay-out	equipment for taking a drug
Lunchbox	children who take drugs
Mainline	injecting into a vein
Matchbox	quarter ounce of marijuana, or six cigarettes
Monkey	drug dependency
Mule	carrier of drugs
Munchies	hunger after smoking marijuana
Nailed	arrested
Nickel bag	$5 worth of drugs
Nix	stranger among the group
Nod	effects of heroin
On ice	in jail
On the bricks	walking the streets
Paper boy	heroin dealer
Pepsi habit	occasional use of drugs
Permafried	effects of long-term use
Perp	fake crack made from baking soda and candle wax
Pinner	small joint of marijuana
Plant	hiding place for drugs
Push, pusher	to sell drugs
Raspberry, rock star	female who trades sex for drugs
Sam	federal narcotics agent
Satch	material saturated with drug solution to smuggle into prison
Set	a place where drugs are sold
Skeegers, skeezers	crack smoking prostitute
Slam	to inject a drug
Slanging, slinging	selling drugs
Stoned	under the influence of drugs
Strung out	heavily addicted to drugs
Teener	one sixteenth of a gram
Toss up	female who trades sex for drugs
Tout	person who introduces buyers to sellers
Tweaking	drug-induced paranoia; using amphetamines
Uncle	federal agents
Zips	one ounce of a drug
Zoomers	person who sells fake crack and then flees

The Business of Illegal Drugs

Producing, marketing, distributing, and selling illegal drugs is an economic activity just like any other business. There is a hierarchy of agents in this business and there are specialists who carry out certain jobs. And as with any business, there are personal and financial risks.

A majority of the illegal drug industry is controlled by a small number of people at the top of an organized crime syndicate. These individuals make the most money and take the fewest risks. They negotiate with people who import drugs from other countries, and arrange to have the drugs refined, diluted, and distributed to local dealers. Very few people are in contact with this echelon. Lower-level people are often killed or imprisoned before they have gained the trust to reach these top individuals. Because the drug trade is so lucrative, organized crime in many countries is assisted by corrupt police who are rewarded for allowing the drug business to continue. In some countries, the Government itself may be involved in the global illegal drug trade.

BASIC ECONOMICS: SUPPLY AND DEMAND

Like any commodity, the price of drugs is determined by supply and demand. This is true everywhere from a small neighborhood up to the international level. If demand is constant, a lower supply will bring an increased price, which in turn will lead to greater criminal activity.

The war on drugs has directed its efforts not on demand but on reducing the supply. As a result, the prices of marijuana, cocaine and heroin have increased to about 100 times more than they would be in a free market,[9] along with a tremendous increase in drug-related crime and the number of people imprisoned. As the price of drugs rises, more people—particularly those who have few other economic opportunities—are drawn into the drug trade. In Washington, Oregon, and northern California, for example, the demise of the logging industry has led unemployed forestry workers to turn to the much more profitable production of marijuana.

 Marijuana is now the largest cash crop in the United States.

Mandatory imprisonment for drug users has not had much effect in stemming the drug business, but it has greatly increased the prison population. It is estimated that about 65 percent of all prisoners are there for drug offenses. Those incarcerated for other reasons are also likely to have used drugs. At least 30 percent of those in jail said that they were using drugs on a daily basis in the month before committing their crime. In Manhattan, New York, 83 percent of arrested males and 84 percent of females tested positive for drugs. In San Antonio, Texas, 51 percent of males and 41 percent of females tested positive. Despite this high rate of imprisonment of drug offenders, trends in drug use and drug-related business do not appear to be sensitive to threats of punishment.

YOUTH EMPLOYMENT

The drug industry favors the employment of young people because they tend to be naïve, have few other employment opportunities, are easily impressed by money and status, and are led to believe that they will be treated leniently if caught.

A typical inner-city drug operation often employs a number of adolescents and children:

Lookouts keep an eye on the street and warn the dealer about police, rival dealers, and gangs.

Spotters are at the sales location, but they don't possess or sell the drugs. The job of spotters is to direct buyers to an ideal location to make the purchase. The dealer usually has an escape route, and might be on a rooftop, passing drugs down on a string, or behind a small opening in a wall. Spotters are visible, work directly with buyers, and are typically among the newest recruits. They therefore have a high risk of being arrested.

Couriers carry drugs around town. Who would suspect a 12-year-old boy or girl on a bicycle of carrying drugs? Most of the time, the kids are not told what is in the bag and told not to look. They are just given five or ten dollars and directed where to take it.

Young dealers sell drugs in small amounts to other adolescents.

Enforcers are usually gang members. Gangs are recruited or created to control certain areas and increase sales territory. They do this by keeping out competition, collecting debts, protecting the dealers, and guarding the operation from theft. Gang members are highly visible to police and very expendable to dealers. They tend to last from one day to two years. Most of them end up injured, imprisoned, or dead.

There is a common belief that that young people are less likely than adults to be punished for crimes. It is actually easier for a person under 18 to be convicted of a crime.[10] A juvenile can be arrested without a warrant in a situation in which a police officer would have to get a warrant to arrest an adult. Adolescents are prosecuted under the same laws as adults and jail time is based on the same penal code. Actual possession of drugs is not necessary to be charged and convicted of drug sales. Simply having a pager and a "pay/owe sheet" or a large amount of cash might be enough.

PROSTITUTION

Prostitution has been linked to psychoactive drug use for thousands of years. Female prostitutes have historically used opiates to disrupt ovulation and provide a form of contraception. Most prostitutes use drugs for more complex reasons, which involve both psychological and practical issues. Opiates and barbiturates have long been a favorite of prostitutes because they numb the person to the experience. These drugs create a dissociation from the body, a detachment that allows the prostitute to survive sexual and physical abuse with less psychological trauma.

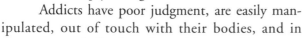

Addicts have poor judgment, are easily manipulated, out of touch with their bodies, and in desperate need of cash or drugs. This combination makes them easy prey for criminal operations. An addicted person will do anything to obtain drugs, and selling the use of his or her body may be the only way to do so. Prostitutes are often called slaves because they are virtually owned by people in the business. They are usually paid in drugs, or a drug-cash combination, and may be lent or traded for services.

SMUGGLING

Drug smuggling has existed as a lucrative profession ever since the first drug laws were enacted. In South America, a person carrying a small load of drugs to the United States can earn as much in a single trip as in an entire lifetime of legitimate wages.

The majority of drugs are smuggled as freight inside, or disguised as, other products. With the volume of international trade, it is impossible to detect more than a tiny fraction of these illegal imports.

An alternative method is to use hired travelers who carry drugs in their luggage or inside their bodies. These couriers are called mules. They typically have little knowledge of the overall operation, and are considered to be expendable by the drug suppliers. To avoid discovery of their drugs, "body stuffers" insert a lubricated package into their rectum

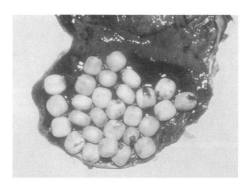

The stomach autopsy of a body packer who died when one of these cocaine-filled condoms burst.

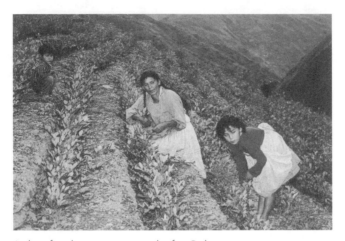

Indian family growing coca leaf in Bolivia

or vagina. In the mid-1980s, a more sophisticated method began with "body packing." The drugs are divided into small packets, usually wrapped in balloons or condoms, and then swallowed. Smugglers may also fill the fingers of latex gloves with drug powder or dozens of tablets, cut each of the fingers off, tie them with dental floss and swallow them. When the journey is complete, the packets are retrieved after being defecated. Up to 1.5 kilograms in a hundred or more packets can be carried this way. For example, in March 2000, customs inspectors caught two men at New York's JFK Airport who had swallowed a total of 2,800 tablets of MDMA contained in sausage-shaped casings called pellets.

Body packing poses severe hazards, such as intestinal obstruction or leaking of the package contents. If a package breaks open inside the body, it will cause a fatal overdose.

WORLD DRUG TRADE

The United States' war on drugs now costs over $18 billion a year and it is estimated that 50 percent of all crimes are drug related. It has spread far beyond American borders to influence other governments, foreign agricultural practices, the migration of people, and the entire global economy.

 World trade in black market drugs is $400 billion per year, about 8 % of the entire global economy.

The annual potential South American production of coca leaf is estimated in excess of 680 million pounds, producing 506 tons of cocaine. Conservative figures indicate that over 1,000,000 people are involved in the growing and harvesting of coca leaves and its conversion into cocaine in Peru, Bolivia, and Colombia. The majority of the cocaine is destined for the United States.

Psychoactive Drugs That Are Not Illegal

The list of substances on Schedules I and II of the Controlled Substances Act does not include many recreational drugs. Some of these are legal to possess, but illegal to manufacture or distribute. A few are restricted in some states but not in others. Most of the following substances, however, are completely unregulated and can be made, grown, or purchased by mail order and over the Internet.

ALCOHOL

Next to tobacco and caffeine, alcohol is the world's most popular drug, and by far the most common cause of disabling intoxication. Alcohol has been produced by the fermentation of fruits and vegetables since the beginning of recorded history. Even animals recognize alcohol, and some appear to get purposefully drunk on fermented berries.

Fermentation allows a maximum alcohol concentration of about 14 percent, after which the alcohol kills the yeasts that produce it. The process of distillation was discovered by Arabs around 800 AD and brought to medieval Europe by 1250. It allowed an increase in the concentration of alcohol to about 50 percent.

Why did alcohol become so popular? Alcohol kills bacteria. Throughout history, the only safe drinks were alcohol preparations such as wine and beer. Most people would rather take the risk of becoming tipsy than the risk of dying from typhoid, cholera, or a number of other types of food poisoning. In many countries, beer and wine became a normal part of a meal, and sometimes it *was* the meal.

Because of general familiarity with its effects and a long tradition of use, alcohol has spread around the world and is now one of the most widely accepted recreational drugs.

 Between 1 AM and 6 AM on weekend mornings, one in every seven drivers is legally drunk.

The impact of alcohol on public health is far worse than all illegal drugs combined. In the United States, it is estimated that alcohol causes at least 200,000 deaths per year (compared with a total of about 8,000 deaths for all illegal drugs), and an untold amount of injury, work loss, and social disruption.

The control of alcohol has served as the model for the control of other recreational drugs, and provided a number of lessons. The two major outcomes of Prohibition, for example, were a shift in consumption from beer to hard liquor and a dramatic increase in organized crime (see *Chapter 3: Prohibition*). From 1802 to 1953, the United States Government outlawed the sale of alcohol to Native Americans. The result was a pattern of binge drinking that was far more socially destructive than in communities where alcohol was readily available.

AMANITA MUSCARIA

The *Amanita muscaria* mushroom grows wild in Europe, Asia, and North America, particularly under birches, firs, and larches, and has been used as a

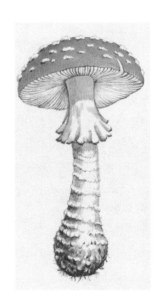

hallucinogen for perhaps 10,000 years. *Amanita* was identified as the *Soma* of ancient India, and some scholars believe that the worship of this mushroom at the base of a fir tree was the origin of the Christmas tree. *Amanita* was used recreationally by Siberian tribes until Russian traders introduced vodka in the 18th century.

This mushroom contains muscimol, ibotenic acid, and muscarine, which led to the discovery of neurotransmitters. *Amanita* is usually eaten after being dried. The drying process changes ibotenic acid to muscimol, the most active constituent. The decarboxylation of ibotenic acid reduces the undesirable side-effects and makes the mushroom five or six times more psychoactive.

As a recreational substance, *Amanita* is a relatively safe drug. Its greatest danger lies in its similarity to other, much more toxic, mushrooms. *Amanita* is not related to psilocybin, a different hallucinogenic mushroom that is illegal.

Amanita mushrooms are chewed, ground and mixed with food or drink, or brewed into a tea. A normal dose is one to five mushrooms. The effects begin within 20 minutes to two hours and last up to about eight hours, bringing increased salivation, increased heart rate, sweating, changes in hearing, touch and visual colors, hot and cold rushes, muscle twitching, occasional hallucinations, and often nausea and vomiting.

AMYL NITRATE

The prescription drug amyl nitrate is a clear, yellow fluid marketed in a glass ampule. It has a fruity odor like rotten apples. It was first synthesized in 1857 and has since been used medically as a muscle relaxant, especially for heart disease.

Recreational use of amyl nitrate "poppers" is common for its pleasant euphoric effects and the breakdown of normal inhibitions. It is especially popular among homosexual men because it relaxes involuntary muscles, including the anal sphincter. Adverse side effects include a visual disturbance of a bright yellow spot with purple radiations.[11]

AYAHUASCA

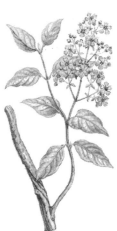

Ayahuasca, a Quechua Indian word meaning "vine of souls," is a psychoactive drug made by combining extracts of a vine, *Banisteriopsis caapi*, and *Psychotria viridis*, both of which grow in the Amazonian forests of South America. The drug is well known throughout tropical South America, and has been in use for at least 4,000 years. The Tupi Indians call it *Yagé*; it is sometimes sold by this name on the Internet. It has also increased in use as a sacrament of Amazonia's many mestizo religious cults of the *Santo Daime Doctrine*. The religious use of ayahuasca has been protected by Brazilian law since 1987.[12]

Recently, American and European drug-seeking travelers have sought out ayahuasca on specially organized tours. One California resident even had the audacity to file an exclusive patent on the drug. Outrage by Amazonian native groups resulted in a dismissal of the patent.

The active ingredients are harmaline and DMT, which together form a powerful hallucinogen that can be readily absorbed. Ayahuasca causes intense vomiting and diarrhea, followed by a dreamlike condition lasting about ten hours.

BETEL NUTS

Hundreds of millions of people in Asian countries chew betel nuts for mild stimulation. The nuts come from the areca palm tree, *Areca catechu*, and are usually mixed with gum from the Malaysian acacia tree and a small amount of burnt lime, which is then wrapped in a betel leaf (*Piper chavica betel*) to be chewed. Some people add nutmeg, turmeric, or cloves for extra flavor.

The active ingredient in betel nuts is arecoline, which is absorbed by saliva and causes central nervous system stimulation. Excessive amounts of betel nuts cause a feeling of intoxication, and possibly dizziness, vomiting, diarrhea, or convulsions. Long-term betel nut chewers have a distinctive dark-red stain of the mouth, teeth, and gums.[13]

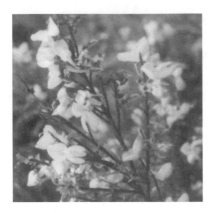

BROOM

Broom, *Cytisus scoparius*, refers to yellow-flowered shrubs grown legally in gardens throughout the United States. When the plant is smoked, it produces a feeling of intoxication and euphoria lasting about two hours. Broom contains cytosine, a chemical similar to nicotine. Like nicotine, it is toxic when eaten but not when smoked.

CAFFEINE

Caffeine-containing tea has been a popular stimulant since it was cultivated in China in the 3rd century BC. Tea was imported to England from China, and then distributed throughout the world following the spread of the British Empire. It is hard to believe that a substance as trivial as tea could dominate global politics, but conflicts ranging from wars in China (see *Chapter 2*) to the American Revolution were instigated by the trade in tea.

The coffee bean was cultivated in Ethiopia in about 600 AD. At first coffee was consumed by chewing the beans, and then by making an infusion of its leaves. Roasting and grinding the beans to make a hot water drink did not begin until the 14th century, by which time it had become the "wine of Islam." It then spread to Europe and led to the creation of coffee houses. American tastes changed to coffee in part as a reaction against the British custom of drinking tea. The American domination of global commerce has helped promote coffee drinking internationally.

Tea and coffee have become the most popular stimulants in the world. Caffeine is also found in other beverages, such as *maté* and chocolate, and it is added to carbonated soft drinks. Many over-the-counter medications and herbal remedies contain caffeine as a key ingredient.

Caffeine is highly addictive, creating both physical and psychological dependence after as little as 100 mg/day. Heavy use of caffeine results in restlessness, nervousness, excitement, insomnia, flushed face, muscle twitching, rapid heart beat, increased urination, and gastrointestinal complaints. Ten grams of caffeine may cause convulsions, respiratory failure, and death. An abrupt withdrawal causes irritability, headache, and restlessness for up to a week.

Amounts of Caffeine (milligrams)

Coffee			
	drip	cup	110-150
	percolated	cup	64-124
	instant	cup	40-108
	decaffeinated	cup	2-5
Tea			
	black	cup	12-50
	green	cup	15
	iced instant	cup	8-15
Soft drinks			
	Jolt	can	72
	Mr. Pibb	can	58
	Mountain Dew	can	54
	Coca-cola	can	46
	Pepsi	can	38
Chocolate drink		can	5
Dark chocolate		bar	20
Milk chocolate		bar	6
Cough and cold remedies		tablet	25-50
Stimulants (e.g., NoDoz)		tablet	100-350
Weight-loss pills		tablet	75-200

CALAMUS

Calamus, *Acorus calamus*, is a wild plant of North America also known as Sweet Flag. It was traditionally used as a hallucinogen by the Cree Indian tribe of northern Alberta, who chewed the root. The plant also grows in Europe and Asia, where it has been used medicinally for at least 2,000 years. In the Biblical Book of Exodus (30:23), it is supposedly the "sweet-smelling cane" used to make the holy anointing oil that the Lord commanded Moses to make and rub on his body when he approached the Tabernacle.

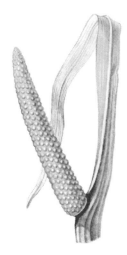

The root was well known to early American settlers and to Walt Whitman, who wrote 45 poems under the title Calamus in *Leaves of Grass*, describing the plant as "leaves of joy."

An iris-like perennial growing five to six feet tall, it is often found among cat-tails near streams and ponds. Calamus is a unique hallucinogen in having both sedating and stimulating properties. The root tastes much like ginger, and a length of about two inches will provide an invigorating and euphoric experience. If a ten-inch length is eaten, the effect is reputed to be like that of LSD.

The active ingredient of calamus is asarone, a chemical similar to mescaline and amphetamine. It is a natural precursor to TMA-2, which has about ten times the potency of mescaline.

CALIFORNIA POPPY

The California Poppy is not an opium poppy, but it has a number of chemicals that are similar to the opiate alkaloids, such as chelerythrine, sanguinarine, protopine, and homochelidonine. The leaves and orange petals can be dried and smoked to produce a mild, marijuana-like intoxication lasting about 30 minutes.

There are no laws against smoking the California Poppy. It is illegal, however, to pick it in California, where it is the official state flower.

CATNIP

Also called catmint, catnip (*Nepeta cataria*) is a strongly scented herb in the mint family, growing wild in Europe and Asia. It is best known for its stimulating effects on cats. The herb can be smoked or made into a tea to produce an effect like that of marijuana, and in high doses it is reputedly similar to LSD.

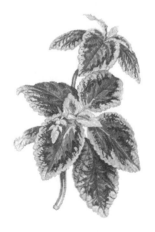

Coleus

COLEUS

Coleus plants, *Coleus blumei* and *Coleus pumila*, are available in gardening stores. They were used as hallucinogens by the Mazatec Indians of southern Mexico. Chewing and swallowing 50 to 75 leaves causes colorful visual hallucinations similar to the effects of psilocybin.

DAMIANA

Damiana, *Turnera diffusa*, is a shrub with sweet-smelling leaves available in gardening stores. Some health-food stores sell the berries. Smoking the dried leaves or berries will bring a mild, marijuana-like intoxication for about an hour.

DATURA

Better known in the United States as Jimson weed, *Datura stramonium*, is a very widespread plant growing wild throughout Asia, Europe, and North America. It has been used throughout history for its hallucinogenic properties, as evidenced by its many names: devil's apple, devil's weed, locoweed, and green dragon. There are references to it in Homer's *Odyssey* and in Shakespeare's *Romeo and*

Juliet and *Antony and Cleopatra*. Datura had ritual use in the religions of ancient China and India. In Tanganyika, Africa, it was added to beer for intoxication, and smoked to relieve asthma.

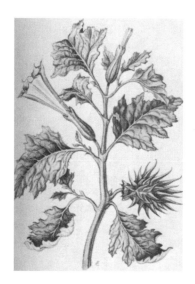

Datura is one of four plants (the others are Henbane, Belladonna, and Mandrake) that formed the basic kit of medieval witches. According to Carlos Castaneda, it was used by Native American witches, *brujos*, as well.

Datura has powerful properties related to atropine, causing dilated pupils, fever, dry mouth, and dramatic hallucinations. Tea made from any part of the plant was used to treat asthma, but excessive use could cause amnesia or permanent brain damage. The seeds are particularly toxic: half a teaspoon can cause death.[14]

The effects can last up to 36 hours, with noticeable effects lasting for several days.

DEXTROMETHORPHAN

This common cough medicine, often referred to as DXM or DM, is found in many popular brands such as Robitussin, Dimetane, and Comtrex. Normally, no more than 120 mg should be taken in a 24-hour period. When taken in larger amounts, 300 mg or more at a time, it may cause euphoria, visual and auditory disturbances, and a loss of coordination.

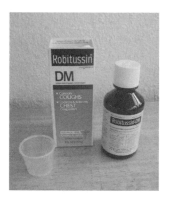

Dextromethorphan is becoming a popular drug of abuse among teenagers who are attracted by its low cost and easy availability. Some say that the effects of high doses, "Robo dosing," are similar to LSD or psilocybin mushrooms.

DOÑA ANA

This small cactus, *Coryphantha macromeris*, grows in southern Texas and northern Mexico. The name is often shortened to Doñana, and it has also been called the "false peyote." It contains macromerine, a phenethylamine hallucinogen similar to mescaline but only about one fifth as potent. A tea made from 8 to 12 fresh cacti will produce a similar experience to mescaline or peyote (see *Peyote and Mescaline*). The psychoactive effects are likely to be accompanied by nausea and vomiting.

EPHEDRA

The *Ephedra* plant has a horse-tail appearance. The plant has a wide global distribution, from Asia to North America, and preparations for medicine have been in use for thousands of years. Ma Huang, the Chinese *Ephedra*, is considered to be among the most potent of all varieties. The principal ingredient is ephedrine, which has all the effects of amphetamines. In large doses, it can be similar to MDMA. A synthetic variant, pseudoephedrine, is common in cough and cold remedies. The herb itself is increasingly popular in capsules and teas as a "natural" alternative to pharmaceutical medications.

Mormon tea, *Ephedra nevadensis*, grows in the western United States. It was used by Mormons as a stimulant tea because their religious beliefs prohibited the use of caffeine-containing drinks.

HAWAIIAN BABY WOOD ROSE

Hawaiian baby wood rose is not from Hawaii and is not a rose. It came by the name because of its appearance and because it grows well in Hawaii, where it was used as a hallucinogen by the Polynesian people.

The flower, *Argyreia nervosa*, is similar to morning glory. It is a woody, climbing vine with silvery foliage and violet flowers. Native to India, it is now cultivated throughout the tropical world. Its large seeds contain lysergic acid amides. Like morning glory, swallowing four to eight seeds will produce a hallucinatory experience.

HENBANE

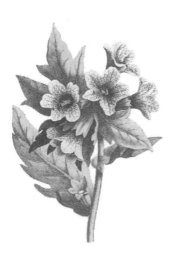

Henbane, *Hyoscyamous niger*, is very similar to *Datura*, with an equally long history of use. The ancient Egyptians described henbane in the Ebers Papyrus of 1500 BC, and it is mentioned in reports of "magic drinks" of ancient Greece and Rome. The prophetic utterances of the Oracle of Delphi were made while intoxicated with the smoke from henbane seeds. In ancient Britain, henbane paste was smeared on the tips of Celtic arrows.[15] Up to present times, the Bedouins smoked the dried leaves for their psychoactive effects.

Also known as Sorcerer's Cherry, Witch's Berry, Devil's Herb, Murderer's Berry, and Dwaleberry (dwale in English deriving from the Scandinavian root meaning "trance"), henbane was a favorite in the potions of medieval witches, who believed it could cause permanent insanity.

Henbane is a hairy, sticky plant with an offensive smell, growing along roadsides and other wastelands. In summer, it produces pale-yellow flowers veined with purple. The active principles are hyoscyamine, atropine and scopolamine. Smoking or eating it can cause dizziness, confusion, nausea, diarrhea, a pounding headache, abrupt loss of consciousness, and amnesia, as well as visual hallucinations and an overall feeling of sedation and intoxication.

HOPS

Hops, *Humulus lupulus*, contain lupuline, which is similar to the THC of marijuana. Hops are cultivated and used as a flavoring and sedating ingredient in alcoholic beverages. The plant also has a long history of use as a medicinal herb, and dried hops were stuffed into pillowcases to alleviate insomnia.[16]

Hops contain lupulin, humulene, and lupulinic acid, which can produce a marijuana-like intoxication. Indeed, many people have smoked hops as an alternative to marijuana. For this reason, hop cuttings are now difficult to obtain and the Government has asked growers not to sell them to the general public.[17]

HYDRANGEA

Hydrangea, *Hydrangea paniculata grandiflora*, is a popular shrub in American gardens. Its leaves can be smoked for a marijuana-like intoxication, but also contain cyanide.

INHALANTS

Inhalants include solvents and cleaning fluids (such as toluene, benzene, methanol, and chloroform), coolants (e.g., Freon), sprays (e.g., canned spray paint), fuels (especially gasoline), gases (butane and propane), and a variety of glues. All of these are rapidly absorbed by inhalation and dissolve in the fatty tissue of the brain, producing intoxication.

Solvent sniffing was recognized as a problem in the 1950s. As more products were developed, sniffing became increasingly common. Surveys show that inhalants are used by 8 percent of middle school students and 15 percent of high school seniors.

"Huffing" is the practice of hyperventilating from a plastic bag with solvent poured into it, or breathing from a cloth or mitt soaked in solvents. The effect is rapid and intense. Solvents are absorbed into the bloodstream and reach the brain within seconds, producing dizziness, disorientation, and light-headedness. As blood levels increase, there may be hallucinations, delusions, muscular incoordination, ringing in the ears, double vision, abdominal pain, flushing of the skin, and vomiting. If inhalation is not stopped, it can result in a loss of reflexes, heart problems, the suppression of breathing, and death.

The most dangerous effect is "sudden sniffing death" due to irregular heart beat, which has occurred with the abuse of coolants, propellants, and fuel gases such as butane and propane. A fatal injury can occur at any time. A British study of 1,000 deaths from inhalant use reported that one-fifth of the fatalities were of first-time users.

Chronic use causes permanent brain damage. A neurological study showed that 65 percent of solvent users had central nervous system damage. Toluene, a common industrial chemical, is especially toxic. About half of toluene users develop damage to the cerebellum, a part of the brain that controls coordination and delicate muscle movements. A final cause of death is suicide, accounting for 28 percent of solvent-related fatalities.

Many gases and solvents are also highly flammable and serious burns have occurred. In one study, 26 percent of deaths from inhalant use were due to such accidents.[18]

KAVA KAVA

Kava kava (also called *waka*) is the name of a drink made from the root pulp and stems of a tall shrub with an odor of lilac, *Piper methysticum*, that grows in the tropical islands of the Pacific Ocean. Missionaries to the islands noted that

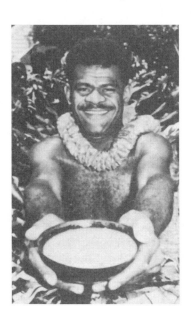

the natives revered this plant and cultivated it religiously. They soon found out why. Kava kava is a remarkable drug that causes talkativeness and euphoria, inducing a peculiar lethargic state of complete alertness and relaxation. The drink was consumed at ritual meetings to discuss family problems, social disagreements, and disputes of any kind, which could then be effectively resolved in an atmosphere of peace and conciliation.

Kava kava is prepared by soaking the crushed roots in water for several hours and straining the pulp. Varieties known as black kava and red kava are reputed to be the most potent. The effects of kava kava are due to kawain, dihydrokawain, methysticin, dihydromethysticin, yangonin, and dihydroyangonin. These compounds are now being studied for medical uses. Excessive use can cause a mild addiction, the loss of appetite and weight, diarrhea, weakened vision, and yellowish skin with rashes and ulcers.

The early missionaries forbid the use of kava kava, hoping to convince islanders to choose a more puritanical lifestyle. Unfortunately, the drug was replaced by alcohol, with far more deleterious consequences. Kava kava is now gradually making a comeback in the Pacific Islands. It is also becoming a popular mainstream herbal preparation, sold in most health food stores and supermarkets.

KETAMINE

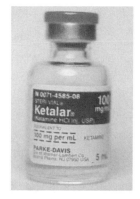

Ketamine was discovered by an American pharmacist, Calvin Stevens, in 1961, as an analog of PCP. It was found to have the same anesthetic qualities of PCP, but less pronounced psychoactive effects.

In 1966, ketamine was marketed by Parke-Davis as a dissociative anesthetic for medical use under the brand name Ketalar, and for veterinary use as Ketajet, Ketaset, and Vetelar. This type of anesthetic is useful because it allows major surgery without paralyzing the muscles for breathing. It achieved recognition in battlefield wound care during the Vietnam War. The medical use of ketamine is limited by a problematic side effect, with patients complaining of bizarre thoughts and hallucinations. This quality, however, has made it popular for recreational use. Like PCP, individuals feel detached or disconnected from their pain and environment, and may have illusions of power and invincibility.

Ketamine powder may be snorted or the liquid form added to drinks. The intoxicating experience lasts 30 to 60 minutes. It is milder than PCP and more is needed for an effect: about 100 milligrams of ketamine are equal to about 25 milligrams of PCP.

The primary use of ketamine is now in veterinary medicine, although it continues to be a useful adjunct in human surgery (and in executions using lethal injection). The green, crystalline substance is usually stolen from medical supplies and sold as Cat Valium, Green, Jet, K, Ket, Kit-Kat, Psychedelic Heroin, Purple, Special K, Super Acid, or Vitamin K. A snorted hit of ketamine is called a "bump," and a person who uses it a lot is a K-Head or Ketter.[19] The trance-like effect is sometimes called the K-Hole or K-Land.

Growing abuse led the DEA to regulate it under Schedule III of the Controlled Substances list in August 1999. Ketamine is now a popular recreational drug around the world. It can be bought on the Internet and is available over the counter in a number of countries, including Mexico and Thailand. Ketamine is especially popular in Russia, where it has become the drug of choice for Moscow teenagers. In New York, a gram of the readily available drug sells for $80 on the street.

LOBELIA

Lobelia, with its red, white, yellow, or blue flowers, grows wild in North America. Native Americans sometimes smoked it for a feeling of mental clarity, euphoria, and marijuana-like intoxication.

The entire plant contains the piperidine alkaloid lobeline, a compound that has found use in treating asthma and bronchitis, and for nicotine withdrawal.

Lobelia smoke is very harsh and acrid; a tea preparation is more tolerable, but causes nausea and vomiting as well as an unpleasant prickly sensation in the mouth.[20]

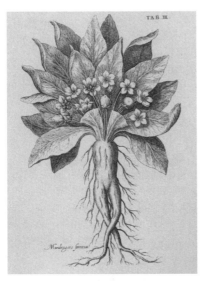

The roots of mandrake were likened to the form of a man or woman, as seen in this early 18th-century engraving

MANDRAKE

Mandrake, *Mandragora officinarum*, grows wild in the stony fields of southern Europe. It causes dizziness, pounding headache, nausea, diarrhea, cramps, confusion, and intense hallucinations. The last quality made it a popular ingredient in potions of medieval witches. Mandrake contains mandragorine as well as atropine, scopolamine, and hyoscyamine.

MORNING GLORY

Seeds of morning glory flowers, *Rivea corymbosa*, were used as hallucinogens in religious rites by the Aztec civilization of ancient Mexico. More recent use has been reported in sacraments by the Zapotecs of the Oaxaca region of Mexico.

Morning glory seeds contain lysergic acid amide. During the 1960s, the seeds were taken as a substitute for LSD. Ingesting the powder of 20 to 50 ground seeds produces restlessness and increased awareness. Taking 100 to 150 seeds causes visual distortions and hallucinations, and 200 to 500 seeds results in intense hallucinations, nausea, vomiting, and abdominal pain.

Since the 1960s, commercial morning glory seed producers have treated their products with a poisonous coating to discourage use as a recreational drug. There are several methods for removing the toxin. While seeds for horticultural purposes are legal, the possession of ground-up seeds, or equipment to extract lysergic acid from the seeds, can be taken as evidence of illegal intent and is therefore a crime.

NITROUS OXIDE

Nitrous oxide was discovered in 1776 by Joseph Priestly, who also discovered oxygen. Priestly apparently never breathed nitrous oxide, but in the same year of its discovery, Sir Humphrey Davy synthesized it and found that a "deep whiff resulted in a riotous state of excitement and glee."[21] For the next 50 years, nitrous oxide became a popular amusement as "laughing gas." In the 1830s, "gas frolics" were a common type of entertainment, and were enjoyed by everyone from country folk to respectable figures such as the philosopher William James.

Nitrous oxide became the first medical anesthetic in the 1840s. It continues to be used in dental anesthesia, for pressurization of whipped cream and other foods, and for recreational purposes.

 "There are no differences but differences of degree between different degrees of difference and no difference."
—*William James, under nitrous oxide, 1882* [22]

Industrial grade nitrous oxide is mixed with hydrogen sulfide; inhaling it will make the user very ill. Medical grade is pure and is usually combined with 20% oxygen. Nitrous oxide is also available as a propellant or frothing agent for whipped cream. Small metal cylinders called whippets are used to charge reusable whipping cream dispensers. The cylinders are sold in some stores for about $1.00 each, and are the most popular method of obtaining nitrous oxide for recreational use.

Long-term use of nitrous oxide can damage bone marrow and the nervous system, deplete the body of vitamin B12, and can cause impaired memory and mental functioning. A further hazard of non-medical nitrous oxide is that it is not mixed with oxygen, and therefore may result in a fatal suffocation.

NUTMEG

Nutmeg is the seed of a tree, *Myristica fragrans*, native to the Moluccas, the spice islands of Indonesia. (The covering of the nutmeg seed produces another spice, mace.) The "narcotic fruit" was introduced to Europe by the Portuguese in 1512, and used for centuries as a snuff. It is now cultivated in Granada and imported to the United States, where it is mainly used to spice Christmas drinks and pastries.

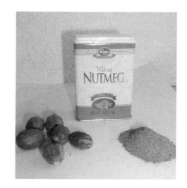

Nutmeg has a small amount of toxin similar to MDMA. Ingestion of two to five whole nutmegs, or a few tablespoons of ground nutmeg, can produce intense nausea and vomiting, facial flushing, dry mouth, and visual hallucinations. Twenty grams of ground nutmeg, about the amount filling a matchbox, contains 210 milligrams of myristicin (similar to MMDA), 70 milligrams elemicin (similar to TMA), and 39 milligrams safrole (similar to MDA). Eating this much nutmeg can produce very severe physical and psychological effects, varying with the person. Most people find it difficult to swallow such a large dose, but those who persist tend to become nauseated during the first 45 minutes. After that, silly feelings and giggling often occur. This is soon followed by dryness of the mouth and throat, flushing of the skin and reddening eyes. Occasionally, a user will feel agitated and hyperactive, but more often he will feel heavy, intoxicated and unable to do anything but lie down. Motor functions may be confused and speech incoherent. Later, the person may enter a euphoric state with a sense of profound peace of mind and dreamy visions.

Sleepless stupor is the most apt description of nutmeg narcosis. This condition may last for 12 hours followed by 24 hours of drowsiness. After-effects are usually quite unpleasant: aching bones, sore muscles, painful eyes, runny nose, tiredness, depression, and headaches.

SALVIA DIVINORUM

One of the newest psychoactive plant discoveries, *Salvia divinorum* ("sage of the diviners"), is a wild member of the mint family. It has large leaves, a hollow,

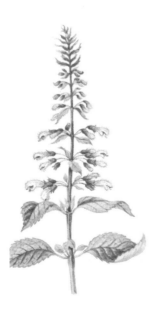

square stem, and light blue flowers reaching a height of about three feet. It has long been used by Mazatec Indians of the Oaxaca region of Mexico, who know it as *Hierba de la Pastora* ("herb of the shepherdess") or *Hierba de la Virgen* ("herb of the virgin"). They crush the leaves on a metate, mix with water, and chew or drink the solution.

Salvia has recently generated much interest as a legal psychoactive substance with effects similar to psilocybin mushrooms, PCP, and ketamine.[23] The active principle appears to be due to several unusual chemical constituents, called salvinorin A[24] and divinorin C.[25] The plant seeds, dried leaves, and purified salvinorin A are all sold over the Internet. An ounce of the dried leaves, enough for about 4 to 12 doses, is sold for $40 to $60.

Like marijuana, people who chew or smoke Salvia leaves (or take the purified extract), may be relatively insensitive to the effects until they have taken it a number of times. About

10 percent of users claim they are quite unaffected by the drug. Others report effects ranging from mild hallucinations to a complete dissociative state, like that of ketamine or PCP,[26] followed by amnesia.[27]

Salvia does not appear to cause noticeable physical harm, withdrawal symptoms, or addiction. However, animal studies have shown that very high doses may cause a type of brain damage (Olmey's lesions), and exacerbate psychiatric illnesses.

SAN PEDRO

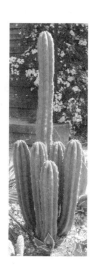

San Pedro, *Tricherocerus pachanoi* (also known as *Echinopsis pachanoi*), is a tall cactus named after St. Peter, the Catholic guardian of the gates of Heaven.[28] It is indigenous to Peru and Ecuador, where it has been used for perhaps 3,000 years. Today, *curanderos* of northern Peru continue to use it in a drink called *cimora*. The cactus, which reaches a height of 10 to 15 feet, is also reported to grow in the southwest United States and is sold in garden stores.

San Pedro contains mescaline, in a lesser concentration than peyote (see *Peyote and Mescaline*). To achieve the same effect, a section of about 6 to 12 inches of the ribbed cactus must be consumed. Since the mescaline is concentrated in the green skin, users eat around the woody core like corn on the cob, or boil the skins for several hours to make a tea.

TOBACCO

Tobacco, *Nicotiana tabacum*, is the most injurious drug in the world today, causing one out of every five premature deaths. In the United States alone, there are about 430,000 deaths every year due to tobacco smoking, and another 50,000 deaths from secondhand smoke. Tobacco smoking causes dozens of different diseases, from heart disease to aging skin. Ninety percent of lung cancers are due to smoking, and fathers who smoke have a 42 percent increased likelihood of having a child with cancer.

 "The use of tobacco is growing greater and conquers men with a certain secret pleasure, so that those who have once become accustomed thereto can later hardly be restrained therefrom."
—*Sir Francis Bacon, 1610*

Now cultivated in many countries, tobacco began as a wild plant in the Americas. Native Americans had used it medicinally and ritually and continue to consider it a sacred plant. Christopher Columbus brought news of tobacco to Europeans who turned the sacred ritual into a casual pastime. Tobacco seeds

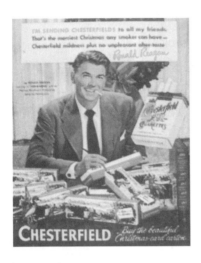

were brought from Brazil to France, leading to cultivation in Europe. At that time, tobacco was called nicotiana, after Jean Nicot, who had described its medicinal properties. In 1828, French chemists isolated the active ingredient in tobacco, which they called nicotine.

Wild tobacco varies in nicotine content, up to 5 percent, as opposed to the 0.5 percent to 2 percent nicotine content of most commercial cigarettes today.

Although tobacco had been smoked in the Americas, Europeans preferred to chew tobacco until the early 1900s, when smoking gradually became more popular. Cigars, which were both smoked and chewed, began the trend. Many historians credit the rapid popularity of cigarettes to soldiers in the First World War, who could not be troubled by a pipe. The easy availability of cigarettes spurred a rapid increase in the use of tobacco throughout the industrial world.

In the United States, tobacco smoking peaked in the 1960s, when an estimated 40 percent of adults were smokers. Since then, advertising restrictions and aggressive educational programs have brought a decline in tobacco use, which has now leveled off at about 25 percent of adults. It is estimated that each day in the U.S. another 3,000 people under the age of 18 will begin smoking.

Studies show that if teenagers smoke more than a single cigarette, they have an 85% chance of becoming addicted.

Tobacco smoke contains about 4,000 different chemicals. Four hundred of these are toxins and 43 are known carcinogens. The most prominent is nicotine, a remarkably potent drug. A dose of 60 milligrams of nicotine taken by mouth would be fatal. Smoked nicotine is somewhat less toxic, but will still cause nausea and lightheadedness until tolerance is developed. An average cigarette has about one milligram of nicotine.

Smoking delivers nicotine to the brain within five to eight seconds, while chewing tobacco takes about five to ten minutes. Nicotine releases the neurotransmitter dopamine, and is therefore addictive. In fact, nicotine is considered to be the most addictive substance ever discovered, far more so than heroin, crack, or other illegal drugs. Nine out of ten smokers say they wish they could quit, and yet they continue to smoke. Even Sigmund Freud, the father of modern psychology, was so addicted to tobacco that he continued to smoke after much of his jaw had been cut away because of mouth cancer.

Other constituents in cigarettes besides tobacco present health risks. Modern cigarettes have about 700 added ingredients, including 13 chemicals considered too toxic to be used in food, 5 of which are classified as hazardous, including the chlorofluorocarbon freon, ethyl 2-furoate, ammonia, and pesticides, all of which can cause damage to the lungs, liver, and nervous system.

TRIHEXYLPHENIDYL

Trihexylphenidyl (Artane) was a prescription drug in the United States, used for Parkinson's Disease until it was replaced by better medications. In larger doses, it causes hallucinations.

Trihexylphenidyl is an uncommon recreational drug. It is found mostly in prisons where the tablets are crushed and mixed with tobacco for a legal, mind-altering smoke.

VIROLA

Related to nutmeg, the *Virola* genus includes about sixty species of vines native to the Amazon region of South America. A dozen of these species have hallucinogenic properties and are traditionally used in Native rituals. The red bark resin is eaten or made into a snuff, *Epená*.

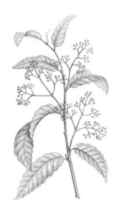

The active principles of virola are a number of DMT analogs, and cause intoxication similar to that of DMT.

Food for Thought

In order to understand the distribution and use of illegal drugs, it is important to know why people use them, what part drugs play in their culture, and what the social consequences are if the drug is removed. Without this understanding, drug laws become a tool for discriminating against social groups instead of a mechanism to improve public health.

Drugs are a part of culture, as closely identified with an ethnic group as their food. In fact, drugs sometimes *are* foods. To the French and Italians (and others) wine is a food, as it was throughout the Mediterranean in Biblical times. To Germans and Australians, beer is a food. To the traditional British, tea is a food (indeed, the afternoon meal is called tea), and to many Americans, coffee is a food (it may constitute their entire breakfast). Khat is a food to Somalis, while coca is a food to the native people of the Andes.

Different ethnic groups have always lived uneasily among neighbors who did not share their prohibitions. Some Islamic people refuse to enter a home in which pork is present, while some Hindus have a similar attitude to beef. Many religious people are offended by alcohol.

An ethnic population can be hurt and discriminated against by attacking its drugs. The opium laws were a thinly disguised attempt to hurt American Chinese immigrants. Cocaine was outlawed only when it became popular among African Americans. In the 1920s, the American prohibition of alcohol was finally successful only with the aid of the anti-German sentiment that swept the U.S. during the First World War. Marijuana, a popular medicinal drug, was made illegal as a racist campaign against Mexican Americans. And the prohibition of peyote was a deliberate policy to hurt Native Americans, even though there was never any evidence that peyote had harmful properties.

Cultures and countries differ in their attitudes and laws about drugs. And over time, in the same country, attitudes and laws can change. Drugs that are legal today (for example, ketamine) may be illegal tomorrow, and currently illegal drugs (marijuana, ibogaine, peyote) may have accepted use in the future.

Cultures and laws can change. The drug itself does not change. In itself, no drug is harmful, no more than the ocean is harmful. It is the lack of respect for the drug that makes it dangerous. A drug used properly may have tremendous benefit. The same drug, if abused, can lead to irreparable harm. One can as easily drown in drug use as one can drown in the ocean. Neither of them, however, is likely to disappear.

PART II

Illegal Drugs
From A to Z

Altering a drug will not make it legal

For each of these drugs, the law also includes "their isomers, esters, ethers, salts, and salts of isomers, esters and ethers, whenever the existence of such isomers, esters, ethers and salts is possible within the specific chemical designation."

Alphabetical List of Drugs Illegal in the United States

Following is a list of all drugs that are illegal in the United States. Only the common names are given here. For alternative chemical names, see the formal listing given in the Controlled Substances Act in *Chapter 3*. For more information on any of these substances, see the *Index* at the end of this book.

The definition of *illegal* used in this book is any drug that is listed on Schedule I or Schedule II of the Controlled Substances Act. The history, current use, chemistry, and effects of each of these drugs are explained in the following chapters. Since many of the drugs are similar, they are grouped together. For example, all drugs related to opium are described in *Opiates*.

For drug ...	See Chapter
Acetorphine	*Opiates*
Acetyl-alpha-methylfentanyl	*Opiates*
Acetyldihydrocodeine	*Opiates*
Acetylmethadol	*Opiates*
AET (Alpha-ethyltryptamine)	*DMT*
Alfentanyl	*Opiates*
Allylprodine	*Opiates*
Alpha-aminopropriophenone	*Cathinone*
Alphacetylmethadol	*Opiates*
Alphameprodine	*Opiates*
Alphamethadol	*Opiates*
Alpha-methylfentanyl	*Opiates*
Alpha-methylthiofentanyl	*Opiates*
Alphaprodine	*Opiates*
Aminohexaphen	*Amphetamines*
Aminorex	*Amphetamines*
Amobarbital	*Barbiturates*
Amphetamine	*Amphetamines*
Anileridine	*Opiates*
Benzethidine	*Opiates*
Benzylfentanyl	*Opiates*
Benzylmorphine	*Opiates*
Betacetylmethadol	*Opiates*
Beta-hydroxyfentanyl	*Opiates*
Beta-hydroxy-3-methylfentanyl	*Opiates*
Betameprodine	*Opiates*
Betamethadol	*Opiates*
Betaprodine	*Opiates*

Bezitramide	*Opiates*
Bufotenine	*DMT*
Carfentanil	*Opiates*
Cathinone	*Cathinone*
Clonitazene	*Opiates*
Coca leaves (unless decocainized)	*Cocaine*
Cocaine	*Cocaine*
Codeine	*Opiates*
Codeine methylbromide	*Opiates*
Codeine-N-Oxide	*Opiates*
Cyclohexamine	*PCP*
Cyprenorphine	*Opiates*
Desomorphine	*Opiates*
DET (Diethyltryptamine)	*DMT*
Dextromoramide	*Opiates*
Dextropropoxyphene	*Opiates*
Diampromide	*Opiates*
Diethylthiambutene	*Opiates*
Difenoxin	*Opiates*
Dihydrocodeine	*Opiates*
Dihydromorphine	*Opiates*
Dimenoxadol	*Opiates*
Dimepheptanol	*Opiates*
Dimethylthiambutene	*Opiates*
Dioxaphetyl butyrate	*Opiates*
Diphenoxylate	*Opiates*
Dipipanone	*Opiates*
DMA (2,5-dimethoxyamphetamine)	*MDMA*
DMT (dimethyltryptamine)	*DMT*
DOET (2,5-dimethoxy-4-ethylamphetamine)	*MDMA*
DOM (4-methyl-2,5-dimethoxy-amphetamine)	*MDMA*
Dronabinol	*Marijuana*
Drotebanol	*Opiates*
Ecgonine	*Cocaine*
Ethylmethylthiambutene	*Opiates*
Ethylmorphine	*Opiates*
Etonitazene	*Opiates*
Etorphine hydrochloride	*Opiates*
Etoxeridine	*Opiates*
Fenethylline	*Amphetamines*
Fentanyl	*Opiates*
Furethidine	*Opiates*
GHB (gamma-hydroxybutyrate)	*GHB*
Glutethimide	*Methaqualone and Glutethimide*
Heroin	*Opiates*
Hydrocodone	*Opiates*
Hydromorphinol	*Opiates*
Hydromorphone	*Opiates*

Hydroxypethidine	*Opiates*
Ibogaine	*Ibogaine*
Isomethadone	*Opiates*
Ketobemidone	*Opiates*
LAAM (levo-alphacetylmethadol)	*Opiates*
Levomethorphan	*Opiates*
Levomoramide	*Opiates*
Levophenacylmorphan	*Opiates*
Levorphanol	*Opiates*
LSD (lysergic acid diethylamide)	*LSD*
Mappine	*DMT*
Marihuana	*Marijuana*
MDA (N-hydroxy-3,4-methylenedioxyamphetamine)	*MDMA*
MDE (3,4-methylenedioxy-N-ethylamphetamine)	*MDMA*
MDMA (3,4-methylenedioxymethamphetamine)	*MDMA*
Mecloqualone	*Methaqualone and Glutethimide*
Mescaline	*Peyote and Mescaline*
Meperidine	*Opiates*
Metazocine	*Opiates*
Methadone	*Opiates*
Methadone-intermediate	*Opiates*
Methamphetamine	*Amphetamines*
Methaqualone	*Methaqualone and Glutethimide*
Methcathinone	*Cathinone*
Methylaminorex	*Amphetamines*
Methyldesorphine	*Opiates*
Methyldihydromorphine	*Opiates*
Methylenedioxymethamphetamine	*MDMA*
3-Methylfentanyl	*Opiates*
Methylphenidate	*Amphetamines*
3-Methylthiofentanyl	*Opiates*
Metopon	*Opiates*
Monase	*DMT*
Moramide-intermediate	*Opiates*
Morpheridine	*Opiates*
Morphine	*Opiates*
Morphine methylbromide	*Opiates*
Morphine methylsulfonate	*Opiates*
Morphine-N-Oxide	*Opiates*
MPPP (1-methyl-4-phenyl-4-propionoxypiperidine)	*Opiates*
Myrophine	*Opiates*
Nabilone	*Marijuana*
N-ethyl-3-piperidyl benzilate	*Cocaine*
N-ethylamphetamine	*MDMA*
N-methyl-3-piperidyl benzilate	*Cocaine*
Nexus (2C-B; 4-bromo-2,5-dimethoxyphenethylamine)	*MDMA*
Nicocodeine	*Opiates*
Nicomorphine	*Opiates*

Noracymethadol	Opiates
Norephedrone	Cathinone
Norlevophanol	Opiates
Normethadone	Opiates
Normophine	Opiates
Norpipanone	Opiates
N,N-dimethylamphetamine	Amphetamines
Opium (raw, extracts, fluid, powdered, granulated, tincture)	Opiates
Opium poppy and poppy straw	Opiates
Oxycodone	Opiates
Oxymorphone	Opiates
P2P (phenylacetone; phenyl-2-propanone)	Amphetamines
Para-fluorofentanyl	Opiates
Parahexyl	MDMA
PCC (1-piperidinocyclohexanecarbonitrile)	PCP
PCE (ethylamine analog of phencyclidine)	PCP
PCP (phencyclidine)	PCP
PCPy (PHP; pyrrolidine analog of phencyclidine)	PCP
Pentobarbital	Barbiturates
PEPAP (1-[-2-phenethyl]-4-phenyl-4-acetoxypiperidine)	Opiates
Pethidine (meperidine)	Opiates
Pethidine-intermediate-A (4-cyano-1-methyl-4-phenylpiperidine)	Opiates
Pethidine-intermediate-B	Opiates
Pethidine-intermediate-C	Opiates
Peyote	Peyote and Mescaline
Phenadoxone	Opiates
Phenampromide	Opiates
Phenazocine	Opiates
Phenmetrazine	Amphetamines
Phenomorphan	Opiates
Phenoperidine	Opiates
Phenylcyclohexylamine	PCP
Pholcodine	Opiates
Piminodine	Opiates
Piritramide	Opiates
PMA (4-methoxyamphetamine)	MDMA
Proheptazine	Opiates
Properidine	Opiates
Propiram	Opiates
Psilocybin	DMT
Psilocyn	DMT
Racemethorphan	Opiates
Racemoramide	Opiates
Racemorphan	Opiates
Remifentanil	Opiates
Secobarbital	Barbiturates
Sufentanil	Opiates
Synhexyl	MDMA

Tabernanthe iboga	*Ibogaine*
TCP (TPCP; thiophene analog of phencyclidine)	*PCP*
TCPy (1-[1-(2-thienyl)cyclohexyl]pyrrolidine)	*PCP*
Tetrahydrocannabinols	*Marijuana*
Thebacon	*Opiates*
Thebaine	*Opiates*
Thenylfentanyl	*Opiates*
Thiofentanyl	*Opiates*
Tilidine	*Opiates*
TMA (3,4,5-trimethoxy amphetamine)	*MDMA*
Trimeperidine	*Opiates*

Amphetamines

In the "fight or flight" response to stress, the adrenal glands produce the hormone adrenaline, making a person feel stimulated, alert, active, and strong—socially engaged and ready to tackle any danger.

Amphetamines are chemically similar to adrenaline, and were invented to achieve the same effects. They are used for alertness, excitation, euphoria, and to suppress appetite.

The Basic Facts

Type of drug	*Stimulant*
How taken	*Injected, smoked, snorted, ingested*
Duration of effect	*2 to 8 hours, depending on type*
Physical danger	*High*
Addiction potential	*High*

Other Names

Amphetamine	*Adderall, amies, amp, bennies, benz, Benzedrine, Biphetamine, black and white, black beauties, black birds, black bombers, black mollies, blacks, blue boy, brain ticklers, brownies, bumblebees, cartwheels, chicken powder, crosstops, Obetrol, pep pills, speed, white*
Dextroamphetamine	*beans, Christmas trees, Dexamyl, Dexedrine, Dextrostat, dexies, Eskatrol*
Dextromethamphetamine	*base, batu (Hawaii, Philippines), bingdu (China), glass, ice, shabu (Japan), yaba (Thailand), yellow rock*
Fenethylline	*Captagon*
Fenfluramine	*Fen-Phen (with phentermine), Pondimin, Redux*
Methamphetamine	*crank, crystal, Desoxyn, Fefamine, meth, Methedrine*
Methamphetamine & crack cocaine	*ice (Florida)*
Methylaminorex	*ice, U4Euh*
Methylphenidate	*Concerta, Metadate, Methylin, pellets, Ritalin*
Methylphenidate & pentazocine	*Ts and Blues (Kansas City)*
Pemoline	*Cylert*
Phendimetrazine	*pink hearts, Preludin*
Phentermine	*Fen-Phen (with fenfluramine), Ionamin*

Speed: The Story of Amphetamines

"You become, after that first hit of speed,
gloriously, brilliantly, vigorously awake."[1]

FROM EPHEDRA TO AMPHETAMINE

The leafless *Ephedra* bush grows throughout the desert regions of Asia and North America. It has a horse-tail appearance, with stems that can be dried and boiled in water to make a stimulating tea. *Ephedra* has been used for thousands of years in China in medicines such as Ma Huang to help treat asthma and other breathing problems. At the same time, other species of *Ephedra* were used by the native Indians of the western United States. When Mormons traveled to Utah in 1847, they discovered the stimulating properties of this beverage and substituted this "Mormon tea" for coffee and tea, which they were not allowed to drink.

In 1892, a team of Japanese and Chinese scientists isolated ephedrine from *Ephedra*, and it was developed for production in the 1920s by the Eli Lilly Company. The new drug soon became the standard treatment for asthma.

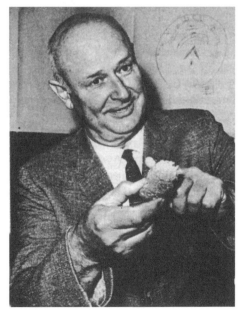

Interest in ephedrine was also kindled by researchers studying adrenaline, the body's natural stimulant. Ephedrine is chemically similar to adrenaline (see *Chapter 6: The Amphetamine Family*), but while adrenaline is an unstable chemical and must be injected — limiting its potential as a medication—ephedrine is very stable and can be taken by mouth.

Research on adrenaline and ephedrine produced a new synthetic drug, amphetamine. It was first discovered in Germany in 1887, but received little attention until 1927, when the UCLA researcher Gordon Alles investigated its therapeutic potential. The good scientist was not averse to using his product. He went on to research, and frequently sample, later amphetamines and variations such as MDA.

"Within a few minutes, I realized that a notable subjective response was going to result."
—Gordon Alles, discoverer of amphetamines, and personal user

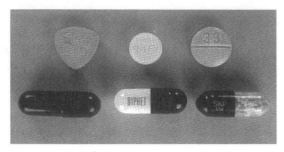
Prescription amphetamines

Amphetamine was first marketed in 1932 as an over-the-counter nasal inhaler, Benzedrine, to treat asthma and to raise low blood pressure. By 1937, amphetamine preparations were also available in tablet form to treat the sleeping disorder narcolepsy, as well as the behavioral syndrome then called minimal brain dysfunction (MBD) and now known as attention deficit hyperactivity disorder (ADHD). People quickly discovered that amphetamines increased energy and took away fatigue, hunger, and the need for sleep. Abuse of the popular new drugs started almost immediately and continued until the FDA banned over-the-counter sales in 1959.

Amphetamine is a combination of two molecular forms that are mirror images of each other. The "left-handed" molecule, *l*-amphetamine (also called levoamphetamine) has effects on the nasal passages but does not enter the brain. The right-handed form, *d*-amphetamine (dextroamphetamine), has very strong effects on the brain. In the 1930s, pure dextroamphetamine was synthesized for medical use as an improved, more stimulating form, of amphetamine. It was followed by the even stronger methylated version, methamphetamine.

The potency of these newer amphetamines became widely appreciated during the Second World War. Pills were handed out along with food and cigarette rations as stimulants to improve endurance and perhaps aggression. Soldiers in the Allied, German, and Japanese forces took amphetamines in enormous amounts. By the end of the war, Japan reported 200,000 cases of amphetamine psychosis among its servicemen.

 The Luftwaffe used amphetamines—"blitz"—to make their pilots as high as their new airplanes could fly.[2]

 Not to be outdone, Americans started packing it into ration kits. Second World War total use amounted to one pill per soldier per day.[3]

It was not only the soldiers who relied on the stimulants, but also their leaders. Churchill used both amphetamines and barbiturates to get himself through the long nights, and Hitler eventually was injecting himself with methamphetamine eight times a day.

After the war, amphetamines were given to factory workers with the intention of making them more productive. The Soviet Union in particular

encouraged their use.[4] But in the long run, as
many countries found, this was ineffective.
Production by workers on amphetamines was
shoddy and uneven as they swung on a hormonal
pendulum from over-stimulation to exhaustion.

Amphetamine use in the military remained
popular. Always looking for a new kick, American
servicemen stationed in Korea and Japan in the
early 1950s invented the "speedball," an injectable
mixture of amphetamines ("splash") and heroin.[5] In
the later stages of the Vietnam War, soldiers
consumed 200 million doses of amphetamines and
more servicemen were evacuated for drug problems
than for battlefield wounds.

On the home front, dozens of amphetamine
preparations were marketed to housewives as diet
pills and for depression. Speed became the drug of
the 1960s. Amphetamines helped truckers to drive
their long hauls without falling asleep, athletes to
push harder and train longer, students to study later,
and many to lose weight and feel more alive.

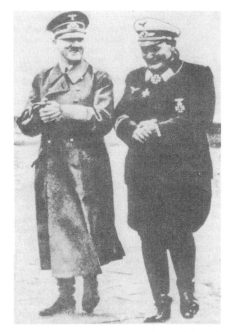

*Both Hitler and Goering were addicted
to methamphetamine*

American annual legal production in 1962 was estimated to be 8 billion
tablets.[6] This eventually peaked in 1971 with 12 billion tablets, much of it diverted
for recreational use.

 Each year in the 1950s, the United States alone produced 50 doses of
amphetamines for every man, woman, and child, and amphetamines
accounted for 20% of all prescriptions.

Most of this production was pushed by the medical industry. As the
use of prescription amphetamines grew, so did their abuse. The speed
epidemic began in California and quickly spread throughout the country.
When the pills were no longer enough, "speed freaks" began to inject powder
("crystal") methamphetamine.

Federal food and drug laws were amended in 1965 to remove many
amphetamine products from the market and to make it more difficult for
doctors to prescribe those that remained. As a result, clandestine laboratories
sprang up to meet the demand, from shady pharmaceutical operations to crude
kitchen-chemistry setups run by motorcycle gangs. On the West Coast, in
particular, methamphetamine laboratories proliferated.

"Crank" came from the Hells Angels' habit of hiding their amphetamines in the crank cases of their Harleys.

Currently, both dextroamphetamine and dextromethamphetamine are Schedule II controlled substances, indicating that they have recognized medical use but also a very high abuse potential. A variant of methamphetamine, *l-*methamphetamine, does not have psychoactive effects, and is the active ingredient in Vicks Inhaler, an over-the-counter nasal decongestant. To avoid confusion, the manufacturer identifies it by the alternative name desoxyephedrine.[7] Other amphetamines are still prescribed to treat narcolepsy, attention deficit disorder, depression, and for the short-term management of obesity.

ICE

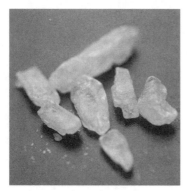

Ice is to methamphetamine as crack is to cocaine[9]

A new form of methamphetamine, a base version of dextromethamphetamine, was made in Asia in 1985. This form gives off vapors when heated, which can produce a rapid and intense intoxication lasting up to 14 hours. It has the appearance of shattered ice or broken glass, and is called ice, glass, batu or shabu. Like crack, ice is usually smoked in a glass pipe or an empty light bulb, leaving a milky or black residue depending on the way it is made.[8] One gram is enough for 10 to 25 hits.

This smokable form of methamphetamine is very popular in Japan and Korea. It spread to Hawaii in 1988, and then to the West Coast of the United States, where distribution is dominated by Asian gangs.

THE RISE OF RITALIN

Methylphenidate is a chemical relative of the amphetamines. Known by the trade name Ritalin, it is used mainly in the treatment of attention deficit hyperactivity disorder (ADHD) or attention deficit disorder (ADD) in children and, increasingly, in adults. About ten percent of boys and three percent of girls in the United States are diagnosed with ADD. It may seem a contradiction, but many stimulating drugs have a calming effect if taken in small doses. (For example, coffee usually makes people more alert, but helps some people calm down or go to sleep.) In children in particular, amphetamines can help focus attention and control hyperactivity. By 1997, 2.5 million schoolchildren were being prescribed Ritalin in the United States, which accounted for 90 percent of the world's production.[10]

Like other amphetamines, methylphenidate may also be abused. Its stimulating effects are similar to those produced by methamphetamine or cocaine. Long-term methylphenidate abuse can also cause a paranoid psychosis identical to that of chronic methamphetamine abuse. As with other amphetamines, people who take Ritalin can become addicted, develop tolerance, and use increasing amounts to try to bring about the same effect. Some users switch to snorting or injecting the crushed pills to try to recapture the original effects.

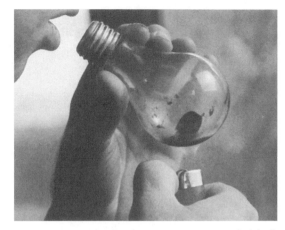

Smoking ice in an empty lightbulb

 Over the Rainbow
Judy Garland was taking 40 Ritalin tabs a day in 1968. The *Wizard of Oz* star died of a drug overdose on June 15, 1969.

OTHER AMPHETAMINE-LIKE DRUGS

Fenethylline, sold as Captagon, was also used to treat hyperactive children. It was marketed internationally for 23 years before the World Health Organization became alarmed at its widespread abuse and discouraged its production.[11] It is now illegal.

Methylaminorex, chemically known as (±)*cis*-4-methylaminorex, was first marketed in 1962 as a weight loss drug. It was followed in 1966 by a derivative, aminorex, which was sold in Europe, also as a weight loss drug. Both of these were withdrawn in 1968 when they were discovered to cause death from pulmonary hypertension, a form of heart-lung disease.[12] After their removal, they were made illegally as designer drugs by clandestine labs, who were less concerned about this side effect.[13] Why would anyone take aminorex or methylaminorex if they are so hazardous? Both drugs produce effects identical to dextroamphetamine. Studies in rats,[14] and monkeys show that they cannot distinguish between aminorex and dextroamphetamine, and become equally addicted to them.[15]

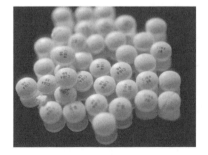

3% to 5% of all school children in the United States are being treated with Ritalin.[16]

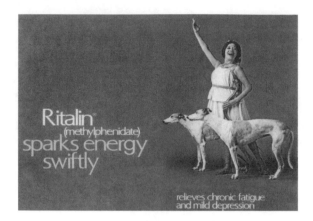

Ritalin®
(methylphenidate)
sparks energy
swiftly

relieves chronic fatigue
and mild depression

Because methylphenidate is readily available by prescription, it is not clandestinely produced.

Phenmetrazine and phendimetrazine are amphetamine-like weight loss drugs. In controlled tests, users cannot tell the difference between these and dextroamphetamine, although they do not appear to have the psychoactive or addictive characteristics of amphetamine.[17] Phenmetrazine continues to be marketed under the trade name Preludin.

 Amphetamines cause weight loss by decreasing appetite. Other weight loss drugs decrease body water or impair the absorption of nutrients. No drugs can "burn fat." Advertisements that make this claim are fraudulent.

YOU CAN NEVER BE TOO THIN

For millions of years, the greatest fear of most people was starving to death. It is still the major concern for about half the world's population. Industrialized countries now face the opposite problem: an epidemic of obesity. It is estimated that almost two-thirds of the American population is overweight, and a large number are clinically obese, meaning they are more than 20 percent above their ideal weight.

Obesity is not just a health problem. Fat people are made fun of, considered unattractive, and discriminated against in many subtle ways. Because of these social issues, fear of obesity has resulted in an obsession with thinness. A 1999 study showed that the winners of the Miss Universe beauty pageant have become progressively thinner over the past decades. Female Hollywood movie stars also are increasingly underweight. By today's standards, Marilyn Monroe seems almost chubby. Her ideal of beauty has been replaced by the anorexic look of Ally McBeal, who would provoke sympathy from a starving African villager.

"You can never be too rich or too thin."—Duchess of Windsor

It is almost impossible to achieve the current ideal of thinness with dieting, unless the person is either extremely masochistic or mentally ill. Using drugs to lessen appetite is a much easier method. Amphetamines began to be promoted as an appetite suppressant during the period of economic affluence after the Second World War. Various formulations were developed as research came closer to targeting the key appetite center in the brain.

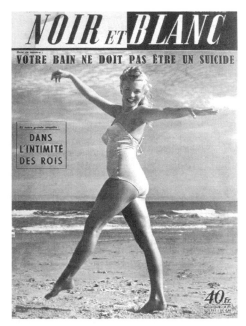

Weight loss drugs hit a peak with the development of fenfluramine and phentermine. Both of these were marketed individually. Then, in the 1990s, their popularity sky-rocketed when they became sold in a combination called Fen-Phen. Clinics popped up everywhere to sell the weight loss combo, even to those not overweight at all— including rail-thin teenage girls who still didn't feel slender enough. With over six million

Marilyn Monroe, an earlier ideal of beauty

users, it became one of the most popular, and undeniably effective, weight loss remedies as long as the user stayed on it. Unfortunately, the weight came back quickly once the user was off the drug.

In September 1997 the bottom fell out of the market: Fen-Phen was discovered to cause heart valve disease and it was immediately withdrawn. It was the product liability lawyers' turn to get rich.

 Fen-Phen was a weight loss sensation—until it was found to cause heart disease. Its manufacturer, American Home Products, has agreed to a $3.75 billion settlement with users.

Who Is Using Amphetamines?

Amphetamines are generally swallowed as a pill, smoked or snorted as a powder, or mixed with water and injected. Powdered methamphetamine is white, yellow, pink, or green, depending on its method of manufacture, and may have an odor of rotten eggs. It is quite easy to make with simple instruments and ingredients.

Amphetamines are used for a wide variety of purposes. Truck drivers, athletes, soldiers, and students use them to increase attention and prolong endurance. Children, and increasingly adults, take them for attention deficit disorder. People struggling to lose weight take them to reduce appetite. Amphetamines are also taken by people who interact poorly in social settings and have difficulty internalizing new experiences. These drugs reduce the need for external stimulation by increasing internal arousal mechanisms.[18]

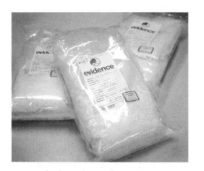

Smuggled methamphetamine

A 1991 survey in the United States showed that seven percent of the total population had used amphetamines for non-medical reasons at some time, with 1.3 percent reporting current use. About two percent of the adult population was addicted to, or had abused, amphetamines at some time in their lives.[19]

Methamphetamine use in the United States is most common in the large western and southwestern cities. The typical user is a male, age 26 to 44, who takes it in combination with alcohol, heroin, cocaine, or other drugs.

Eighty percent of all methamphetamine now sold in the United States is either manufactured in Mexico or produced in the U.S. by Mexican drug traffickers. The rest of the production comes from unskilled chemists ranging from individual addicts to motorcycle clubs, Asian and Mexican gangs, and organized crime syndicates.

 "The drug is like a companion telling you that you're good enough, handsome enough and smart enough, banishing all the little insecurities to your subconscious, liberating you from self doubts yet making you feel totally and completely alive." [20]

Internationally, methamphetamine has become the drug of choice for young people, particularly in nightclubs, throughout Southeast and East Asia. It is produced by large drug trafficking organizations in Myanmar (Burma), Thailand, and Laos. In February and March 2000, several shipments of over 20,000 Southeast Asian methamphetamine tablets were seized in Sacramento. The small reddish-brown tablets had been sent by mail from Laos, heralding a new trend of inexpensive methamphetamine imports to the United States. These tablets have an average weight of 90 milligrams (about one fourth the size of an aspirin), and contain 23 milligrams of methamphetamine and 45 to 65 milligrams of caffeine. Some also contain theophylline, a caffeine-like stimulant.

In Thailand, the wholesale price is about U.S. 50 cents per tablet, and consumers pay about $3 per tablet. Once the shipment has reached the United States, the price has increased to $5-$10 per tablet.

METH LABS

The production of methamphetamine in small home operations—"meth labs"—first began in California in the 1950s and proliferated throughout the Southwest in the 1960s. By 1999, manufacturing was taking place in most states, and new labs were discovered in Massachusetts and New York.

> Ephedrine and pseudoephedrine are structurally mirror-images of each other, and both can be used to manufacture methamphetamine.

Clandestine labs are sprinkled throughout urban and rural areas of the West but, for some reason, they are most common in the straight-laced state of Utah. Every year, 250 to 300 labs are busted at a cost of millions of dollars. A minor industry has grown up in Salt Lake City just to dispose of the leftover hazardous chemicals, which include highly flammable ether, acetone, red phosphorous, caustic sodium hydroxide, cancer-causing chloroform, and extremely poisonous chemicals such as mercuric chloride, phosphane gas, hydrochloric and sulfuric acids, iodine gas, and cyanide gas.

Methamphetamine is easily made from recipes learned from friends or taken off the Internet. Until 1980, most illegal methamphetamine was made by the P2P amalgam method, using phenyl-2-propanone (P2P) and methylamine as the primary precursors, along with mercuric chloride, hydrochloric acid, aluminum, isopropanol, and sodium hydroxide. P2P can be made by reacting lead acetate with phenylacetic acid. This material can cause severe lead poisoning,[21] with symptoms such as abdominal pain, nausea, vomiting, weakness, weight loss, or lower back and leg pain.

In 1980, P2P was designated a Schedule II drug and became very difficult to obtain. Now, the most common method uses the reduction of ephedrine or pseudoephedrine. In this process, over-the-counter cold and allergy tablets containing ephedrine or pseudoephedrine (for example, Sudafed) are placed in water, alcohol, or another solvent for a few hours until they dissolve. Hydrogen chloride gas is then used to chemically reduce the

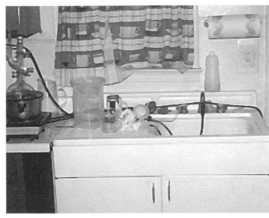

2,155 meth labs were raided in the year 1999[22]

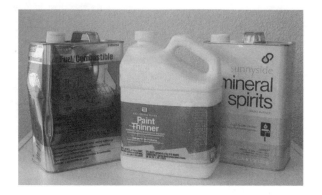

ephedrine (or pseudoephedrine) to methamphetamine.

The entire process can be done using only common household products and utensils. Certain brands of drain cleaner, for example, have a high concentration of sulfuric acid. When this powder is mixed with table salt or rock salt, hydrogen chloride gas is produced.

The final product often shows how it was made. Pink methamphetamine indicates that red-colored pseudoephedrine tablets were used. A bluish tint may come from the use of Coleman camper fuel. Green meth was probably made from green gun scrubber, purchased in sporting goods and hardware stores.

Meth lab chemicals ...	are obtained from[23]
Ephedrine	cold and allergy medicine
Pseudoephedrine	cold and allergy medicine
Alcohol	rubbing alcohol
Toluene	brake cleaner
Ether	engine starter
Sulfuric acid	drain cleaner
Methanol	gasoline additive
Lithium	camera batteries
Trichloroethane	gun scrubber
Anhydrous ammonia	farm fertilizer
Sodium hydroxide	lye
Red phosphorous	matches
Iodine	veterinary products
Sodium metal	can be made from lye

Other materials	
	Table salt or rock salt
	Kerosene
	Gasoline
	Muriatic acid
	Campfire fuel
	Paint thinner
	Acetone
	MSM (cutting agent)

Because the materials for methamphetamine are so readily available, it is difficult to control its manufacture. In 1992, less than two percent of seized amphetamine laboratories used pseudoephedrine, but this had grown to 55 percent by 1996. To plug this loophole, Congress passed the Comprehensive Methamphetamine Control Act of 1996, placing pseudoephedrine under the same regulations that apply to ephedrine. A single sale is limited to 24 grams of pseudoephedrine. Some stores, such as Wal-Mart, limit sales of all cold medicines to three packages per customer. A loophole to these restrictions in buying quantities of ephedrine or pseudoephedrine is to buy "herbal extract" pills. They may be loaded with ephedrine but do not come under the regulations because they are herbs.[24]

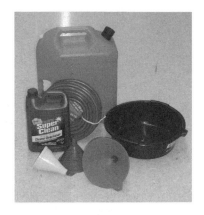

 "These folks are biohazards in and of themselves. They have open sores, chemical burns, higher incidences of HIV, TB, and hepatitis. They even sweat the by-products of these drugs."—Meth lab investigator [25]

The law also amended the Chemical Diversion and Trafficking Act to restrict the sale of iodine, red phosphorus, and hydrochloric gas. These three chemicals are used to make hydriolic acid, a key ingredient in the ephedrine reduction method of making methamphetamine.

PURE SPEED?

Meth lab operators tend to be uneducated and usually have a very poor understanding of chemistry or quality control. Amphetamine by-products and other drug variants such as N-methamphetamine (MA) and N,N-dimethyl-amphetamine (NNDMA) sometimes appear in police confiscations.[26] They are synthesized unintentionally by sloppy manufacturing.

Many of these meth lab "cooks" are violent because they use their own product. Addicts can go without sleep for up to 15 days, making them delusional and aggressive. Police have been attacked with scissors, chain saws, and even fire bombs.

Methamphetamine is generally a white to tan powder. Drug seizures show an average purity of 54 percent, diluted with ingredients such as baking soda, lactose, Epsom salts, quinine, mannitol, procaine, ether, insecticides, MSG, photo developer, and strychnine. Heavy speed users may even prefer these additives because the impurities can give a more intense rush.[27]

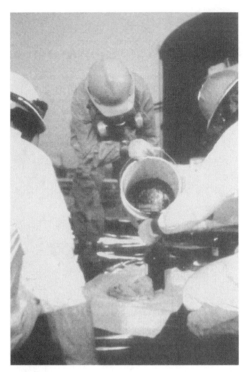

Busting meth labs is a hazardous occupation. According to a DEA spokesman, at least 40 percent of these labs are booby-trapped with explosives and nerve agents.

Some addicts crush prescription amphetamine pills and inject them. Beside the general hazards of intravenous drug use, this practice can cause additional physical problems. Amphetamine pills are often combined with other substances that are not meant to be injected. For example, some tablets use insoluble fillers that do not disperse in the bloodstream. Crushed tablets may look like a solution in water, but are in fact a mixture of tiny hard particles. When injected, these particles can block small blood vessels and cause serious damage throughout the body, especially in the lungs and the retina of the eye[28] (see *Chapter 4: Intravenous Drug Use*).

Chemical Characteristics

The effects of amphetamines, especially methamphetamine, are similar to those of cocaine, but their onset is slower and they last longer. Like cocaine, amphetamines cause a rapid release of serotonin and dopamine from nerve terminals. In high doses, amphetamines can injure the serotonin nerve endings, and up to 50 percent of the dopamine producing cells, with the possibility of long-term brain damage.

The seemingly additional energy provided by amphetamines actually comes from using up the stores of neurotransmitters in the central nervous system. Rather than being released in short bursts as needed for the body's "fight or flight" response, amphetamines cause an enormous amount to be released at once. This release is inevitably followed by the feeling caused by depletion of these neurotransmitters—the sluggishness of withdrawal.

A single amphetamine dose may increase attention and performance, but exhaustion eventually takes over and performance deteriorates as the effects wear off. The worker on amphetamines is often nervous, suspicious, and hyperactive. His sense of increased work performance may actually be due to impaired judgment, rather than to increased intellectual ability. To others, he may appear to be a hard, aggressive worker, but at the same time he is on the brink of collapse.

The appetite-inhibiting effects of amphetamine probably result from the release of norepinephrine and serotonin. Amphetamines that release mainly serotonin—for example, dexfenfluramine—can effectively suppress appetite without producing addiction. However, serotonin-specific amphetamines have proved to be dangerous to the heart and taken off the market.

Amphetamines, particularly methylphenidate, also affect the dopamine-producing nerves. Small doses block the reuptake of dopamine, but a higher dose may also block the dopamine receptors, resulting in mindless or jerky body movements. These movement disorders usually resolve after the drug has worn off.

Smokable amphetamines are stronger and more addictive than the snorted or the injected forms. When methamphetamine is smoked, other products can be formed by combustion. The smoke contains 14.5 percent of the initial methamphetamine. It also contains phenylacetone (3.1%), N-cyanomethylmethamphetamine (1.9%), trans-beta-methylstyrene (1.7%), N,N-dimethylamphetamine, and trans-beta-methylstyrene—all of which are intoxicating drugs on their own.[29] Together they make a distinctive, potent combination.

TESTING FOR AMPHETAMINES

Amphetamines are well absorbed from the nasal cavity, the lungs, and the gastrointestinal tract. When methamphetamine is used, nearly half of the dose is excreted in the urine unchanged, but a small percentage is demethylated to amphetamine. Therefore, tests will show both amphetamine and methamphetamine in the urine even though only methamphetamine might have been taken. This may have important legal implications if the user is suspected of taking amphetamines.

The natural excretion of amphetamines from the body can be speeded up by certain diets. For example, consumption of large amounts of vitamin C, vinegar, and acidic fruit juices can increase the rate of amphetamine excretion. Amphetamines are chemically basic compounds. When the urine is acidic, amphetamines are leached out of the blood and absorbed by the urine and therefore excreted more quickly. With normal urine, about 30 percent of an amphetamine dose appears in the urine unchanged. But this can rise to 70 percent if the urine is acidic and can be as low as 1 percent if the urine is alkaline. Some illicit drug users drink vinegar or cranberry juice to acidify their urine and "cleanse" themselves of amphetamine. Even so, ten milligrams of amphetamines

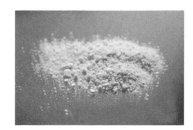

Methamphetamine

generally produces a positive urine test for about 24 hours, depending on the individual. High-dose abusers can have positive urines for two to four days after the last use.[30]

LEGAL AND ILLEGAL AMPHETAMINES

Both amphetamine and methamphetamine can exist in two molecular forms: one has psychoactive effects and the other does not. The two forms are known as *d-* (dextro) and *l-* (levo) enantiomers, or stereoisomers. These molecules are mirror images of each other. The designators *d-* and *l-* can be remembered as "drug" and "legal", but they actually indicate the direction (*d*=right and *l*=left) in which each enantiomer rotates a beam of polarized light. The *d*-isomer has a strong stimulant effect on the central nervous system, while the *l*-isomer acts primarily on the peripheral nerves (for example, it reduces nasal stuffiness but does not affect the brain). If a test for amphetamines is positive, a further test can be ordered to distinguish between *d-* and *l-* forms to see if the positive result was due to the use of an illegal or legal form.

The *d*-form of amphetamine in a positive test does not always indicate the use of illegal drugs, but can be due to a legal prescription of amphetamines. A number of medications metabolize to amphetamine or methamphetamine in the body. These include amphetaminil, benzphetamine, clobenzorex, deprenyl, dimethylamphetamine, ethylamphetamine, famprofazone, fencamine, fenethylline, fenproporex, furfenorex, mefenorex, mesocarb, and prenylamine, and can cause a misinterpretation of the test results.[31]

Because amphetamine-like drugs contain such a wide variety of structurally similar chemicals, amphetamine immunoassay tests are often wrong. False-positive tests can result from the use of nonprescription drugs that contain ephedrine, pseudoephedrine, and phenylpropanolamine (e.g., Alka-Seltzer Plus, Dexatrim, Primatene Tablets, Triaminic) and the prescription drug Ritalin. If there is any question of the meaning of the test results, a Medical Review Officer (MRO) should be consulted.

Withdrawal Signs

A medical dose of amphetamines seldom exceeds 60 mg per day, and is unlikely to cause serious withdrawal symptoms when it is stopped. In contrast, "speed freaks" develop a tolerance to the effects and may need a dose up to 100 times greater than the original one. They may take more than 5,000 mg a day during a speed run lasting three to five days and then crash, to sleep for one or two days. Withdrawal causes a state of depression which may last for weeks unless more amphetamines are taken, resulting in a speed run/crash cycle.

Withdrawal from amphetamines generally produces the opposite of the stimulating effects. Physically, there can be muscular aches, abdominal pain, chills, tremors, and voracious hunger. Apathy, long periods of sleep, increased appetite, fatigue, and a sense of sluggishness are common. Reaction times are slower and the whole body is less alert and responsive. There may also be irritability or agitation, disorientation, insomnia, and vivid and unpleasant dreams. Most users experience depression and some are brought to the point of suicide.

Amphetamine effect and ...	the withdrawal symptom[32]
Stimulation	becomes sluggishness
Strength	becomes fatigue
Alertness	becomes apathy
Concentration	becomes disorientation
Loss of appetite	becomes voracious hunger
Euphoria	becomes depression
Feeling of vitality	becomes aches and pains

These withdrawal effects are not harmful to the body, and disappear within days. One particularly unpleasant symptom of amphetamine withdrawal—that may *not* disappear as quickly—is anhedonia, or the inability to feel pleasure. When a stimulating drug is removed, so is its artificial stimulation of the brain's pleasure center. The result is a suppression of dopamine neuron activity during the withdrawal period, which can cause a very disagreeable feeling that can last for weeks, depending on the severity of the addiction. Even the memory of the good feelings associated with the drug, and the bad feelings away from it, can be enough to drive the user back to the drug.

 "No one ever died from a few days without pleasure, but in the absence of any positive feelings, the temptation to use the drug to feel better becomes stronger and stronger. Anhedonia is thought to be a major reason why people start using stimulants after a period of attempted abstinence....the craving can last for months."[33]

Long-term Health Problems

With repeated use, tolerance to the drug develops, and attempts to reduce the dose result in depression and lethargy. Eventually, users are caught between being overly stimulated when using the drug, and overly depressed if they have not taken enough. It is impossible to maintain a satisfactory balance.

Frequent use of amphetamines can produce a psychosis that resembles schizophrenia. This "amphetamine psychosis" is characterized by paranoia, picking at the skin, preoccupation with one's own thoughts, and auditory and visual hallucinations. Violent and erratic behavior is often seen among chronic abusers.[34] Long-term users may get the feeling that bugs or insects are crawling under the skin, a sensation called formication. Picking at these imaginary bugs can lead to large wounds that become infected. Addicts have almost died trying to cut these "speed bugs" or "crank bugs" out of their skin.

Dopamine-related effects account for the odd behavior of some amphetamine addicts. As use increases, the bizarre, repetitive, stereotyped movements become more extreme. They can be very self-directed behaviors, such as saying the same thing over and over, or repeatedly assembling and taking apart equipment.

On a biological level, long-term amphetamine use alters the sensitivity of the post-synaptic membrane receptors in the central nervous system, eventually leading to neurochemical exhaustion. If only low doses are taken, nerve receptors will eventually regain their sensitivity when amphetamine use is stopped. High doses of amphetamine—methamphetamine in particular—cause permanent damage to the nerve endings of serotonin and dopamine neurons. The nerves do not die, but the nerve endings are "pruned" or cut back, leaving a permanent deficit in the density of nerve terminals and the amount of dopamine and serotonin. The effect of this may not be immediately obvious, since there are billions of such nerves. However, as people get older and experience the normal aging-related loss of dopamine and serotonin neurons, this deficit can start to become noticeable in the form of movement disorders such as Parkinson's Disease, or mood disorders such as depression.

What To Do If There Is An Overdose

Thousands of people have died from amphetamine overdose. It is an emergency that requires immediate medical attention. Death most often has resulted from seizures or an irregular heart beat causing heart failure.

It can be difficult to detect an overdose in a long-term user, as the signs of normal use and the signs of overdose are quite similar. The high energy and alertness can become jitteriness or even paranoia and hostility. The increased movement can become repetitive aimless activity, such as drawing closely spaced lines, taking watches apart and putting them back together, or talking constantly without listening. A mild increase in the pulse can become palpitations or chest pains as the heart rhythm is disturbed, and the skin becomes flushed as body temperature rises. Other overdose symptoms include headaches, from the amphetamine effects on blood vessels, and nausea and vomiting, usually from the impurities taken along with the drug.

Physical signs of overdose	Fever
	Rapid or irregular heart beat
	Shallow breathing
	High blood pressure
	Enlarged pupils
	Dry mouth
	Sweating
	Tremors
	Stroke
	Heart failure

Mental signs of overdose	Confusion
	Agitation
	Paranoia
	Hallucinations
	Impulsive behavior
	Hyperactivity
	Unresponsive coma

If there are only mild symptoms, drinking solutions of ascorbic acid (vitamin C) or ammonium chloride can help the body to get rid of the amphetamines by making the urine more acidic. Other stimulating medications should be avoided, including coffee or soft drinks with caffeine.

 Amphetamine overdose can be fatal. If you suspect an overdose, call 911 or get to an Emergency Department.

Anxiety reactions without the physical signs of an overdose can be managed by reassurance. The user should recover within a few hours. Chronic anxiety reactions, particularly during the withdrawal period, may be helped by sedative medications, but this should be done under medical supervision.

If there is a fever or high blood pressure, the amphetamine user should be taken to the Emergency Department *immediately*. Doctors may use blocking agents such as propanolol or phentolamine, and may treat psychotic reactions with haloperidol (Haldol). Without these treatments, amphetamine overdose can cause permanent brain damage or be fatal.

Barbiturates

Barbiturates are sedating drugs that cause sleepiness, numbness, and a relief from anxiety. Some barbiturates are used medically as sleeping pills, for headaches and anesthesia, and to prevent seizures. Others are used recreationally for an alcohol-like intoxication.

Until recently about 3,000 people a year died from barbiturates, about half of them suicides. By far the greatest risk of death due to illegal drugs is from barbiturate abuse.

The Basic Facts

Type of drug	*Depressant*
How taken	*Ingested, injected*
Duration of effect	*5 to 8 hours*
Physical danger	*High*
Addiction potential	*High*

Other Names

Amobarbital	*Amytal, blue dolls, blues*
Aprobarbital	*Alurate*
Butabarbital	*Butisol*
Butalbital	*Fioricet, Fiorinal*
Mephobarbital	*Mebaral*
Methohexital	*Brevital*
Pentobarbital	*nebbies, Nembutal, yellow jackets, yellows*
Phenobarbital	*Luminal, purple hearts*
Phenobarbital and theophylline	*Bronkolizer, Bronkotabs, Primatene-P, Tedrigen*
Secobarbital	*reds, red devils, red birds, Seccy, Seconal*
Talbutal	*Lotusate*
Thiamylal	*Surital*
Thiopental	*Pentothal*
Tuinal (amobarbital and secobarbital)	*Tooeys, double trouble, rainbows*

Dolls and Devils: The Story of Barbiturates

Barbiturates are stable compounds of barbituric acid, discovered in 1864 by the German pharmaceutical firm of Dr. Adolph Von Bayer. The first marketed barbiturate, barbital, was promoted as a sleeping pill in 1903. It was followed in 1912 by phenobarbital, a drug that is still in medical use.

More than 2,500 kinds of barbiturates have been synthesized. By the 1950s, at the height of their popularity, about 50 were marketed for human use. Many others were designed for the veterinary treatment of animals. Today, a total of only about a dozen are still available.

Barbiturates have many different medical uses, depending on the strength and the particular chemical characteristics of the individual compound. They produce a wide spectrum of central nervous system depression and cause effects ranging from mild sedation to severe coma. This damping-down action is the opposite of stimulant medications, and makes barbiturates useful as sedatives, sleeping pills, anesthetics, and anticonvulsants.

THREE TYPES OF BARBITURATES

Barbiturates are usually grouped into three categories, roughly based on the length of effect:

Long-acting barbiturates

With effects lasting from 12 to 24 hours, these include the original barbital, phenobarbital, and mephobarbital. They are useful for daytime sedation, and for the treatment of mild anxiety or seizure disorders. A combination of phenobarbital and theophylline was sold in several over-the-counter preparations, but was discontinued after a 1995 FDA ruling against over-the-counter sales of theophylline, which is hazardous in overdose.[1]

Intermediate or short-acting barbiturates

With effects typically lasting six to seven hours, these include pentobarbital, secobarbital, butalbital, butabarbital, talbutal and aprobarbital. Short-acting barbiturates behave much like alcohol, producing light excitement in a small dose, giving pleasant feelings in moderation, and causing a heavy, stupor-like condition in high doses. Medical use is primarily for the short-term treatment of insomnia, although there are much better medications now available for this condition, and as a sedative before operations. Veterinarians use pentobarbital as a painless way to kill animals.

Very short-acting barbiturates

When injected, these have effects within about one minute and cause almost immediate unconsciousness. They are used medically for anesthesia, and include methohexital, thiamylal, and thiopental.[2]

VALLEY OF THE DOLLS

"Doll" or "dollie" was the original slang for Dolophine (methadone), but over time the word came to mean nearly any pill that put one into a stoned-out state—particularly Seconal, the numbing drug of choice. Barbiturates became especially popular among movie actors and others in the entertainment industry; they were a way to cope with the uncertainty and stress of an intensely competitive profession.

"Anxiety and tension melt into peaceful, calm relaxation. Cares vanish into a blurry intoxication, where nothing really matters. The user staggers through his altered universe, speech slurred, muscles like rubber. Reaction time slows to a zombie pace."—*Recreational Drugs* [3]

In 1967, the pulp fiction book *Valley of the Dolls* caught the mood perfectly and sold millions of copies. Its main character, Neely, was helplessly addicted to Seconal. Barbiturates were an escape, an inner retreat from sexual abuse and loneliness and the personal loss of identity of the country girl in the big city. *Valley* was a metaphor for her refuge, as well as her descent into hell.

Carole Landis, the original "sweater girl" of the silver screen and the star of *One Million B.C.* (1940), died in 1948 after gulping a bottle of Seconal. She was 29 years old.

DOWNSIDE OF THE DOWNERS

Barbiturates are often called "downers," as opposed to the stimulant "uppers." The downside of these downers is that, in medical terms, they have a very narrow therapeutic ratio. This means that the amount needed for an effect is close to an amount that is dangerous or even lethal. The result is an extraordinarily high tendency to overdose. In fact, by far the greatest risk of death due to illegal drugs is from barbiturate abuse. Lethal amounts may be taken unknowingly by someone already drugged who is unable to remember how much he has previously ingested. This confused mental state is called "drug automatism."[4] For example, a user may take one or two barbiturate pills. Pleasantly sedated, and with some loss of judgment, he may take a couple more to increase the effect. By then, he might have forgotten how many he had taken and swallow a few more. Because of the delay in absorption, an overdose results.

The list of celebrity deaths due to barbiturates would fill pages. One was Elvis Presley. His use of drugs ranged far beyond barbiturates, however (see *Methaqualone*).

In recent years, barbiturates in medical use have largely been replaced by the benzodiazepines, including Librium, Valium, Xanax, and Halcion. Unlike barbiturates, benzodiazepines have a very *wide* therapeutic ratio, making them less likely to cause a fatal overdose, and they are much safer overall.

In addition to the ready availability of the newer benzodiazepines, the many celebrity deaths from barbiturates brought about a gradual decline in their popularity. Both use and abuse are now less common.

Who Is Using Barbiturates?

About four percent of the U.S. population has taken barbiturates for non-medical purposes. Although illicit use has largely fallen out of fashion, many people like to take barbiturates to counteract the stimulant effects of amphetamines, or to enhance the effects of heroin.

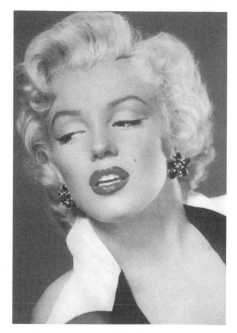

Marilyn Monroe was found dead on August 5, 1962, lying in bed with her hand gripping the telephone, and 47 Nembutal tablets in her stomach

THE CHOICE OF SUICIDES

Barbiturates have recently entered the news again as a painless way to commit suicide. They are recommended in the popular suicide handbook, *Final Exit*,[5] and have been used by a number of suicide cults.

 Thirty-nine Heaven's Gate cult members committed suicide on March 26, 1997, by overdosing on phenobarbital, their "Hand of Death."

Chemical Characteristics

Barbiturates are rapidly and completely absorbed when taken by mouth, and begin to have an effect within 10 to 60 minutes. Barbiturates bind to the GABA receptors in the central nervous system. GABA inhibits the transmission of nerve impulses so that the system is not overloaded by excitatory signals. An overdose of barbiturates provides so much inhibition that the person may enter a coma, stop breathing, or die.

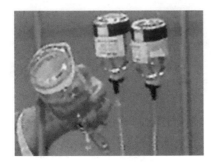

Jack Kevorkian's "Suicide Machine" consisted of three bottles hung from an aluminum frame and a small electric motor. One bottle holds a saline solution, and a second holds a mixture of potassium chloride and succinylcholine. The third holds sodium pentothal, a widely available barbiturate.

At therapeutic doses, barbiturates do not noticeably affect basic physical abilities but performance is impaired on tasks that require concentration or coordination. The intoxication syndrome is quite similar for all types of barbiturates and generally resembles that of alcohol. Slurred speech, disorientation, and uninhibited behavior are common. The drugged person appears drunk, but without the conspicuous odor of alcohol. High doses may cause extreme mood swings, aggressiveness, unsteady walk, jerky eye movement, impaired judgment, and loss of physical control.

"The barbiturate addict presents a shocking spectacle. He cannot coordinate, he staggers, falls off bar stools, goes to sleep in the middle of a sentence, drops food out of his mouth. He is confused, quarrelsome, and stupid. Barbiturate users are looked down on in addict society: 'Goofball bums. They got no class to them.'"—*William Burroughs, Naked Lunch, 1959*

The time to recovery from barbiturates depends on the type used. Elimination half-lives—the time it takes for half the dose to be eliminated from the body—typically is about 24 hours. Complete recovery can therefore take several days. Elimination is faster with repeated use and in younger people.

Elimination half-lives of common barbiturates[6]

Generic name	Trade Name	Elimination half-life
Amobarbital	Amytal	8-42 hours
Pentobarbital	Nembutal	15-48 hours
Phenobarbital	Donnatal	24-140 hours
Secobarbital	Seconal	19-34 hours

TESTING FOR BARBITURATES

Short-acting barbiturates can be detected by common urine tests for a couple of days after use. Intermediate-acting barbiturates such as secobarbital may be detected for up to four days. Long-acting barbiturates such as phenobarbital can be detected for several weeks after chronic use.[7]

With repeated use, the previous doses may not have time to metabolize and barbiturates can accumulate in the body. An overdose, or dangerous interaction with other drugs, then becomes increasingly likely.

Withdrawal Signs

Withdrawal from barbiturates is characterized by anxiety, irritability, nervousness, tremor, progressive weakness, fatigue, nausea and vomiting, loss of appetite and weight, sweating, fever, spastic blinking, headache, muscle twitching or aching, and insomnia. There may also be feelings of depersonalization, disorientation, and abnormal perception or sensation of movement. Withdrawal from a severe addiction can result in delirium, convulsions, shock, and death.

 Abrupt withdrawal from a barbiturate addiction can be fatal.

Withdrawal should never be attempted alone. In a medically supervised withdrawal program, which can last up to two weeks, the addict is first given the equivalent of his usual dose. This dose is then reduced by ten percent each day until the addict is drug free. Alcohol may also be used for a recovering addict, as there is cross-tolerance to both drugs.

Long-term Health Problems

Long-term use of barbiturates can result in continual drowsiness and sluggishness, shortened memory and attention span, loss of coordination and awareness, emotional instability, rashes, nausea, anxiety and nervousness, involuntary eye movements, staggering gait, slurred speech, and trembling hands. Paranoid delusions and increased hostility may lead to a barbiturate trademark—violence.

Tolerance to barbiturates develops gradually, but disappears after about one or two weeks of abstinence.

What To Do If There Is An Overdose

Barbiturate overdose causes a shock syndrome: cold and sweaty skin, weak and rapid pulse, and either very slow or very rapid and shallow breathing. Deep coma may follow, as well as respiratory and kidney failure. Since barbiturates reduce the amount of oxygen reaching the brain, the overdosing person who survives may be left with permanent brain damage.

Physical signs of overdose[8]   Slow breathing
Low blood pressure
Slurred speech
Difficulty walking
Jerky eye movement

Mental signs of overdose   Confusion
Drowsiness
Delirium
Impulsive behavior
Hyperactivity
Unresponsive coma

The progression of overdose symptoms is typically …

Drowsiness and muscular incoordination with slurring of speech
↘
Deep sleep from which the person cannot be easily aroused
↘
Loss of reflexes such as eye blink, gag, and reacting to pain
↘
Suppressed breathing
↘
Death

A person can overdose on even small amounts of barbiturates if a number of depressant drugs are taken at the same time—for example, the combined effect of barbiturates taken with alcohol or Valium can easily cause an overdose.

If a person has taken a barbiturate and cannot be aroused, get medical attention immediately.

Any overdose should be treated in a hospital. In the meantime, avoid letting the user fall asleep. Keep the person walking and, if possible, force vomiting by sticking a finger down the throat. Do not give coffee as this breaks up the barbiturates in the stomach, causing them to be dispersed even more. Do not give amphetamines—the combination may be fatal.

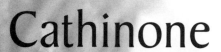

Cathinone

Cathinone is a natural amphetamine-like substance found in khat leaves, used for centuries in Africa as a stimulating drug.

Methcathinone is a newer, more potent, synthetic version of the drug, popular in Russia.

The Basic Facts

Type of drug	*Stimulant*
How taken	
Cathinone	*Smoked, ingested*
Methcathinone	*Smoked, snorted, ingested, injected*
Duration of effect	*Up to 6 days*
Physical danger	*Moderate*
Addiction potential	*High*

Other Names

Cathinone	*Abyssinian tea, chat, goob, khat, miraa, qat, shat*
Methcathinone	*bathtub speed, cat, gagers, gaggers, go-fast, Jeff, sniff, star, wild cat, wonder star*

Nine Lives of Cat: The Story of Cathinone

When the United States sent troops to Somalia in 1992, they were surprised to find a large part of the population in a pleasantly drugged state. People of all ages and social status had a regular of habit of chewing the leaves, twigs, and young stems of the khat bush. From the Arabian peninsula down to Kenya, up to half of the population appeared to be addicted to khat, and it was not unusual for homes in that region to have a room dedicated to khat chewing. In Yemen, where it is especially popular, many people spend over one-third of their family income on the drug.[1]

Khat (pronounced "cot") may be new to Americans, but it has been around since at least the 13th century, when Arab scribes documented its use. Khat comes from a North African shrub, *Catha edulis*, which grows to 10 or 20 feet and is widely cultivated in the region. The leaves and tender stems are picked fresh, with a preference for the youngest leaves near the top of the plant. After harvesting, they are often wrapped in banana leaves and sprinkled with water to preserve their potency.

Khat leaves are chewed for a few minutes, after which the soft mass is kept tucked in the cheek as a ball and then slowly munched or swallowed. Dried leaves and twigs may be crushed and steeped in water for tea or made into a paste for chewing.

When taken in moderation, khat acts much like caffeine, reducing appetite and providing a mild stimulation. Excessive use may result in overstimulation with manic behavior, grandiose delusions or paranoia, and even hallucinations.

The active principle in khat is cathinone, a drug stronger than cocaine and with similar effects.[2] Only fresh leaves contain pure cathinone. As they mature or dry, the cathinone is converted to cathine, a less stimulating compound about one tenth as potent.[3]

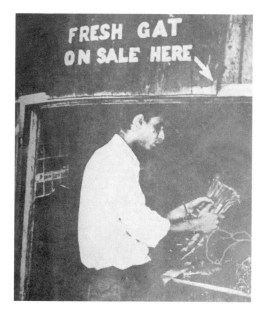

A typical khat shop in Nairobi, Kenya

MIGRATION OF PEOPLE AND THEIR DRUGS

During the Cold War between the Soviet Union and the United States, the countries of northeastern Africa shifted alliances between the superpowers. For decades, Egypt and Ethiopia fell into the Soviet sphere while Somalia, Djibouti, and Kenya were allied with the United States. When workers and students of the African countries traveled to Russia or America, they brought khat with them.

As the drug left Africa, it became more refined and more potent. Both in the Soviet Union and in America, khat underwent an evolution from fresh leaves to a more convenient, manufactured synthetic substance. First, the leaves were replaced by a smokable khat paste, which could be shipped easily and innocuously. Then, in the United States, khat paste gave way to illegally manufactured pure cathinone.

METHCATHINONE

Methcathinone was patented as a wholly synthetic drug by the pharmaceutical firm Parke-Davis in 1957. However, Parke-Davis did not market the drug because of its numerous adverse side effects. Soviet chemists discovered the formula. They spread word of this substance, which they called ephedrone, and how it could be synthesized as easily as methamphetamine (see *Amphetamines: Meth labs*). The new, powerful designer drug could be snorted or injected, and made from simple drugstore precursors. By 1982, methcathinone was cooked up in the kitchens of countless tiny apartments in Moscow, Leningrad and other cities. It quickly became a favorite of the underground drug scene. Drug abuse has increased since the dismantling of the Soviet Union, and it is now estimated that 20 percent of illicit drug users in Russia are addicted to methcathinone.

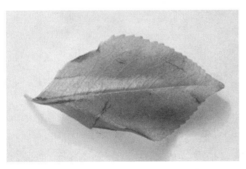

Khat has been around longer than coffee, and is used for much the same reason—to get a pleasant, stimulating buzz in a socially acceptable way

Russians immigrating to the United States brought methcathinone to the Midwestern cities of America. It was spread by motorcycle gangs and had hit most rural areas by 1991. The DEA believed that methcathinone would be the up and coming drug of the 1990s, but its popularity has mysteriously declined. It is likely that the drug was largely replaced by methamphetamine, which is similar and more readily available, and by MDMA.

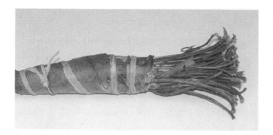

In fiscal 1998, U.S. Customs seized 62,000 lbs of khat, most of which was destined for the ethnic markets, restaurants, and shops of New York, Boston, Detroit, Dallas, and Washington, D.C.

Methcathinone was listed as a Schedule I controlled substance on May 1, 1993.[4] Making it illegal, of course, did not put an end to its use. By 1994, a total of 34 methcathinone labs had been raided in Michigan, 22 in Indiana, 8 in Wisconsin, and many more in other states.

Methcathinone is considerably more potent and addictive than cathinone. The yellowish-white powder looks like cocaine and produces the same euphoria as crack. Both its chemical structure and stimulating effects, however, are more similar to those of methamphetamine.

Methcathinone is easy to make and the chemicals used are inexpensive. As with methamphetamine, ephedrine is a key ingredient. The ephedrine is extracted from commercially available tablets or capsules and then oxidized by adding chromium salts, such as sodium chromate or potassium dichromate. The final product is an off-white, yellowish, or brownish powder.

Cat powder is usually snorted, or dissolved in water and then drunk or injected. It may also be smoked for a particularly intense and rapid intoxication. A typical dose is a half-gram to one gram per day.

Who Is Using Cathinone?

Khat is popular in the countries of North Africa, where it is used during holidays and celebrations such as birthdays and weddings. The stimulant makes it easier to fast during the month-long Muslim holy period of Ramadan, when food should not be taken during the day.

Khat is legal in Great Britain and many other European countries, where it is imported by East Africans. In Europe, couriers may be employed to smuggle it to the United States. The couriers are typically paid between $150 and $500 plus expenses per trip, and often have the mistaken belief that khat is not illegal and their supplies will merely be confiscated if they are caught. (Like many natural substances that contain a drug, *Catha edulis* is not prohibited in itself, but its use for cathinone is illegal.) A bundle of 40 twigs, 12 to 16 inches in length, has a street value of $30 to $60 per kilogram.

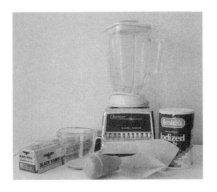

CAT CONTAMINANTS

Illegally manufactured methcathinone is synthesized from ephedrine, sulfuric acid, sodium hydroxide, Epsom salts, toluene, muriatic acid, acetone, sodium dichromate, and distilled water. The equipment needed is quite simple, consisting of coffee filters, a pipette, funnel, auto stirrer, tubing, glass jars, and a stove.

Most methcathinone contains a number of adulterants from incomplete processing, including ephedrine, sulfuric acid, and more hazardous substances such as toluene, which is toxic to the heart, kidneys, skin, and brain. Potassium permanganate and sodium dichromate can cause severe burns and chromium toxicity. Many users of poorly processed "green cat" get sick from these ingredients.

Other adulterants may be deliberately added to increase volume and mimic the effects, such as caffeine, laxatives, and ephedrine.

$CH_2-CH-NH-CH_3$
CH_3

Methamphetamine

O
$CH_2-CH-NH-CH_3$
CH_3

Methcathinone

Chemical Characteristics

Cathinone is chemically known as S(-)-alpha-aminopropiophenone, and is indistinguishable from amphetamine in its effects on the central nervous system. Experiments with drug-conditioned animals show that they cannot tell the difference between cathinone and amphetamine. Cathinone operates through the same mechanism as amphetamine, by causing a release of dopamine and other neurotransmitters from the presynaptic storage sites.[5]

Methcathinone is much like methamphetamine, giving a feeling of limitless energy, alertness and speeding of the mind, a sense of invincibility, and a euphoric high with reports of increased sexuality, creativity, and garrulousness. Some less pleasant effects include anxiety, tremor, insomnia, weight loss, dehydration, sweating, stomach pains, pounding heart, nose bleeds and body aches. Toxic levels may produce convulsions, paranoia, and hallucinations. Like other central nervous system stimulants, methcathinone binges are usually followed by a "crash" with fatigue and depression.[6]

Withdrawal Signs

Cathinone and methcathinone are physically and mentally addictive. Abrupt withdrawal of these stimulants can cause fatigue, irritability, pinpoint pupils, runny nose, and a craving for sweets. It also may result in muscle aches and spasms, joint pain (especially in the knees), and heart failure.[7]

Long-term Health Problems

Mild use of khat is tolerated well, even over the long term, but frequent use of cathinone or methcathinone can cause problems similar to those of chronic amphetamine use. Common features include a decline in personal hygiene, loss of appetite, muscle-wasting, overly enlarged taste buds, blue fingers and toes, acne, enlarged liver, antisocial behavior, and signs of Parkinson's Disease. Anxiety and disorientation can progress to a complete paranoid psychosis.

 Chronic use of methcathinone also causes a distinctive, very disagreeable body odor as the metabolic breakdown products are exuded from the skin.

What To Do If There Is An Overdose

Signs of methcathinone overdose include visual and auditory hallucinations, fever, and a rapid heart rate. This may be followed after 6 to 12 hours by an overly slow heart rate and low blood pressure. A more severe overdose will appear as enlarged pupils, jerky eyes, flushing, sweating palms, and convulsions leading to death.

 There are no good tests for methcathinone. If an overdose is suspected and medical attention is needed, it is important to explain what drug has been taken. Antipsychotic medications may be necessary.[8]

Physical signs of overdose	Fever
	Rapid or irregular heart beat
	Low blood pressure
	Enlarged pupils
	Sweating
	Tremors
	Stroke
Mental signs of overdose	Confusion
	Agitation
	Paranoia
	Hallucinations
	Hyperactivity
	Unresponsive coma

Cocaine

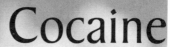

Cocaine is extracted from the leaves of the coca plant, which grows in South America. Crack is a more addictive, smokable version of cocaine.

After processing, cocaine is shipped to the United States, where it is one of the most prominent drugs of abuse.

The Basic Facts

Type of drug	*Stimulant*
How taken	
Powder	*Ingested, snorted, injected, applied*
Crack	*Smoked*
Freebase	*Smoked*
Duration of effect	*1 to 2 hours*
Physical danger	*Moderate*
Addiction potential	*High*

Other Names

Powder cocaine	*All-American drug, Angie, blow, booger, bouncing powder, buger sugar, C, cabello, California cornflakes, caine, candy, Carrie Nation, cecil, chick, coke, dust, flake, Florida snow, girl, la dama blanca, lady, nose candy, snow, toot*
Crack or freebase cocaine	*apple jacks, B. J., baby T, bad, ball, basay, base, baseball, basuco, bazooka, bazulco, bebe, beemers, big eight (one-eighth kilogram of crack), bings, biscuit (50 rocks), black rock, blowcaine (diluted with cocaine), bobo, bolo, bonecrusher, bones, botray, boubou, boulder, boulya, breakfast of champions, bullion, caviar, hubba, pasta, pestillos rock*
Cocaine and heroin	*Belushi, speedball*

Flake: The Story of Cocaine

For thousands of years, natives of the Andes chewed or brewed coca leaves into a tea for refreshment and to relieve fatigue, similar to modern customs of chewing tobacco and drinking tea or coffee. The Indians considered the leaf to be sacred and essential to life.

When the Spaniards conquered the Inca Empire in the 16th century, they attempted to ban coca chewing. They relented when they discovered that Indians working in the silver mines would work harder if given their daily allotment of coca. Coca leaf chewing remains even now an important part of traditional Andean culture and nutrition.

The coca bush can grow to a height of 30 feet but is usually pruned down to about 6 feet for easy collection of the leaves. Leaves are harvested three times a year, but up to six times in some areas.

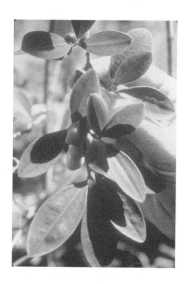

 According to Indian legend, coca was brought from heaven by Manco Capac, the first Inca Emperor: "a gift from the gods to satisfy the hungry, fortify the weary, and make the unfortunate forget their sorrows."[1]

There are four major varieties of coca, *Erythroxylum coca*, *E. ipadu*, *E. novogratense*, and *E. truxillense*, but *E. coca* accounts for about 95 percent of the total production. The leaves of the different varieties have a taste ranging from green tea to a mint-like flavor. About 0.5 percent of the weight of the leaf is cocaine, but can range from 0.1 percent and 0.8 percent depending on environmental factors. Coca plants grown at higher altitudes contain a higher percentage of cocaine. The leaf also contains smaller concentrations of 14 other drugs, which seem to modify the stimulating effect of the cocaine, as well as many vitamins and minerals, which are a significant part of the Indians' diet.

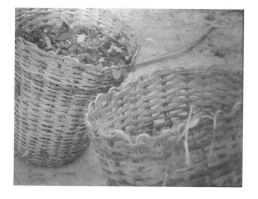

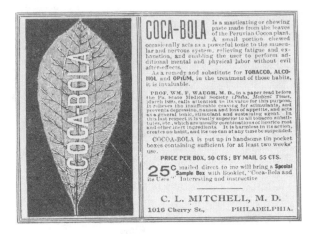

CHEWING COCA

Coca leaves are chewed fresh or dry. They are mixed with a small amount of alkaline substance such as ash, lime, or powdered seashells, and the whole wad is sucked on for a half hour or so. Saliva, mixed with the alkaline powder, leaches the drugs from the leaves and is swallowed. Eventually, the leftover residue is spit out.

Chewing the leaves has little psychological effect other than a mild stimulation, similar to that of coffee but soothing rather than irritating the stomach. There is also a tingly, numbing sensation in the mouth and throat.

COCA BECOMES POWDER COCAINE

Soon after its refinement in the 19th century, cocaine was prescribed for almost any illness. It effectively became a recreational drug, as much of its early medical use was more likely a matter of abuse or addiction. Cocaine wines and cocaine soft drinks (including Coca-Cola) became extremely popular. When its addictive potential was realized, however, cocaine was made illegal. Now, only cocaine hydrochloride remains medically available for very restricted use.

 In the 1980s, it was estimated that six million Americans used cocaine regularly.

Illegal cocaine is usually distributed as a white crystalline powder or as an off-white chunky material. The powder, cocaine hydrochloride, is often diluted with a variety of substances, the most common being sugars such as lactose, inositol or mannitol, and local anesthetics such as lidocaine. This adulteration increases the volume and therefore multiplies profits. Powder cocaine is generally snorted or dissolved in water and injected.

Powder cocaine surged in popularity in the 1970s. It was called the champagne of drugs because it was expensive and thought to have no serious consequences. It was also known as the yuppie drug because it appealed to young urban professionals. Cocaine fit in well with this affluent and prosperous class—they liked the stimulation and euphoric high, and they had the money to buy it. Having cocaine, particularly high-purity cocaine, became a status symbol among this competitive group, and the choice method of snorting it was with a rolled-up $100 bill. Its use was prominent among entertainment and political figures, to the point that it became almost an icon of the moneyed life. The demand for cocaine and the extreme amounts of cash involved to supply it created a gigantic illegal drug industry.

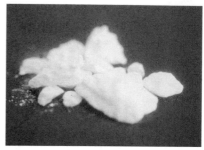

Not surprisingly, cocaine use spread to people who were not quite so wealthy. Cocaine addiction was a health problem for those who could afford it. For those who couldn't, it often led to economic ruin.

 By 1996, an analysis of U.S. $1 bills showed that 79% of them contained residues of cocaine.[2]

Much as the alcohol prohibition of the 1920s led to the growth of the mafia, the demand for cocaine created a criminal network to supply it. By 1980, the cocaine crime industry was so pervasive in the United States that it was dramatized in its own TV shows such as *Miami Vice*. The criminal syndicates also had a devastating impact on the countries that supplied cocaine. The authority of the governments of Colombia, Bolivia, and Peru was undermined by the economic power of the cocaine cartels, resulting in a virtual drug economy— lawless, corrupt, and bankrupt. These countries are still suffering from the demand caused by the continuing American addiction.

POWDER COCAINE BECOMES FREEBASE

Powder cocaine is usually snorted, with the fine powder absorbed by the mucosal membranes of the nasal passages. This is much more effective than simply ingesting cocaine. The absorption of snorted cocaine is still not as fast as smoking it, however, because the small nasal blood vessels are constricted by the drug. But powder cocaine cannot be smoked because it is destroyed by the high temperature of combustion. In order to make a smokable form of cocaine, it was chemically modified into a substance called freebase.

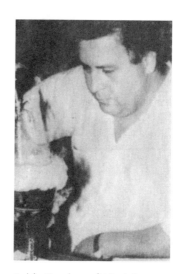

Freebase cocaine is made by heating cocaine hydrochloride in water and adding a base, usually sodium bicarbonate or buffered ammonia. This base "frees" the

Pablo Escobar of Medellín, Colombia, dominated the cocaine trade in the 1980s. Before his death, he amassed a personal fortune of $5 billion.

cocaine from the hydrochloric acid used in its initial production. An organic solvent (usually diethyl ether or acetone) is then added and the solution is shaken vigorously. The liquid separates into two layers, with cocaine dissolved in ether in the top layer. This can be drawn off with an eye dropper and placed into a dish to evaporate, leaving almost pure cocaine crystals. The result is an alkaloid—the base—which is both resistant to heat and is also very fat-soluble, meaning that it can enter the brain easily. Since ether is extremely flammable, freebase users must be careful to wait until all the ether has evaporated before smoking the crystals to avoid explosive burns.

 Richard Pryor ended a career as one of the most famous and successful comedians when he suffered severe burns to his face from an explosion of freebase cocaine.

Freebase cocaine was developed around 1976 and caused another upsurge in cocaine abuse. It was purer, and therefore more potent, than the typical powder cocaine, and it could be smoked, allowing a large amount of cocaine to quickly enter the bloodstream from the lungs and go directly to the brain. (Although the nose seems close to the brain, in fact snorted cocaine takes a while to reach the brain. It is first absorbed into venous blood and then sent to the heart before it makes its way to the brain—see *Chapter 6*). The effects of freebase were faster and more potent, making freebase more highly addictive than powder cocaine.

Until the mid-1980s, freebasing grew in popularity to the extent that about 10 to 20 percent of all cocaine was used in this way.

"My other car went up my nose."—*Bumper sticker of the 1980s*

FREEBASE BECOMES CRACK

The danger of using extremely flammable chemicals such as ether presents a major problem in making freebase. The solution is a technique that is simpler than freebase, called "dirty basing." Rather than extracting pure cocaine, the crude powder is simply dissolved in baking soda and water. The mixture is then boiled or put in a microwave oven to speed up the chemical reaction, after which it is removed and cooled quickly by putting it into a refrigerator or pan of ice water. The solid settles out at the bottom and is removed and dried. The result is a yellowish-white material that looks like pieces of soap or plaster. These can be broken into smaller chunks, usually about one tenth to one half of a gram. When these "rocks" are heated, they make a popping, cracking sound—hence the name, crack.

Crack appeared in 1985 as a simple, much cheaper way to get the benefits of freebase cocaine. A single rock, enough for a 15-minute buzz, could be bought for just a few dollars. Crack was actually more expensive than powder cocaine, but it seemed cheaper because it was sold and used in much smaller amounts. By 1986, crack use had become a full-blown epidemic.

 1.8% of the U.S. population over age 12 has used crack.

Crack created a wave of fear in the United States. Until crack came along, hard drug use was limited by its high cost and the risk of disease. The public has always tolerated a limited amount of drug abuse, especially when it is largely restricted to the eccentric, wealthy, or politically well-connected. But crack pushed the limits of this tolerance. It was too close to home. It was cheap, did not require needle injection (avoiding hepatitis or AIDS), did not use flammable liquids such as ether, and it could be easily hidden or stored. Crack was a low-cost, highly addictive form of cocaine and it spread most rapidly into the inner city and minority neighborhoods.

The Government responded with severe penalties, about 100 times greater than those for possession or sale of an equivalent amount of powder cocaine. Current Federal sentencing guidelines stipulate that conviction for the sale of 5 grams of crack cocaine brings a minimum sentence of 5 years, but it takes the sale of 500 grams of powder cocaine for the same sentence.[3] In 1994 year, 3,588 defendants were sentenced under this regulation: 90 percent were black and 4 percent white.[4] Critics have pointed out that a local dealer (who is most often black) will likely serve more jail time for selling a small amount of crack than the regional supplier (who is most often white) who sold him larger amounts of powder cocaine.

Whether justified or not, crack is currently viewed as the single most worrisome illegal drug.

 Before his death with Diana, Princess of Wales in a car accident, Dodi Fayed was said to have spent $15,000 per week on cocaine, and many have speculated that the drug was a factor in the crash.[5]

Who is Using Cocaine?

Cocaine is one of the few drugs that is used by three completely different groups of people: traditional users, medical users, and recreational users. In the United States, only medical use under direction of an appropriately licensed physician is legal.

Yet another, entirely unrelated, use of coca involves the extraction of flavoring agents used in soft drinks. In 1994, the United States imported 730,000 pounds of coca leaf from Bolivia and Peru for this purpose.[6]

 On March 20, 1994, Vice-President Al Gore visited Bolivia. He was honored by a collar of coca leaves, the traditional welcome to the country.[7]

TRADITIONAL USE: COQUEROS

In South America, coca leaf chewing continues for dietary and ritual purposes, much as it has for thousands of years. It is legal in Bolivia and Peru, where it is used by millions of people. In La Paz, Bolivia, for example, coca is sold openly in the markets. One can also buy a number of products made from it, including coca tea (the national beverage, see *Chapter 5*), syrups, jam, chewing gum, and toothpastes.[8]

It is perhaps incorrect to refer to this as a type of cocaine use, because it is the complete leaf, rather than the isolated cocaine, that is used. Chewing coca leaf does not cause social problems, economic ruin, health problems, or addiction.[9]

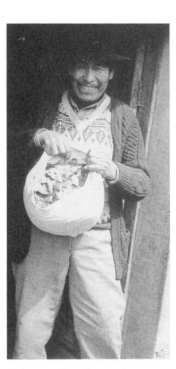

Bolivian seller of coca leaves

The inhabitants of South America are not immune to the psychoactive effects of coca, however. Coca paste (coca leaves mashed with alkali, kerosene, and sulfuric acid) is used as a recreational drug in many South American countries, where it is called *basulca*. This crude form is further refined to powder before shipment to the United States.

MEDICAL USE

Cocaine is listed as a Schedule II controlled substance, indicating that it has recognized medical use as well as a high abuse potential. Physicians use cocaine in the Emergency Department and for several types of surgery, particularly on the nose and throat. Every year, cocaine is used for about 200,000 such operations in the United States.

Some physicians prefer to use TAC (a combination of *t*etracaine, *a*drenaline, and 12 percent *c*ocaine) in a liquid applied to skin to anesthetize lacerations in children. It is much less frightening and painful than a needle injection.

Cocaine is also used to control severe chronic pain, usually in terminal illness. The combination of cocaine with morphine or methadone, a "Brompton's Cocktail," allows a greater dose of narcotic while the stimulating properties of cocaine preserve the patient's mental functioning.

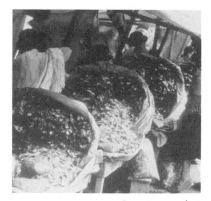

Peruvian market

RECREATIONAL USE

Recreational users of cocaine usually take it in one of three ways: snorting cocaine powder, smoking freebase or crack, or by intravenous injection of dissolved powder cocaine. Pure cocaine hydrochloride can also be absorbed through other mucous membranes, and some users apply it to the inside of the mouth, rectum, penis, or vagina.

 In a 1985 NIDA survey, 5% of employed people age 20 to 40 had used cocaine in the past month.

 It is estimated that Americans spend $32 billion a year on cocaine, but the true figure may be much higher.

Cocaine and crack are used by a wide spectrum of people in the United States—everyone from the poorest inhabitants of urban ghettos to major entertainment and political figures. Cocaine was reportedly used by current President George W. Bush, and crack was smoked by Washington, D.C., Mayor Marion Barry, even as he led rallies for schoolchildren against drugs. Professional athletes are especially drawn to it because of the intense stimulation and feelings of power.

 "Cocaine often stirs feelings of hatred and aggression. Some athletes rely on it to get them into the proper 'kill-or-be-killed' state of mind."[10]

About 75 percent of cocaine users snort it. To get a more intense effect, cocaine addicts may progress to smoking (either freebase or crack) or intravenous injection.

Snorted cocaine is prepared by pouring a small quantity of the powder on a smooth surface such as a mirror. A sharp-edged tool, such as a credit card or razor blade, is used to chop the larger chunks into a fine, uniform powder. The powder is then formed into thin lines, sometimes called rails, about an eighth inch wide and one to two inches long. An average line of relatively pure material contains 10 to 35 milligrams of cocaine. The drug is snorted by holding a tube, such as a straw or rolled up dollar bill, to one nostril and sniffing as the tube is moved along the line. Cocaine is also sometimes snorted from a tiny "coke spoon" held up to the nostril.

Cocaine numbers in the United States[11]

3,000,000	Occasional users (less than monthly) This is down from 8.1 million in 1985
1,300,000	Used cocaine in last month
582,000	Weekly users (mostly crack) About the same as in the 1980s

THE COLOMBIAN CARTELS

About 35 percent of the world's coca leaf is grown in Colombia, mostly in the southern rain forests and eastern lowlands of the country, in the Departments of Guaviare, Caqueta, and Putumayo. The remainder is cultivated in the neighboring countries, particularly Bolivia and Peru. Because coca leaf is cultivated only in one region of the world, the cocaine trade is dominated by relatively small groups of traffickers in tightly knit cartels.

The cartels control the movement of coca leaf and paste from the jungles of Bolivia and Peru to the large cocaine conversion laboratories in southern Colombia. This area is under the military control of insurgents and beyond the reach of Colombian Government forces, who face tremendous difficulty in stopping the drug trade.

Cocaine conversion laboratories range from small "family" operations, to large facilities employing dozens of workers. Once cocaine hydrochloride is manufactured, it is shipped to Mexico, or the Caribbean Islands, and on to the real market—the United States. The most common entry points are Puerto Rico, Miami, and New York, accounting for about one third of the imported cocaine. The remainder is smuggled across the lengthy U.S.-Mexico border.

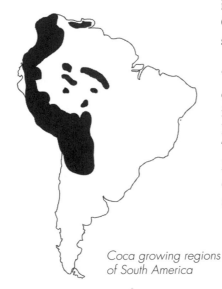

Coca growing regions of South America

FROM FIELD TO FLAKE: THE MAKING OF COCAINE

The majority of coca leaf is grown in small, family plots. The cash crop is often grown along with other vegetables and provides a much-needed source of income for poor farmers. The farmers themselves are seldom involved in the coca trade and only sell the fresh leaves.

The development process begins when the leaves are dried and taken to a "pasta" lab, which is usually located in the growing region. The leaves are shredded or mashed and dumped into a pit. Water and a strong alkali, such as lime, are added to dissolve the leaves and release the cocaine. This maceration pit can be as small as a plastic bucket or steel drum, or as large as a 40-foot long plastic-lined pit. The whole mixture is left to soak for a few days, after which a solvent such as kerosene or gasoline is added to further dissolve the cocaine.

Sulfuric acid is then added to the mixture. This causes the cocaine to bind to the sulfuric acid and precipitate as cocaine sulfate. The cocaine sulfate is filtered out and dried, forming a crude cake-like form of cocaine known as *pasta* ("paste").

The paste is normally transported to Colombia for further processing in a "base" lab. There, it is dissolved in water. Sulfuric acid and potassium permanganate are added to remove impurities, and an alkali is added to precipitate the cocaine. The cocaine once again is filtered out of the solution and dried, and is now known as *basulca* ("base").

For further processing, the cocaine base is shipped to a "crystal lab," usually still in Colombia. There, the cocaine is first dissolved in acetone, and then hydrochloric acid, which converts the cocaine base to cocaine hydrochloride. Ethanol is then added to precipitate the cocaine hydrochloride,

Spreading out coca leaves to dry, before further processing

After drying, the leaves are placed in a plastic-lined maceration pit to release the cocaine

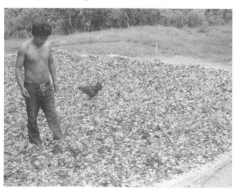

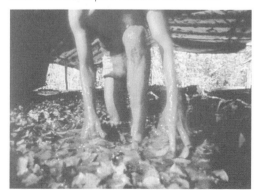

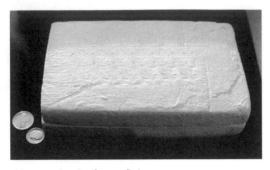

Kilogram brick of pure flake cocaine

which is filtered out and dried. The resulting "flake" cocaine hydrochloride can be snorted or dissolved in water and injected intravenously.

The cartels typically ship cocaine hydrochloride with a purity of up to 90 percent, but professional quality control in the jungle labs is unknown. Under the pressure of an illegal operation, shortcuts may be taken to speed up production, resulting in an off-color, less pure product.

The output of these primitive labs is tremendous: the U.S. Government estimates the potential cocaine production in Peru, Bolivia, and Colombia at about 2,200,000 lbs per year. The majority of this is destined for American consumption.

From coca to cocaine[12]

Coca leaves (chewed) less than 2 percent cocaine

➔   *Kerosene, sulfuric acid, alkali*

Coca paste (occasionally smoked) 20 to 85 percent cocaine

➔   *hydrochloric acid*

Cocaine hydrochloride (snorted, injected) 90 percent cocaine

➔   *baking soda*   ➔   *ether or acetone*

Crack (smoked)   Freebase cocaine (smoked)
95 percent cocaine   95 percent cocaine

ECONOMICS OF CRACK

Crack is about 75 to 90 percent cocaine. Pure powder cocaine is actually a combination of cocaine and hydrochloric acid. This makes it water-soluble. When the hydrochloric acid is removed, the powder is no longer water-soluble and forms the waxy, rock-like material of crack. With the loss of the hydrochloride component, one gram of pure cocaine will convert to an average of 0.89 gram of crack cocaine.

Crack is broken into rocks, which may be sold individually on the street for $5 to $20. Crack is usually smoked in a glass pipe fitted with a fine mesh screen on which the rock is placed. The smoker heats the side of the pipe bowl with a flame and the heat causes the cocaine base to vaporize. Some users sprinkle crack into cigarettes to smoke it. The result is a small, brief dose of very pure cocaine.

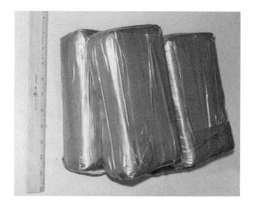

Confiscated kilos of powder cocaine

From $50 to $50,000: the economics of a pound of crack cocaine[13]

Harvesting: In Bolivia one 100 lb cargo of leaves costs about $50
↘
  Refining: After refining in South America, one pound of powder is about $500
  ↘
    Shipping: Shippers charge American connections about $5,000 per pound
    ↘
      Wholesaling: In the United States, imported cocaine is resold
                 in 1-ounce packets, about $15,000 per pound
      ↘
        Retailing: Converted to crack, a pound broken into rocks
                 is about $50,000, or $100,000 if diluted.

Pure coke?

Virtually all cocaine comes from leaves grown and processed in South America. As the leaves are processed into coca paste, and the paste refined, impurities may enter the product. Once the cocaine reaches the United States, it is usually diluted with cheaper substitutes. While the average import purity of cocaine is about 83 percent, by the time it gets to the street, the average purity has dropped to about 61 percent. The remainder consists of other white powders, such as cornstarch, talcum powder, lactose, or mannitol. Sometimes, dealers will add specific substances to fool users into believing that they are getting the pure stuff. Caffeine and amphetamines mimic the stimulating effects of cocaine. Inexpensive and easily obtained anesthetic drugs such as lidocaine or procaine will give a similar numbing sensation.

It is possible to remove some of these impurities by "washing" the cocaine in acetone.[14] The acetone does not dissolve cocaine but it does dissolve many of the more common substances used to cut cocaine. An acetone wash is performed by mixing cocaine with acetone in a glass container and pouring the solution through filter paper. The acetone and the dissolved impurities will flow through the paper but the cocaine collects on the filter and is allowed to dry. The process can be repeated, further improving purity each time. Acetone also removes the yellowish color present in much cocaine, and results in a much whiter substance.

Sophisticated cocaine buyers have a number of ways to check the purity of the product:

Appearance
Cocaine hydrochloride appears in four basic forms: liquid, powder, flake, and rock (not to be confused with rocks of crack). Liquid cocaine is generally only sold for medical use, and is very pure. Flake and rock cocaine are also very pure, but seldom found on the street. It is difficult to dilute them without altering their look. Pure cocaine has an iridescent, pearly, light-scattering appearance. This is noticeably different from the diluting powders, which tend to be a plain, dull white.

Taste
When a small amount is put on the tongue, pure cocaine has a slight chemical taste and causes a gradual numbing. Anesthetics such as lidocaine and procaine cause a stronger, more immediate numbing, and other diluting substances may have a different taste altogether.

Feel
When a small amount of pure cocaine is rubbed between the thumb and forefinger, it will dissolve smoothly and quickly. Other substances will not dissolve so readily, or feel gritty.

Foil or flame test
When pure cocaine is placed on a sheet of aluminum foil and held over a flame, it will melt and vaporize, leaving an amber-colored residue.

Water, Clorox, and methanol tests
Because cocaine is water-soluble, it will dissolve immediately when mixed with water. Most of the other substances used to cut cocaine are less water- soluble, or do not dissolve at all. The same is true of cocaine dissolved in Clorox bleach or methanol.

Hotbox test

Cocaine hydrochloride melts at the very specific temperature of 187° Celsius. In comparison, lidocaine melts at 127°, lactose at 203°, and baking soda at 270°. A hotbox can be used to determine not only what other substances are present, but their relative amounts (see *Chapter 6: Testing Drug Purity*). This simple apparatus can be used to establish the purity within five percent.

Chemical Characteristics

The intensity of the psychological effects of cocaine depends on how quickly, and how much of, the drug reaches the brain. Snorted cocaine reaches the brain in one to three minutes and produces a high that lasts for half an hour or so. Intravenous injection of cocaine takes only 15 to 30 seconds to produce its effect, which peaks in 3 to 5 minutes and lasts for 15 to 20 minutes. Smoking is even faster, producing an effect within 10 seconds and a peak in 3 to 5 minutes, which lasts about 15 minutes. Because the high of smoked cocaine is so short and intense, it is especially addictive.

Cocaine has both euphoric and stimulating properties, much like the amphetamines, but they do not last long. There is increased alertness, excitation, and a feeling of confidence and well-being. There is also an increased pulse rate and blood pressure, insomnia, and a loss of appetite. The euphoric effect is often followed by a dysphoric crash—a disagreeable feeling of fatigue, depression, and anxiety. To avoid this, another dose is usually taken; and the cycle continues until the supply of cocaine is used up.

Animal research on the effects of cocaine demonstrates the strength of the addiction. Most animals will not willingly take dangerous amounts of alcohol, nicotine, or heroin, but once the animals are familiar with cocaine they will take it until they kill themselves. When rats and monkeys, for example, are trained to press a lever to deliver an intravenous dose of cocaine, they will keep pressing the lever up to 300 times just to get a single injection. If the animals are given free access to cocaine, they will keep taking it until they collapse in convulsions. Humans are not much different.

Both the euphoric and addictive properties of cocaine come from stimulating the D_1 dopamine receptors in the mesolimbic part of the brain. This part of the brain produces short changes in mood and is active in the stimulant-reward cycle, and is therefore considered to be responsible for addictive behavior (see *Chapter 6*).[15] Cocaine also interferes with the normal re-uptake of norepinephrine, serotonin, and dopamine at the nucleus accumbens, so that these neurotransmitters are increased and intensely stimulate this "pleasure center" of the brain.

When cocaine is smoked, as freebase or crack, it is broken down into a number of combustion products, including methyl-4-(3-pyridyl) benzoate isomers of anhydro-ecgonine methyl ester (AEME). AEME is related to N-ethyl-3-piperidyl benzilate and N-methyl-3-piperidyl benzilate, both of which are classified as hallucinogenic substances under Schedule I of the Controlled Substances Act. It appears, therefore, that smoked cocaine has psychological effects that go beyond snorted powder cocaine. The effects of these burned forms of cocaine are not completely understood.

Usually the only thing that stops a serious addict during a binge is running out of cocaine.[16]

COCAINE AND ALCOHOL

When cocaine and alcohol are used together, a new chemical, cocaethylene (cocaine and ethanol), is formed in the liver.[17] This compound crosses the blood-brain barrier and produces a longer and more intensely euphoric high.[18] Cocaethylene stimulates the brain's D_1 dopamine receptors more effectively than cocaine alone, and intensifies addiction and withdrawal symptoms.

The risk of sudden death is 25 times greater in those who abuse both alcohol and cocaine than in those who use only cocaine.[19]

TESTING FOR COCAINE

Once absorbed into the bloodstream, cocaine is quickly and almost completely metabolized by liver and plasma enzymes. The major metabolic products are benzoyl-ecgonine and ecgonine methyl ester, along with a small amount of norcocaine. These metabolites are excreted into the urine along with a fraction (less than one percent) of non-metabolized cocaine.

Drug testing for cocaine looks for these metabolites as well as actual cocaine. The metabolite benzoyl-ecgonine has the longest biologic half-life (the time it takes to reduce the concentration in the body by half) and can be detected in the urine for up to three days after a single dose. It does not significantly accumulate in the body, meaning that any benzoyl-ecgonine detected in the urine suggests recent use and is not the result of heavy use a long time ago.[20]

Half-lives of cocaine metabolites in the body

benzoyl-ecgonine	7.5 hours
ecgonine methyl ester	3.6 hours
cocaine	1.5 hours

Extensive contact of bare skin with cocaine can result in low urine concentrations of benzoyl-ecognine. One study reported a concentration of 72 ng/mL in an individual 12 hours after the person had handled money that had been immersed in coca paste.[21] This amount was not enough to make the person test positive under the Federal drug testing guidelines, but it does show that cocaine can be absorbed in other ways beside deliberate use.

Medical cocaine is restricted to clinical procedures and is not given to a patient by prescription. The use of cocaine as a topical anesthetic can lead to positive urine test results. In this case, the physician performing the procedure should document the application of cocaine in the patient's medical record. Topical "caine" anesthetics such as procaine (Novocaine), lidocaine (Xylocaine), bupivacaine (Marcaine), and benzocaine (Cetacaine) have no structural similarity to cocaine or its metabolites and do not cause cocaine-positive drug test results.

A small amount of cocaine is excreted in semen. This excuse has even been used by some creative people to explain how they managed to test positive for the drug. However, the amount of absorbed cocaine from exposure to semen from a cocaine-using male partner is not enough to cause positive drug results when the Federal cutoff values are used.[22]

Withdrawal Signs

Like all stimulants, the longer cocaine is used, the more the user needs to achieve the same level of excitement and euphoria. In the meantime, the unpleasant effects of anxiety, insomnia, and overall discomfort begin to accumulate. Long-term users say that although cocaine no longer produces much of a "high," they still cannot stay away from it. There is a persistent, unsettling sense of craving the drug.

Withdrawal from cocaine produces the opposite of the high. After a cocaine binge, the user has feelings of apathy, irritability, depression, and disorientation. He or she may sleep for long periods, be lethargic and drowsy, ravenously hungry, and have vivid dreams. These symptoms usually abate in a few days or weeks.

Physical signs of withdrawal include muscular aches, abdominal pain, chills, tremors, and complete exhaustion. Abrupt withdrawal from a long binge can cause the "Cocaine Washout Syndrome"—a state of decreased consciousness to the extent that the user can be aroused only after vigorous stimulation, and even then may be too exhausted even to speak or make any movement.[23]

Cocaine withdrawal phases[24]

Phase	Time	Symptoms
Initial crash	immediately after binge	Dysphoria, depression, anxiety, and agitation
Middle crash	1 to 4 hours after binge	Craving is replaced by desire for sleep
Late crash	3 to 4 days after binge	Increased appetite and constant sleepiness
Craving	6 to 18 weeks later	Depression, lethargy, and lack of ability to feel pleasure
Recovery	months to years later	Gradual return of mood, interest in environment, and ability to experience pleasure; gradual loss of craving episodes.

Long-term Health Problems

Cocaine affects virtually every part of the body, and long-term use can cause a number of problems, ranging from minor irritations to fatal injuries. Long-term snorting of cocaine can result in stomach ulcers or damage to the intestines, but the most common problems are as follows:

Percent complaints of hotline callers to 1-800-COCAINE[25]

85% Severe depression
78% Irritability
65% Chest congestion
65% Paranoia
58% Loss of sexual desire
40% Memory lapses
40% Chronic cough
31% Violent behavior
18% Suicide attempts
 7% Seizures with loss of consciousness

COCAINE NOSE

Powder cocaine is an effective vasoconstrictor, shrinking the small blood vessels. While this effect is medically useful to stop bleeding, overuse of cocaine starves the tissues of blood and causes a chronic irritation leading to ulcers. Snorting damages the nasal tissues. The telltale runny nose of the "horner" is due to irritation of the mucous membranes lining the nose. Prolonged snorting leads to nasal ulcers and a perforated septum.

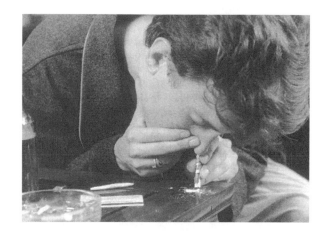

Use of powder cocaine on any other mucosal area will cause the same ulcers as in the nose. For example, some cocaine users apply the powder to the inside of the penis believing that it will enhance sexual performance. The result can be necrosis and even amputation of the penis.

 Police used to finger the nose of a suspected cocaine addict—if he screamed in pain, it was an obvious giveaway.

COCAINE LUNGS

Smoking crack or freebase can cause bleeding in the lungs when the small blood vessels burst. Many crack smokers develop a cough and chest pain that worsens with deep breathing. They may cough up phlegm that is black or tinged with blood. Both powder cocaine and crack can also cause the lungs to fill with fluid (pulmonary edema) from injury to the small vessels lining the air sacs.

Crack smokers are sometimes identified by the "Cocaine Callus"—a thick, hard skin on the inner right thumb from constant rubbing on the serrated wheel of a lighter.

COCAINE AND THE HEART

Cocaine has dramatic, even fatal, effects on the heart. Even mild cocaine use may cause palpitations—an awareness of the heart beat, or sense of a skipped beat.

Cocaine increases the effect of the natural stimulants in the body. In the heart, cocaine increases the cellular production of norepinephrine and inhibits its reabsorption, flooding the tissues with this stimulating hormone.[26] The result is an accelerated pulse and increased blood pressure. Sustained high levels of norepinephrine can cause inflammation of the heart.

Cocaine also has a direct vasoconstrictive effect on vascular smooth muscle, including the heart. It not only shrinks the blood vessels supplying the heart, but some researchers believe that it injures the heart muscle directly— it kills the heart muscle cells. Chronic use of cocaine may therefore lead to myocardial fibrosis, a condition in which the normal heart muscle is replaced by fibrous tissue, resulting in constriction bands on the heart so that it can no longer pump effectively.

Both cocaine and marijuana increase the heart rate. Taking the two together can increase it up to fifty beats per minute.[27]

Cocaine causes clumping of blood platelets as well (by increased thromboxane production) and blood clots (by a temporary depletion of protein C and antithrombin III).

All of these effects can cause heart muscle damage, an irregular heart beat, and make chronic users much more likely to suffer a heart attack.

At 22 years of age, Len Bias was an outstanding basketball star and the All American choice at the University of Maryland. In June 1986, he was drafted by the Boston Celtics, the NBA champions at the time. His future looked brilliant. Minutes after smoking freebase cocaine, possibly for the first time, he was dead of a massive heart attack.

COCAINE AND THE BRAIN

Chronic users of cocaine often develop a peculiar habit of little spastic jerks. These multifocal tics are thought to be due to the effect of cocaine on the brain's dopamine production.

The theory of the cause of these tics is as follows:

Chronic use of cocaine causes a depletion of pre-synaptic dopamine. This results in an increased sensitivity of the post-synaptic dopamine receptors, as they try to make up for the shortage. A cocaine binge then floods the synapse with dopamine causing the neurons to be overwhelmed, and resulting in the chaotic muscle spasms known as multifocal tics.[28]

COCAINE PARANOIA

The psychological hazards of cocaine were noticed over a century ago, and led to the drug becoming illegal. The degree of addiction and psychosis depended on the way in which cocaine was used. When cocaine was drunk as a wine, long-term users complained of exhaustion, lethargy, and mental depression. Increasing refinement of the drug led to more dramatic psychological problems. In South America, smoking coca paste led to a distinctive psychosis called the "coca paste syndrome," characterized by dysphoria, hallucinations, and paranoia.

With the development of powder cocaine, paranoid psychosis became a common feature of long-term users. The delusions can be extreme, with wild hallucinations and irrational behavior. A peculiar characteristic of the cocaine psychosis is formication, the hallucination that ants, insects, or snakes are crawling on or under the skin. People have used a knife or tweezers to cut out the "coke bugs" or "snow bugs." Long-term users have even bled to death in an attempt to escape the imagined infestation.

 Sigmund Freud was an early enthusiast of cocaine, calling it a "magical drug" and "cure-all." He later turned against it when he saw the paranoid psychosis it caused in his friend.

COCAINE BABIES

Two to three percent of all women who give birth, and up to 30 percent of women in some inner-city hospitals, have used cocaine during their pregnancy. These women tend to have poor access to health care, and most of them also smoke cigarettes and drink alcohol, so it is difficult to isolate the effects of cocaine on the health of the baby.

Many cocaine-exposed babies are born prematurely and with low birth weight. These infants tend to be jittery, cranky, and overly sensitive to any form of sensory stimulus. A few have experienced strokes even before they were born. Cocaine use can cause a premature separation of the placenta from the uterus, a condition that can cut off the baby's blood supply and result in brain damage or death.

What To Do If There Is An Overdose

An overdose of cocaine may cause seizures, respiratory failure, stroke, cerebral hemorrhage or heart failure. Death can result from any of these. There is no specific antidote for cocaine overdose.

It is impossible to determine the amount of cocaine needed for an overdose; it can be caused by snorting as little as one fiftieth of a gram. Between two and ten percent of those taken to the hospital for a cocaine overdose have seizures, which can occur as long as 12 hours later. Seizures can happen at any time, with the first use, the twentieth, or the hundredth, and will eventually strike most users.[29]

Cocaine is sometimes used in combination with heroin or other opiates, because the edginess caused by the first is mellowed by the dreamy effects of the second. The combination can be especially dangerous. People who are taking cocaine normally back off on their use when the jitteriness gets too great, but in the presence of heroin the shaky feelings are not so obvious and they tend to take more cocaine, increasing the risk of an overdose. On the other hand, heroin users who would normally back off when they feel they have had enough sedation might take more because of the stimulation from cocaine, resulting in a heroin overdose.

John Belushi, the star of *Saturday Night Live*, died at age 33 in the Chateau Marmont Hotel on March 5, 1982. He had been injected with heroin and cocaine 20 times that day by his girlfriend, who later went to prison for involuntary manslaughter.

One cause of heart attacks in cocaine users has been called the "Sex-Cocaine Syndrome." The surge in heart rate during intercourse combined with cocaine can cause an irregular heart beat, heart failure, and death.

Physical signs of overdose[30]	Fever
	Rapid or irregular heart beat
	Shallow breathing
	High blood pressure
	Enlarged pupils
	Dry mouth
	Sweating
	Tremors
	Stroke
	Heart failure

Mental signs of overdose	Confusion
	Agitation
	Paranoia
	Hallucinations
	Impulsive behavior
	Hyperactivity
	Unresponsive coma

With any sign of cocaine overdose, the user should be taken immediately to a hospital. Monitoring may be required even if the person appears to have recovered, since seizures can occur hours later.

In the hospital, cocaine users may be checked for signs of other toxic drugs. Crack or powder cocaine is sometimes cut with arsenic. The user may experience nausea, vomiting, diarrhea, and neuropathy (a loss of strength or feeling in the limbs). Cocaine may also be laced with phenytoin, an anti-convulsant. If there is lethargy, nystagmus, or ataxia, it may be useful to get a blood phenytoin level.

A cocaine abuser will probably be kept in the hospital until he or she is past the early withdrawal stage. There are several standard detoxification protocols, including medications such as bromocriptine (Parlodel) and desipramine (Norpramin or Pertofane).[31] Psychotic reactions may be treated with haloperidol (Haldol).

DMT, Bufotenine, and Psilocybin

DMT, dimethyltryptamine, is an intensely visual hallucinogen that is found in many substances, including trees, vines, grasses, mushrooms, and the venom of a large toad. Chemically synthesized DMT was briefly popular as a recreational drug in the 1960s.

Bufotenine is a non-psychoactive variant of DMT first discovered in toad venom. It was made illegal because of a mistaken concern that it might become a drug of abuse.

Psilocybin is a variant of DMT found in hallucinogenic mushrooms. It was used for thousands of years for religious purposes and now is popular as a relatively safe recreational drug.

The Basic Facts

Type of drug	*Hallucinogen*
How taken	*Smoked, ingested, injected*
Duration of effect	
DMT	*1 hour*
Bufotenine	*4 to 12 hours*
Psilocybin	*3 to 6 hours*
Physical danger	*Low*
Addiction potential	*None*

Other Names

Alpha-ethyltryptamine	*alpha-ET, love pearls, love pills*
Bufotenine	*toad, yopo*
DMT	*AMT, businessman's high, fantasia*
Psilocybin	*Alice, boomers, hombrecitos, las mujercitas, magic mushrooms, musk, shrooms*

Businessman's High: The Story of DMT

On the second voyage of Columbus to the New World, his naturalist, the friar Ramón Paul, reported a strange new drug. He described how the Tairo Indians of what is now Haiti used a snuff to communicate with the spirit world.

 "This powder they draw up through the nose and it intoxicates them to such an extent that when they are under its influence, they know not what they do."— Ramón Paul [1]

The snuff was called *cohoba*, used throughout Central and South America, and made from seeds of the yopo tree (*Anadenantherea peregrina*). The main psychoactive components of this snuff were identified in 1955 as DMT (N,N-dimethyl-tryptamine) and 5-methoxy-DMT, chemicals which had first been synthesized in 1931. DMT and related hallucinogenic compounds were soon found to be widespread in nature: present in trees, vines, grasses, mushrooms, toads, and even moth larvae, grubs, and fish. [2]

DMT was synthesized and illicitly manufactured in the 1960s, when it became a popular recreational drug. Unlike LSD and other hallucinogens, DMT is quickly destroyed by stomach acids and is ineffective if taken by mouth. When smoked or injected, it produces a very brief experience lasting no more than 15 to 30 minutes. Users could have a wild psychedelic trip but get back to normal a half hour later. They called it the "businessman's high."

 "Initiates, after taking a toke, have often started to say they weren't feeling anything and then suddenly become silent in mid-sentence." [3]

DMT hallucinations typically are described as a visual pattern of overlapping small rhomboid elements in vivid hues of red, yellow, green, and blue, sometimes referred to as the "chrysanthemum pattern." [4] The overall experience is much more intense than that of most other hallucinogens. Even veteran drug users such as Allen Ginsburg and Richard Alpert (who gained notoriety for his popularization of LSD), found DMT to be too powerful and uncontrollable for enjoyment. Many users would later say that they had had "the most terrifying three minutes of my life." Some reported a feeling that they were melting or fusing into the floor, that their heart was stopping, or that their life-force was ebbing away.

By the 1970s, DMT had fallen out of favor among recreational drug users. It is now rarely found; the few illicit samples available usually prove to be LSD.

Who Is Using DMT?

In its pure form, DMT is sold as a white powder that smells like mothballs. If it has not been completely purified, it may have a tan or brownish color, or an orange, waxy appearance. When smoked in pipes or mixed with marijuana, it is reported to taste and smell like burning plastic. A single inhalation is usually enough to produce a five- or ten-minute intense hallucinatory experience.

The usual dose is 20 to 50 mg, injected or smoked, although as little as 5 mg will have a significant effect. A dose of 75 mg or more will result in a loss of consciousness.

Very little synthetic DMT is available on the black market, and it appears to have been replaced by the milder, natural forms of DMT such as are found in hallucinogenic mushrooms.

A number of other hallucinogens similar to DMT have been synthesized, including the somewhat less potent DET (N,N-diethyltryptamine), AET (alpha-ethyltryptamine)[5] and DPT (N,N-dipropyltryptamine). These are rarely available on the black market and are not in common use.

Smoking Toad: The Story of Bufotenine

Bufotenine is a compound found in a number of South American plants and in secretions from the many species of Bufo toads. It is a form of DMT (5-hydroxy-DMT) that in itself is not hallucinogenic, probably because it does not cross the blood-brain barrier. However, bufotenine may be changed by combustion or other preparation to a form of DMT that is hallucinogenic.

Bufotenine was first isolated in the 1950s from *Bufo marinus*, a toad with some very peculiar characteristics.[6] This toad, the world's largest, lives in marshy areas in the southern United States from Mexico to Florida, and down through the Caribbean coastlands to South America. It measures about ten inches across and weighs up to seven pounds. The toad has no teeth, cannot breathe with its mouth open, and periodically sheds its skin. It is also known for its bizarre mating habits. A group of frenzied males may completely cover a single female and attempt to copulate with her even after she is dead and decomposed.

The *Bufo* toad has large parotid glands at the back of its head, secreting a thick, milky venom. In addition to bufotenine, toad venom also has at least 25 other biologically active compounds, including bufotoxin and bufogenin, which are not hallucinogenic but highly toxic.

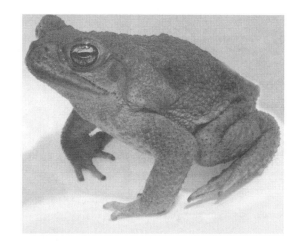

TOXINS AND TOADSTOOLS

The fact that DMT is found in both mushrooms and toads is reflected in many languages and cultural associations, from the Chinese *ha-ma-chun* ("toad mushroom"), the French *pain de crapaud* ("toad's bread"), the Norwegian *paddehut* ("toad's hat") and, of course, toadstool, the English word for poisonous mushroom, which first appeared in 1398.[7]

Toads around the world have been known to have drugs in their skin, and these have long been used for medicines. By boiling the toad in olive oil, the skin secretions could be skimmed off and concentrated. Historically, extracts from toads were used in Europe and China as remedies for a number of sores and illnesses, including toothache, sinus and gum inflammations.

 "Classical German violinists used to handle toads before their performances because the toxins reduced the sweat on their palms." [8]

Toad extracts were also valued as poisons, and used in witches' potions. The poisonous power of toad venom was believed to be so potent that it was even mixed with gunpowder and added to cannon shells. In 17th-century England, traveling salesmen sold medicines that could protect against toad poison. To demonstrate the effectiveness of their product, they would have an assistant swallow a live toad. The term "toad swallower" eventually degenerated to "toady" meaning a creepy person willing to do anything for the boss.[9]

MAYAN TOAD STATUES

The ancient use of toad extracts was apparently common in the Americas as well. By the time of the Spanish conquest of Central America, the Mayan civilization had long passed into history. However, from their myths, carved drawings, and the many statues of toads, it was clear that they held the toad in special regard. Speculation that the Maya might have used the toad in religious intoxications was borne out when anthropologists discovered remains of *Bufo marinus* in their sacred sites.

The Maya may have had the most prolific toad art, but they were not the only ancient Americans to use toads. The Olmec and even older central American cultures showed a worship of toads as long ago as 2000 BC. Toads were also widely used in North America. A Cherokee Indian burial site in South Carolina revealed the skeletal remains of 10,000 toads.

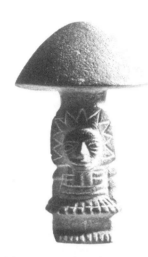

Mayan sacred mushroom statue, often found with toad icons

The fact that toads do not have much nutritional value, and most of the art suggests a more religious use, indicates that these people were well aware of the hallucinogenic property of the venom. But how could they ingest it without also suffering from the other toxins in the toad secretions? Some anthropologists suggest that the Mayans fed the toad to ducks, which can eat them safely, and then ate the duck meat. This method of using an animal intermediary to remove toxic compounds is not unique: Siberian shamans would feed *Amanita* mushrooms to deer, and then eat the deer meat, or drink the deer urine, to appreciate the hallucinogenic effects while avoiding the mushroom toxins. In any event, it is not certain how the Maya used *Bufo marinus*, but this has not stopped others from experimenting with the toad secretions.

TOAD LICKING IN AUSTRALIA

In 1935, the *Bufo marinus* toad was introduced to Australia in the hope that it would consume the greyback beetles which were destroying the sugarcane fields. As it turned out, one of the few things in Australia that the toads did not eat was this beetle. Cane toads, as they came to be called, turned into an enormous pest themselves, littering the lawns and roads with their carcasses, and poisoning local animals that mouthed them.

The 1960s saw a confluence of an interest in psychedelic drugs, a tremendous popularization of anthropology, and a discovery of ancient mind-altering practices. Bufotenine came to attention as a possible source of DMT. An Australian newspaper jokingly reported that toad slime was hallucinogenic and young people had taken to toad licking when other drugs were not available. In a bizarre development, the story inspired a few Australians to try licking live toads.[10] The Australian Government responded by making cane toad slime an illegal substance under their Drug Misuse Act. This only encouraged even more people to try it, thinking that, if the Government banned it, it *had* to be good. The practice spread to the United States, where the Haight Ashbury Clinic reported that a few people had become violently ill from licking live toads,[11] and the U.S. Government followed by making bufotenine illegal in 1967.

 "Inevitably, reality imitated fiction"—Scientific American, review of toad licking

Toad smoking in America

Anyone who tried toad licking quickly discovered that a government ban was hardly necessary—all they got out of it was intense drooling, frightening heart palpitations, and a splitting headache.

Not easily deterred, the "toad kissers" experimented with another method: smoking the secretions. The heat of combustion, they discovered, destroys some of the dangerous chemicals while keeping the hallucinogenic ones, and even increases the overall intoxication by allowing more rapid absorption through the lungs. In the 1980s, toad smoking developed a small following. They preferred a different species, *Bufo alvarius*, found only in the Sonoran Desert from southeastern California to Arizona and northern Mexico, and more commonly known as the Colorado River toad. Not much notice had been taken of this toad before, because it hides in the sand and only appears with the summer rains. It is, however, commonly available from pet stores. The Colorado River toad glands secrete a milky white venom, which turns to brown as it dries, containing at least 26 biologically active compounds. It is also unique among other *Bufo* species because its venom has an enzyme, O-methyl-transferase, which converts bufotenine into 5-MeO-DMT, one of the most potent hallucinogens known. Up to 15 percent of the dry weight of the Colorado River toad parotid glands may be 5-MeO-DMT.

Smoking toad, however, proved to be too powerful an experience for most people. Besides the obvious difficulty of getting and handling the toad, the intoxication was too intense, with too many physical side effects, to achieve any real popularity.

 "I can't imagine why anyone would do it [to get high]. It's just too heavy. It's too harsh physically."—psychedelic drug researcher Tom Lyttle

Who Is Using Bufotenine?

Bufotenine, an illegal Schedule I substance, is not psychoactive and is not a recreational drug. The secretions from Colorado River toads contain a variant of bufotenine, 5-MeO-DMT. This substance is legal, and is occasionally used as a recreational hallucinogen. In 1984, Albert Most revealed his methods of milking the toad secretions, drying them, and smoking them.[12] He formed The Church of The Toad of Light to justify his use in a manner similar to the religious consumption of peyote. This informal "church" was never legally recognized and has all but disappeared.

"There's not much of a street market for it."—High Times Magazine

For the few adventurous individuals willing to use 5-MeO-DMT, the process begins with collecting the toad venom. A mature Colorado River toad, *Bufo alvarius*, can be purchased from pet shops for about $50. The parotid glands at the back of the head are gently squeezed and the venom scraped onto a glass surface. Great care must to be taken in handling the venom, as it is quite toxic. The expressed venom is allowed to dry, turning from an off-white color to light brown.

The venom powder is then smoked, either by vaporizing it in a glass pipe with a flame, or by sprinkling it in parsley or marijuana and smoking the mixture.

The legal status of the toad or 5-MeO-DMT is questionable and varies from state to state. Although possession of the toad is legal, in general, extraction of the venom could be a criminal offense under laws forbidding use as a psychoactive analog. In the same way, 5-MeO-DMT is not specifically forbidden but could be considered illegal as an analog of DMT.

In 1994, a 41-year-old teacher was arrested in California with several Bufo specimens. He was the first person to be charged with possessing a toad for illicit purposes since 1579, when a British woman was declared a witch and executed.[13]

Magic Mushrooms: The Story of Psilocybin

Psilocybin is a hallucinogen found in three genera of mushrooms, *Psilocybe*, *Panaeolus*, and *Conocybe*, with a total of about 100 different species.[14] The most commonly used species in the United States are *Psilocybe mexicana*, *Psilocybe cyanescens* (often called "wavy caps," and reputedly the most potent of the many psilocybe varieties), and the closely related *Stropharia cubensis* (often listed as *Psilocybe cubensis*).

In North America, there is evidence that psilocybin-containing mushrooms were used for ritual purposes as long ago as 1000 BC. The first recorded use was by the Aztecs for the coronation of Montezuma in 1502. They called it *Teonanacatl*, the divine flesh. Dr. Francisco Hernandez, the personal physician to the King of Spain, wrote that three kinds of narcotic mushrooms were worshipped and "when eaten cause an uncontrolled laughter ... and others which bring before the eyes all kinds of things, such as the likeness of demons."

The use of hallucinogenic mushrooms was little known and largely confined to esoteric shamanic practices until 1953. Then, interest was kindled by the research of R. Gordon Wasson, a wealthy New York banker fascinated by mushroom lore. His extensive discoveries included evidence of the ritual use of psychoactive mushrooms throughout European, Asian, and North American history, going back 10,000 years (see *Chapter 2*), and

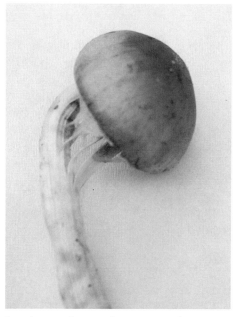

Stropharia cubensis, the most popular hallucinogenic mushroom, purchased legally in Amsterdam

continuing up to the present in Mexican mushroom cults. Wasson may have contributed to the burgeoning interest in hallucinogens in the 1960s, and led to their widespread popularity in the drug culture. Albert Hofmann, the discoverer of LSD, was intrigued by Wasson's reports, and analyzed the Mexican mushroom to extract psilocybin and psilocin. His employer, the pharmaceutical firm Sandoz, manufactured synthetic psilocybin for psychiatric use and marketed it as Indocybin until 1965, when it became illegal.

 Psilocybin comes from the Greek words "psilo" (bald) and "cybe" (head). Looking for a catchy title for a cover story, a *LIFE* Magazine editor called it the Magic Mushroom.

Despite the lack of any evidence that these mushrooms caused injury, concern over their recreational use led the Government to include psilocybin and psilocin on the list of Schedule I drugs in the Controlled Substances Act of 1970. Technically, possession of the mushroom itself is not illegal, but its content is illegal. Therefore, possession of the mushroom is a criminal offense if it is intended for use as a drug.

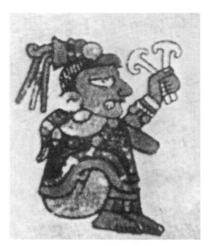

This page from the Codex Vindobonensis (Florentino) clearly shows the use of mushrooms in pairs, a ritual continued to the present by Mazatec Indians of Oaxaca

Who Is Using Psilocybin?

Most users of psilocybin are relatively affluent young people experimenting with hallucinogens. Psilocybin is widely regarded as a natural, harmless, non-addictive drug that does not require paraphernalia such as pipes or needles.

The mushroom can easily be grown from spores. Complete kits containing the spores and all materials and instructions may be bought by mail-order or over the Internet. Enough spores to grow dozens of crops may be purchased for about ten dollars. The spores are legal because they do not contain psilocybin or other psychoactive substances (an exception is California, where anti-spore laws were enacted in 1985 specifically to close this loophole). Psilocybin mushrooms themselves are also technically legal if it can be shown that they are used for legitimate purposes such as studying mushroom cultivation or mycology. However, anyone growing psilocybin mushrooms for the purpose of producing psilocybin or psilocin may be found guilty of "manufacturing" these substances.

With the easy availability of spores, most users obtain psilocybin from friends or grow the mushrooms at home. Because there is not much of a market for the drug, there is very little criminal activity involved.

The most popular and easily grown variety is *Stropharia cubensis*, which was originally collected in Cuba in 1904. Spores are sold in a water solution in a ten milliliter syringe. The spores are injected into a mixture of vermiculite, brown rice flour, and water. After four to six days, a white growth appears. This is the early growth of the mycelium, known botanically as the primordia knots of the mushrooms. It is followed by primordia pinheads, plump yellow growths with brown tips. About three weeks after the spores are planted, the mycelium can produce fruiting bodies. Another three weeks or so are required before mature mushrooms begin to appear, which may then be harvested weekly for about two months.

Psilocybin mushrooms may also be harvested wild, particularly in the wet northwest coastal region from California to British Columbia, where they are prevalent. The major danger in "shroom" harvesting is mistaking poisonous mushrooms for those containing psilocybin. Some toxic mushrooms (for example, *Amanita phalloides*) can cause death or permanent liver damage within hours of ingestion. There is no way to tell that a mushroom is poisonous by its taste or initial physical effects. With many mushroom poisons, liver damage is insidious and may show no symptoms until the liver is already seriously injured.

Both psilocybin and psilocin can be produced synthetically,[15] but this form of the drug is not often found. Most street drugs sold as psilocybin prove to be another substance. Some are normal grocery-bought mushrooms laced with LSD or PCP. In an 11-year study, 886 samples that were said to be psilocybin were analyzed. Only 28 percent of these were hallucinogenic mushrooms, while 35 percent were other drugs, mostly LSD or PCP, and 37 percent contained no drug at all.[16]

Chemical Characteristics

DMT

DMT is an indole hallucinogen, sharing a chemical structure with LSD and other hallucinogens (see *Chapter 6*). DMT is found naturally in the blood, brain, and cerebrospinal fluid, where its function is not well known. When DMT (or its variants) are taken, they probably bind not only to the brain's DMT receptors, but also to acetylcholine and serotonin. It is likely that these additional bindings produce the diverse psychological effects.

DMT is easily broken down and does not survive in the stomach acids if it is ingested. When DMT is injected, effects begin in 2 to 5 minutes, last for about 10 to 15 minutes, and resolve within 15 to 30 minutes. When smoked, the effects occur within seconds, producing intense, very visual and auditory hallucinations. There may also be extreme shifts in mood and a sense of bodily dissociation. The peak lasts for three to ten minutes and resolves quickly.

Synthesized 5-methoxy-DMT is about five times stronger than DMT when smoked and very short acting. The user experiences a "rush" similar to that from amyl nitrate. There is little in the way of visuals, just intense thoughts and bodily sensations that last for five to ten minutes.

DMT is not psychoactive when taken orally because the mono-amine oxidase (MAO) enzymes of the body destroy it. Curiously, many of the South American plants which contain DMT also contain harmala alkaloids which inhibit MAO (see, for example, *Chapter 7: Ayahuasca*). When MAO is inhibited, DMT taken orally becomes a very potent hallucinogen.

BUFOTENINE

Over 200 species of the *Bufo* toad have been identified. All of them have parotid glands on their backs, producing a wide variety of biologically active compounds including dopamine, epinephrine, norepinephrine, serotonin,[17] and bufotenine (5-hydroxy-DMT). The only species that produces 5-MeO-DMT (5-methoxy-DMT) is the Colorado River toad *Bufo alvarius*.[18]

The venom of the other toads, including *Bufo vulgaris*, *Bufo bufo bufo* (the European toad), *Bufo gargarizans*, and *Bufo marinus* (the Cane toad, or American Tropical toad in Florida), are also reported to be used as hallucinogens. However, many of these venoms are extremely toxic to the body.

Bufotenine is chemically very similar to DMT, psilocybin, and to serotonin (see *Chapter 6: The Indole Hallucinogens*). It is likely that the resemblance to serotonin is responsible for most distinctive effects.

The most well-known tryptamines are:

psilocin   = 4-hydroxy-DMT
psilocybin   = 4-phosphoryloxy-DMT
bufotenine   = 5-hydroxy-DMT
5-MeO-DMT   = 5-methoxy-DMT

PSILOCYBIN

Psilocybin is found in over 100 species of mushrooms, in varying amounts. The most potent is *Psilocybe azurescens*, where it can exceed two percent of the dried mushroom by weight. The most popular recreational mushroom, *Strophoria cubensis*, has about one percent psilocybin. However, the potency of both wild and cultivated psilocybin mushrooms can vary greatly.

Mushrooms are composed of chitin, carbohydrates, proteinaceous matter, and mineral salts, but are mostly water—about 90 percent of fresh mushrooms. By drying mushrooms, in other words, the psilocybin concentration is increased about ten-fold. When the mushroom is eaten, the psilocybin is dephosphorylated by the liver to form psilocin. Only psilocin actually enters the brain.

Psilocybin (4-phosphoryloxy-N,N-DMT) and psilocin (4-hydroxy-N,N-DMT) cause effects that are difficult to distinguish from those of LSD or mescaline. They have a potency of about one percent that of LSD. A typical dose is about ten to twenty milligrams of synthetic psilocybin, or two to four mushrooms.

If the mushrooms are chewed well and kept in the mouth, effects may be seen within seven or eight minutes. It takes longer if the mushrooms are rapidly swallowed, about 30 to 45 minutes. The initial experience is yawning, without sleepiness, and a sense of restlessness or malaise. Some people feel chills, weak in the legs, stomach discomfort, or nausea. These feelings are replaced within an hour or two with heightened visual imagery and often a comical sense of wanting to laugh. The symptoms gradually resolve and are over in four to six hours.

Withdrawal Signs

Like most hallucinogens, DMT and its variants rapidly produce tolerance, such that further doses have little or no effect. The user has to wait for days and as long as a week to become fully susceptible again to the drug's effects.

There is cross-tolerance of DMT to LSD (and to some extent with other hallucinogens), so that if one of these drugs is taken, there is reduced intoxication from the other.

There are no known withdrawal signs from DMT, other than fatigue.

Long-term Health Problems

Other than isolated case reports, there is very little knowledge of the long-term hazards of DMT-type substances. It is possible that the use of DMT or its variants may cause psychotic reactions such as those reported for other hallucinogens such as LSD. Certainly, there is a risk of exacerbations of pre-existing mental illness.

Unlike LSD, post-hallucinogen perceptual disorder, or "flashbacks," has not been reported.

What To Do If There Is An Overdose

DMT is relatively nontoxic; for example, it is estimated that at least 50 lbs of psilocybin mushrooms would need to be ingested for a fatal dose. A more likely outcome of overdose is a psychotic or panic reaction. This may appear extreme but it is likely to be brief and resolve spontaneously.

There is no easy way to remove the drug from the body. The best management for a disturbed user is simply to put him or her into a safe, quiet, supportive environment in the company of a trusted friend. The user should recover within a few hours, without further problems.

   Probably the greatest danger of using these substances comes from poisoning with the other, more toxic variants of DMT drugs, such as components of toad excretions, mistakenly identified mushrooms, or from adulterants in synthetic preparations.

   People who use anti-depressant medications may be at risk of a serotonin-overload syndrome, which can be very hazardous. If there is difficulty breathing, irregular heart beat, fever, or the person cannot be aroused, medical attention should be sought immediately.

Physical signs of overdose[19]

Fever
Fast pulse
High blood pressure
Enlarged pupils
Drooling
Blank stare
Jerky eyes
Muscle rigidity
Difficulty walking

Mental signs of overdose

Anxiety
Panic
Paranoia
Amnesia
Loss of ability to speak

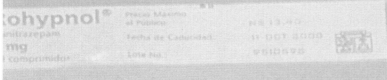

Flunitrazepam

Flunitrazepam is a potent sedative sold internationally under the trade name Rohypnol. It is illegal in the United States, where it has been associated with date rape.

The Basic Facts

Type of drug	*Depressant*
How taken	*Ingested, snorted*
Duration of effect	*6 to 12 hours*
Physical danger	*Moderate*
Addiction potential	*Moderate*

Other Names

circles, Mexican valium, R-2, rib, roaches, Rohypnol, roofies, roopies, rope, Rophy

Roofies, Rape, and Robbery: The Story of Flunitrazepam

In the 1950s, a new category of sedative drugs, benzodiazepines, was developed that did not have the danger of barbiturates. One of the first of these new drugs, diazepam (Valium) was very useful for anxiety, pain, muscle tension, and insomnia. For the next few years, it became the most widely prescribed drug in the world.

> In the 1960s, Valium was the number one prescribed drug. In the 1970s, the top spot went to the anti-ulcer drug cimetidine (Tagamet), and in the 1990s to the antidepressant fluoxetine (Prozac).
> This may say something about our society: the most common complaint being anxiety, ulcers, and then depression.

Valium was soon joined by similar drugs, including such commonly prescribed medications as alprazolam (Xanax), temazepam (Restoril) and triazolam (Halcion). All these names end in "am", indicating that they are benzodiazepines.

Flunitrazepam (Rohypnol) is an unusually potent benzodiazepine with a very rapid onset. Its maker, Hoffman-La Roche, marketed it in 160 countries for anesthesia, the treatment of anxiety, sleep disorders, and alcohol withdrawal.[1] Although it is widely used in Europe, Central America, and South America, it was never approved for sale in the United States.

All benzodiazepine drugs cause muscle relaxation and forgetfulness. For both of these, Rohypnol is extremely potent, with effects about ten times stronger than Valium. It can cause paralysis or unconsciousness, and short-term amnesia such that the user has no memory of what happened in the past few hours. In South America, where it is very popular and can even be bought over the counter in some countries, it is often called *La Rocha* after the manufacturer.

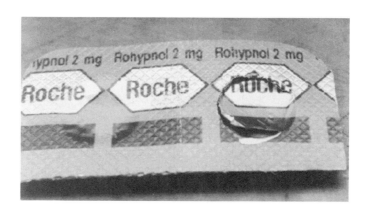

Rohypnol first showed up in the United States in 1989 when it was imported from South America to Florida.

THE "FORGET-ME" PILL

In 1996, an alarming number of news reports began to appear about a new drug involved with non-violent rape, particularly among college students, in nightclubs, and in other social settings. "Date rape," as this came to be known, is not new. It typically involves taking advantage of a partner who is drunk and has weakened inhibition or judgment, or is too intoxicated to fight back.

Flunitrazepam is especially effective in date rape. A tiny amount can disappear in a drink without affecting the taste. Two milligrams of Rohypnol, the standard dose, is equivalent to 20 mg of Valium, enough to put most people into a dreamy stupor. The effect is compounded by alcohol, so that the victim may slip into a helpless, comatose state, with no recollection the next day of what happened after taking the drink.

Rohypnol, rapists learned, was the perfect drug to use to take advantage of an unwilling partner: there was no resistance, and no memory of what happened. Both of these made it difficult to prosecute the offender under the rape laws, which require that the victim tried to fight back and can give accurate testimony.

Rohypnol is the ideal rape drug: the victim has no resistance and no memory of the event.

EASY PREY

While Rohypnol came to attention in the United States as a rape drug, it is better known in other countries as a drug used in robbery. An unsuspecting victim is not only powerless to resist, but also has a poor recollection of the event afterward, making it very difficult to explain what happened or make a convincing accusation against the thieves.

In South America, victims have been known to wake up in the street, without a wallet or any idea of what happened after that last drink in the bar, bought by a friendly stranger.

LA ROCHA BECOMES ILLEGAL

In 1995, as a result of increasing worldwide abuse and trafficking, the United Nations Commission on Narcotic Drugs transferred flunitrazepam from Schedule IV to Schedule III of the Convention of Psychotropic Substances, increasing restrictions on its sale. Rohypnol was the first benzodiazepine to require more rigid controls in its distribution.

The following year, concern increased in the United States over the reports of rape and robbery associated with the drug. The DEA banned the import of flunitrazepam and Congress passed the Drug-Induced Rape Prevention and Punishment Act of 1996. This law calls for harsher penalties when a drug is given to someone without his or her consent and with the intent to commit a crime. The law specifically imposes imprisonment of up to 20 years for the distribution or importation of one gram or more of Rohypnol.[2]

The Drug-Induced Rape Prevention and Punishment Act

Crime...	... and punishment
Give someone an illegal drug, with the intent to commit a crime	maximum 20 years
Simple possession of Rohypnol	maximum 3 years
Import/export Rohypnol	maximum 20 years
... with prior drug conviction	maximum 30 years
Cause injury or death by giving Rohypnol	minimum 20 years maximum life

Who Is Using Flunitrazepam?

Flunitrazepam is neither manufactured nor legally sold in the United States. It continues to be produced and sold by prescription in Europe and Latin America under the trade name Rohypnol.[3]

Although flunitrazepam is legal in many countries, concern about abuse is increasing. In Germany, Roche recently removed the two-milligram dose from retail distribution and has restricted Rohypnol to hospital use only.

Not only criminals use Rohypnol. In Spain and Malaysia addicts use flunitrazepam to relieve withdrawal symptoms from other drugs, or as a "parachute" remedy for the depression that follows a stimulant high. In many of the countries where it is legal, as well as in the United States, Rohypnol is a party drug—a cheap, easy method of getting intoxicated without the side effects of alcohol.

Despite its illegal status in the United States, flunitrazepam abuse is increasing, particularly in southern states from California to Florida. In Texas, most of the supply comes from Mexico. The Texas Border Patrol has seized individual shipments of more than 50,000 tablets, often combined with other drugs such as marijuana, cocaine, and heroin. In Florida, fluni-trazepam is mainly imported from South America. Packages seized in Miami are often shipped by overnight mail from Cali, Colombia, and contain up to 11,000 tablets.

WHY ARE ROOFIES POPULAR?

Rohypnol is popular among young people in part because it is cheaper than most other drugs. A two-milligram pill costs about $5, in comparison to $40 or so for MDMA and other party drugs.

Besides providing an economical high, highschool students are attracted to Rohypnol for two reasons—both of them wrong.

First, many believe that the drug is safe because it is produced by a large, well-known pharmaceutical company and it is legally sold in other countries. It comes in a pre-sealed plastic bubble pack and does not look like other illegal drugs. Roofies look reassuringly like a normal prescription drug, and not like an illegal substance made by unprofessional chemists. Despite its appearance, however, flunitrazepam is a powerful substance that can be fatal.

Second, many people think that Rohypnol use cannot be detected, so they have no fear of being caught. In fact, flunitrazepam is easily detected in urine.

To young people, getting "roached out" is a novel, seemingly benign way of getting high, different from the marijuana, cocaine, and heroin of the older generation. The fact that this drug's main effect is heavy sedation—and not euphoria, stimulation, or hallucinations—is an interesting commentary on the life of the modern highschool student.

Chemical Characteristics

Flunitrazepam is similar chemically to other benzodiazepines such as Valium. It differs by having a short onset, in as little as ten minutes, and a very powerful sedative and amnestic (memory loss) effect.

The most common dose of flunitrazepam is the two-milligram pill, which lasts 4 to 6 hours and has some residual effect for up to 12 hours. Higher doses, or combination with alcohol or other drugs, can cause severe intoxication with an unresponsive coma lasting several days.

Flunitrazepam acts by binding to the GABA receptors in the brain. GABA neurons work by inhibiting nervous impulses—relaxing the body, dulling sensations, and slowing mental functions. Flunitrazepam floods these receptors, effectively damping down the entire brain.

The usual effects of flunitrazepam are decreased blood pressure, memory impairment, drowsiness, visual disturbances, dizziness, and confusion. Some users also complain of constipation and difficulty urinating.

Rarely, flunitrazepam can cause the opposite reaction in a user, and result in excitable or aggressive behavior.

TESTING

The use of flunitrazepam can be determined by both blood and urine tests. It has a half-life of 16 to 35 hours,[4] meaning that it can be detected for days; the actual length of time that users test positive will depend on how much they have taken and for how long. The test results may also be affected by the use of other benzodiazepine medications, or by contaminating the urine with Visine eye drops, hand soap, Drano, or bleach.

Withdrawal Signs

Repeated use of flunitrazepam brings a tolerance to its effects. There is also a moderate degree of both physical and psychological dependence. Once dependence has developed, withdrawal causes a number of symptoms, including headache, muscle pain, extreme anxiety, tension, restlessness, confusion, and irritability. There may also be a sensation of numbness or tingling in the limbs, a feeling of loss of identity, hallucinations, and delirium. Rarely, shock and heart failure have been observed, as well as seizures, which can occur a week or more after use has ended.

 A combination of Rohypnol and champagne put musician Kurt Cobain into a coma one month before his suicide.

The treatment for flunitrazepam addiction is a gradual, tapering use, best managed by a physician who may prescribe other, less toxic, medications.

Long-term Health Problems

Long-term use of flunitrazepam presents problems similar to the extended use of any benzodiazepine, such as Valium. It may cause impaired mental functioning, depression, and a wide variety of other symptoms. Physical dependence is the major concern, requiring a tapering withdrawal under medical supervision.

What To Do If There Is An Overdose

Death from overdose has occurred after the ingestion of 7 to 14 tablets.[5] Most fatalities have occurred when flunitrazepam was combined with other depressant drugs such as alcohol or heroin.

If the user is unresponsive, or stops breathing, medical attention should be sought immediately. The standard antidote is flumazenil, given intravenously in the Emergency Department.

Physical signs of overdose
Slow breathing
Low blood pressure
Irregular heart beat
Slurred speech
Difficulty walking

Mental signs of overdose
Confusion
Drowsiness
Delirium
Unresponsive coma

GHB

GHB, gamma-hydroxybutyric acid, is a depressant drug recently added to the list of illegal substances. Although it is relatively safe, high doses cause a coma-like state that has resulted in fatalities.

The Basic Facts

Type of drug	*Depressant*
How taken	*Ingested*
Duration of effect	*2 to 4 hours*
Physical danger	*Moderate*
Addiction potential	*Low*

Other Names

GHB	*cherry meth, Eclipse, Fantasy, G-riffic, Georgia homeboy, grievous bodily harm, growth hormone booster, liquid ecstasy, liquid G, liquid X, scoop, Serenity, Somatomax*
GHB and amphetamine	*max*
GBL	*Blue Nitro, Fire Water, Gamma G, GH Revitalizer, Remforce, Renewtrient, Revivarant*
BD (1,4-butanediol)	*Sucol B, Zen*

Dancehall Depressant: The Story of GHB

GHB was first synthesized in France in 1960 by Dr. Henri Laborit, a researcher looking for a better anesthetic. Laborit knew that the major inhibitor of the central nervous system was GABA. He wanted to create a GABA-like substance that could be taken by mouth and penetrate the brain.

 GHB is very similar to GABA:

GHB   = gamma-*hydroxy*-butyric acid
GABA = gamma-*amino*-butyric acid

The first studies of GHB showed that it might have some promise as an anesthetic. It rapidly put patients into a deep coma. Unfortunately, it did not prevent pain and it seemed to cause neurological problems, which dampened enthusiasm for its use in the operating room. Its ability to cause deep sleep, however, made the drug attractive to those suffering from insomnia. GHB became popular in Europe as a non-addictive sleeping aid that was available without prescription.

In the United States, GHB was sold at health food stores, gyms, and by mail order, as a "natural" sleeping aid and nutritional supplement. Body-builders believed that GHB was an artificial variant of growth hormone that helped them increase muscle mass. Others took it for its euphoric or dreamy effects, and it became a popular dance-club drug.

Along with the increased use came reports of people slipping into an odd, comatose state, and of deaths from overdose. Emergency Departments were mystified by drugged patients who seemed to be in the deepest life-threatening coma but who, just hours later, woke up and could walk out.

On November 8, 1990, the U.S. Food and Drug Administration warned consumers against the use of GHB, and prohibited its manufacture and sale. Its sales restriction did not do much to hamper its popularity, particularly in the southeast and western states. Increasing reports of overdose and deaths contributed to concern about this new drug.[1] The ability of GHB

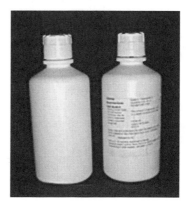

GHB is easily made from GBL, a common industrial solvent

to cause a rapid, deep sleep also resulted in its use in "date rape" (see *Flunitrazepam*). Because of this, the DEA added GHB on March 13, 2000, to the list of Schedule I drugs under the Controlled Substances Act, indicating that it has no acceptable medical use and a very high abuse potential.

 March, 2000: In one of the first trials involving a death from a date-rape drug, three Michigan men were found guilty of involuntary manslaughter after giving a fatal dose of GHB to a 15-year-old girl.

BODY BUILDERS

In the 1980s, GHB became popular in the United States as a nutritional supplement sold in health clubs. The sellers claimed that it would stimulate the brain's production of growth hormone, building muscle and reducing body fat. Both body builders and dieters eagerly sought out the drug.

In laboratory and clinical studies, GHB does indeed show an increase in growth hormone in rats and perhaps humans. However, no study has ever demonstrated that GHB causes weight loss or increased muscle growth.[2] Regardless, many body builders are convinced that GHB helps build muscle mass. Some researchers speculate that there may actually be some truth to the claim, though not directly. Growth hormone is produced mainly during deep slow-wave sleep. If GHB increases the amount of this type of sleep, it may also lengthen the time that the body produces growth hormone.

RAVES

Raves began in 1987 on the Spanish island of Ibiza, when young people from Britain began to hold all-night parties during their holidays. The dance parties were easily arranged—just a simple sound system blasting out propulsive, trance-inducing, heavily electronic music. Drugs were plentiful, to help get into the mood and to keep going all night.

The ravers brought the dances home to nightclubs in Britain, and then, to avoid police harassment, to empty warehouses and open fields. Even though raves were kept secret until the last moment, the word always managed to get out to enough people. Some London raves had as many as 30,000 dancers.

The phenomenon spread throughout Europe and in 1991 came to California, where one of the first raves in San Francisco was held by a group called Toontown. By the mid-90s, there were as many as a dozen raves in San Francisco and Los Angeles each weekend night.

GHB became a common drug at raves for the same reason that dancers take alcohol or Ecstasy (see *MDMA*). In small amounts it produces a sense of relaxation, reducing anxiety and making people feel more sociable. The euphoria caused by GHB is very similar to the feeling given by MDMA, and it is often called "liquid ecstasy," or "liquid X". GHB also produces a sense of drunkenness very much like that of alcohol, but without the subsequent hangover.

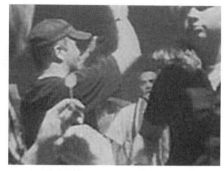

Like alcohol and MDMA, GHB can also be conveniently taken on the dance floor. It is hot in dance clubs and many people have water bottles. The salty GHB powder is dissolved in water or juice and can be easily carried and passed around. Because it is odorless and colorless, it is difficult to detect.

"It is super, euphoric, like getting drunk, but you don't wake up the next morning feeling hammered."—21-year-old Web designer, Salt Lake City

GBL

When GHB became illegal, users turned to a related substance that had the same effect. GBL is gamma-butyrolactone, also known as furanone di-hydro or by its chemical name 2(3h)-furanose di-hydro. It is a solvent available in floor cleaning products, nail polish, and glue removers. People who had been using GHB found that GBL is more potent and longer lasting. It quickly became a popular substitute, and was sold as an herbal remedy in "health" shops, in gyms, and over the Internet. The DEA prohibited the illicit use of GBL as an analog of GHB, but could not make the substance itself illegal because it has so many industrial applications. By this loophole, Internet sites continue to sell GBL "as a solvent only," even though it is advertised on body-building sites and is clearly intended for drug use.

 In December 1999, NBA basketball player Tom Gugliotta went into respiratory failure and almost died from an herbal remedy containing GBL.[3]

GBL is a List I chemical, meaning that special regulations apply to the purchase of large quantities. In some states GBL is illegal.

BD

BD—1,4-butanediol—is also an industrial solvent. When it is ingested, it is quickly converted to GHB.[4] Because BD is metabolized by alcohol dehydrogenase, the same enzyme used to metabolize alcohol, taking BD together with alcohol increases the effects of both, and adds to the risk of damage to the liver or kidneys.

Who Is Using GHB?

GHB is popular in most industrialized countries, particularly in Britain and Australia, where it is legal or available by prescription. In these countries, GHB is used for medical purposes or self-medication in drug addiction as well as a recreational drug.

In the United States, GHB is most common in Florida, Texas, California, and Georgia, but use is increasing throughout the country. The typical user is white (94 percent) and male (79 percent) 18 to 25 years old, and either a body builder or someone attending a rave or party.

Before the new laws to restrict GHB came into effect, many users stockpiled the drug, buying as much as they could from gyms and health food stores. Some of this supply is still available. However, most GHB in the United States comes from illicit manufacture using legal materials and instructions available over the Internet.

The typical dose of pure GHB powder is one to three grams, taken as a drink when the powder is dissolved in water or fruit juice. Some people use as much as four or five grams, particularly if they use it often and have developed a tolerance to it.

Illegally made GHB powder is cheap, at $10 to $50 for 100 grams. This is usually sold in smaller units as a powder or mixed with water. One gram of powder can be dissolved in a bottle of water or in as little as one milliliter of water (one fifth of a teaspoon). Consequently, once GHB is dissolved it is difficult to know what the concentration is unless the user knows both the purity of the original powder and the amount of liquid for the mixture.

A highly concentrated street form is available in small plastic bottles, the size and shape of hotel shampoo bottles. These are sold for about ten dollars and contain about ten average doses. An individual hit might be sold at a dance club for two dollars.

MAKING GHB

GHB is a popular drug in part because it is so easy to produce. The chemical process for making GHB is quite simple. The only supplies needed are the industrial solvent GBL, and a minimum of other ingredients and equipment.

GHB recipes are very simple:

Ingredients	Equipment
GBL	Pyrex bowl
hydroxide	pH papers
water	microwave oven
	hot plate

When GBL is combined with a strong base such as lye from drain cleaner (sodium hydroxide), it undergoes a chemical process of saponification to become GHB. Other strong bases may also be used for this conversion, such as potassium hydroxide, magnesium hydroxide (the key ingredient in Milk of Magnesia), or calcium hydroxide. Even laundry detergent and baking soda have been used to convert GBL to GHB.

MEDICAL USES

Despite its legal status as a drug with no acceptable medical use, GHB does have a number of recognized medical applications. It continues to be used in Europe as a general anesthetic, sleeping aid, and as a treatment for anxiety and stress. It is also a common treatment of alcohol and opiate addiction and withdrawal. Perhaps most remarkable is its use in childbirth. In France and Italy, GHB is used to calm anxious mothers about to give birth, to accelerate the dilation of the cervix, and to protect the baby from hypoxic injury.

GHB appears to prevent damage to cells from the lack of oxygen. Hypoxic cellular damage is the mechanism of injury in a number of conditions, including hemorrhagic shock, sepsis, strokes, mesenteric ischemia, heart attacks, and organ transplant rejection. In Europe, GHB has been used for women in labor and for many surgical operations, including aortic and heart surgery, cataract surgery, and emergency laparotomy for hemorrhagic shock. How GHB can protect hypoxic cell injury is not known. It may prevent damage from free radicals or from the immune response, and it has also been shown to be protective in radiation exposure.

Although GHB is illegal in the United States, experimental medical use may continue under research applications for an Investigational New Drug (IND). At this time, INDs have been filed for the use of GHB in the following conditions:

1. Improving sleep patterns and maintaining daytime alertness in narcolepsy
2. Reducing schizophrenic symptoms
3. Stabilizing Parkinson's Disease
4. Reducing nocturnal myoclonus
5. Improving memory
6. Stimulating natural growth hormone release
7. Decreasing pain and improving sleep in fibromyalgia
8. Relieving symptoms in Huntington's Chorea
9. Regulating muscle tone in dystonia musculorum deformans
10. Controlling tardive dyskinesia symptoms
11. Decreasing alcohol and opiate withdrawal symptoms
12. Decreasing hyperactivity and learning disabilities in children
13. Sedation and tranquilization
14. Relieving anxiety
15. Lowering cholesterol

Only the first of these has been approved by the FDA, as research on GHB has shown considerable promise in treating narcolepsy. The drug is produced under a federal exemption by Orphan Medical Inc., of Minneapolis, and distributed to research programs under the trade name Xyrem. Orphan plans to begin marketing Xyrem in 2002.[5]

Chemical Characteristics

GHB is a very simple substance with a chemical structure similar to the neurotransmitter GABA. It is found naturally in all animal and human cells and also in cerebrospinal fluid. Most natural GHB in the body apparently is from the breakdown of GABA, and it is also reformed back into GABA.[6] In addition, GHB is made in the body from naturally occurring GBL.

In the brain, the action of GHB is very complex.[7] It binds to GABA-B receptors and interferes with dopamine transmission, inhibits noradrenaline release in the hypothalamus and mediates the release of an opiate-like substance in the striatum. It produces a biphasic dopamine response, increasing its release at high doses and inhibiting its release at lower doses. Binding sites are present in the cortex, midbrain, substantia nigra, basal ganglia and, most predominantly, in the hippocampus—the location where memory is formed. The result of all this complex activity is that most of the functions of GHB are still largely unknown.[8]

When GBH is used as a drug, it is taken as the sodium or potassium salt of gamma-hydroxybutyric acid. In other words, the actual drug is either Na-GHB or K-GHB, respectively. Both of these variants have an identical appearance, as an odorless, salty substance, which may also have a bitter taste.

GHB is rapidly absorbed after swallowing, especially on an empty stomach. The maximum blood concentration is reached in 20 to 30 minutes with a typical dose, or longer with a larger dose or if it is mixed with food. The effect is usually felt within 15 minutes or so, with a peak at about 40 minutes. People vary unpredictably in their response to it, and the same person may react differently to the same dose on different occasions.[9] The major effects last for one to two hours, followed by an additional period of about two hours with more subtle effects.[10] This pattern is much the same as alcohol, and some users take it in the same way—sipping it slowly over an evening rather than gulping the full dose at once.

A dose of GHB is distributed throughout the body in the blood and easily crosses the blood-brain barrier. It also crosses the placental barrier, so that unborn children are exposed to its action.

The elimination half-life—the time it takes to decrease the amount in the blood by half—is 27 minutes. The body metabolizes GHB to carbon dioxide, which is then exhaled.

EFFECTS ON THE NERVOUS SYSTEM

The hallmark of GHB use is central nervous system depression. The onset of action is very rapid. If too much is taken, unconsciousness can occur after 15 minutes and lead to a coma within 30 to 40 minutes.

A mild dose of one gram or so will cause relaxation with a subtle drop in muscle tone. There may be mild euphoria, heightened sexual interest, short-term forgetfulness, and a loss of inhibition, making people feel more sociable. A moderate dose of two to three grams produces drowsiness and sleep. After swallowing a large dose of four to five grams (about one teaspoonful), a very deep sleep and coma can result. This can occur in as little as 10 to 15 minutes if a very large dose is taken on an empty stomach.

 Like "a drowning swimmer flailing for air"—*typical appearance of a GHB reaction*

The neurologic effects of GHB range from mild symptoms, such as blurred vision, dizziness, and stumbling, to severe impairment, including respiratory failure, coma, and death. Typically, the user experiences a short period of euphoria followed by a rapid and profound decline in the level of consciousness. Along with sleepiness, there may be spastic jerks and flailing limbs.

At higher doses, GHB produces lightheadedness, vertigo, drowsiness, slurred speech, and muscle incoordination, which may progress to uncontrolled movements, a coma-like state, and arrested breathing. Although most people recover within a few hours, GHB can be fatal, especially if combined with alcohol or other drugs that compound the effect.

GHB AND SLEEP

The ability of GHB to bring about a deep sleep accounted for its early popularity in Europe. It rapidly initiates delta wave and REM (dreaming) sleep, and specifically enhances Stage 3 and Stage 4 sleep. These stages are the deepest part of the sleep cycle, that portion which is most often decreased in insomnia sufferers and in elderly people who complain that they don't get enough "restful" sleep. The improvement of Stage 4 sleep probably accounts for its benefit in patients with narcolepsy, a disorder characterized by excessive daytime sleepiness and a tendency to suddenly fall asleep even during stimulating activities.

GHB's ability to lengthen the deepest part of sleep may explain why some people believe that it increases growth hormone production, which occurs naturally during deep sleep.

GLASGOW COMA SCALE

The most dramatic feature of GHB is its ability to cause a coma-like state that can be very frightening to friends or caretakers (the user himself is probably not only oblivious to the effects, but won't remember any of it).

Coma is a condition of unresponsiveness in which the person cannot be aroused.[11] The most common assessment used to determine the degree of coma is the Glasgow Coma Scale (GCS), which gives a score to the amount of eye opening, verbal response, and muscle response. The GCS ranges from a maximum of 15, which is normal, to a minimum of 3, which indicates the deepest coma and often represents brain death. Anything less than 9 or 8 is considered by most hospital Emergency Departments to indicate a serious condition that will probably require intubation and mechanical ventilation. A recent study showed that two-thirds of GHB overdose patients had a GCS of less than 9, and one-third had a GCS of 3.

Glascow Coma Scale

Eyes	opens spontaneously	4
	opens only when asked	3
	opens only to pain	2
	does not open	1
Movement	obeys request	6
	moves only to pain	5
	withdraws from pain	4
	rigid flexion	3
	rigid extension	2
	none	1
Talking	talks and oriented	5
	talks and disoriented	4
	mixed up words	3
	unrecognizable sounds	2
	no response	1
TOTAL	normal =	15
	mild coma =	8
	deepest coma =	3

There are some peculiar aspects to the GHB coma, however:

?   Even though the GHB user may be in a deep coma, he or she can suddenly become completely awake, be very combative and agitated, and then slip back into the coma. This may be very surprising to physicians or paramedics who are not familiar with GHB.

?   The coma usually resolves completely and spontaneously within one to four hours. It is unusual to have such a complete recovery from such a profound condition.

?   During the onset of the coma, and when coming out of it, there may be spastic movements and seizures.

EFFECTS ON THE HEART

Approximately 36 percent of GHB ingestions are accompanied by extreme slowing of the heart. In about ten percent, there is also unusually low blood pressure. Other heart conditions are less common, but include irregular heartbeat, first-degree heart block, atrial fibrillation, right-bundle branch block, and ventricular ectopy. In one study, about 70 percent of GHB users had U waves on the ECG, a condition thought to result from the effect of GHB on the blood potassium balance, which has a strong effect on the heart. Many of these characteristics may be due to the combination of GHB with alcohol or other drugs.[12]

EFFECTS ON THE LUNGS

GHB slows and deepens respiration. This effect lasts about an hour, but if GHB has been mixed with alcohol or other drugs, the slowed breathing may last up to five hours or longer.

The decrease in breathing rate can be extreme, to the point that breathing stops entirely. In some unusual cases, mechanical ventilation has been required for up to 13 hours. At least five deaths have been reported due to respiratory failure.

OTHER EFFECTS

Some users have caustic burns to the lips and mouth from the concentrated powder, or from poorly mixed GHB.

In about 70 percent of users, there is an abnormally low body temperature.

Nausea and vomiting are common with GHB ingestion and often occur when a user comes out of the deep sleep.

Some people feel an urge for a bowel movement after taking GHB. This may be due to the relaxing effect on the intestinal muscles.

Finally, contamination of home-made GHB with other substances is common. Depending on the method used, the GHB may contain various amounts of unconverted GBL, solvents, heavy metals, and polyester derivatives,[13] all of which are toxic and can cause serious illness.

TESTING

GHB can be detected in the urine and blood by a test using gas chromatography-mass spectrometry. After ingestion, the test will be positive for about 4 to 8 hours in the blood and 12 hours in the urine. However, most hospitals do not have this specific test for GHB and rely on outside information to know what the patient has taken.[14]

Withdrawal Signs

Most users recover spontaneously and completely, without withdrawal symptoms. In some cases, dizziness has continued up to 14 days after GHB use. Other withdrawal symptoms that have been reported include drowsiness, headache, nausea, vomiting, diarrhea, incontinence, trouble breathing, uncontrollable shaking, temporary amnesia, and seizures,[15] but it is not clear how many of these are due to GHB, to other drugs, or to impurities in the substance. Most withdrawal signs appear within hours after the last dose.

Daily use of GHB can lead to addiction, with both physical and mental dependence in a small percentage of users.

Long-term Health Problems

Some advocates of GHB claim that it can be used for years, or even decades, without any bad effects. There have not been any good medical studies on long-term use. It is difficult to separate the possible effects of GHB from the effects of other drugs or psychological conditions in long-term users.

GHB has been noted to cause changes suggesting epilepsy in the electroencephalograph (EEG) in animals, although studies in humans do not show an increase in epilepsy. Some researchers believe that the muscle spasms of users recovering from the drug are a form of epilepsy. Further research is needed to see if this is the case.

What To Do If There Is An Overdose

Along with the growing use of GHB is a surge of visits to hospital Emergency Departments, which increased from 20 in 1992 to 629 in 1996. About 60 percent of these cases involved multiple drug use. GHB was taken in combination with alcohol in 76 percent, cocaine in 6 percent, marijuana in 5 percent, and MDMA in 4 percent. In a one-year period ending September 1996, there were 69 overdoses and one death due to GHB use in Texas and New York.[16]

Because the liquid concentration of GHB is difficult to determine, it is relatively common for people to accidentally take a larger dose of GHB than they intended. An amount only slightly larger than the normal recreational dose can cause unconsciousness, and this is compounded by alcohol.

At higher overdose levels, GHB can produce both unconsciousness and vomiting—an extremely dangerous combination. Vomiting while unconscious can lead to inhaling the vomit and death by suffocation.

The usual form of overdose of GHB is an unresponsive coma. Since 1990, the DEA and Poison Control Centers have documented at least 7,100 overdoses and 66 deaths, although many more have gone unreported.[17]

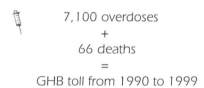

7,100 overdoses
+
66 deaths
=
GHB toll from 1990 to 1999

The typical appearance of overdose is an abrupt loss of consciousness, seizures, or slipping into a coma. Other reactions to GHB include vomiting, drowsiness, vertigo, confusion, agitation, and hallucinations.[18] Because GHB results in memory loss, users don't remember what happened when they wake up in the hospital.[19]

Care for someone who has taken too much GHB is primarily supportive.[20] Attention should be paid first and foremost to making sure that there is no difficulty breathing. If unconsciousness is prolonged, or there is any other concern about the person's condition, he or she should be taken to an Emergency Department. It is very important to notify medical personnel about the use of GHB, since many are not familiar with its effects and most hospitals are not able to test for it.[21]

EMERGENCY DEPARTMENT CARE

Since GHB is rapidly absorbed, there is little need for pumping the stomach unless other drugs have been taken as well. Oxygen should be given, and the patient intubated if necessary. Although naloxone, an opiate antidote, does not improve GHB toxicity, it is usually given to any patient who has respiratory impairment requiring intubation.

Because of the risk of irregular heartbeat, the patient should be placed on a heart monitor. If the heart rate is too slow, atropine may be given.

There is a controversy about the best method to reverse central nervous system depression from GHB. Most patients recover spontaneously, without the need for medical intervention. Physostigmine has been shown to be effective in bringing the patient out of the coma, but most experts currently believe that the risks of its use outweigh the benefits in most GHB ingestions and that it should be reserved for selected cases, if used at all.

Once the patient comes out of the coma, he or she may be confused and agitated. In this case, a mild sedative may be helpful.

Patients who are in stable condition and whose symptoms completely resolve may be released from the Emergency Department after six hours, when it is likely that they will have fully recovered.

Physical signs of overdose	Slow breathing
	Low blood pressure
	Vomiting
	Irregular heart beat
	Slurred speech
	Difficulty walking
Mental signs of overdose	Confusion
	Agitation
	Drowsiness
	Vertigo
	Hallucinations
	Delirium
	Unresponsive coma

Ibogaine

Ibogaine is a natural hallucinogen used in West Africa. Little is known about this drug, and it is rarely found in the United States.

The Basic Facts

Type of drug	*Hallucinogen*
How taken	*Ingested*
Duration of effect	*30 hours*
Physical danger	*Low*
Addiction potential	*None*

Other Names   *Endabuse*

Out of Africa: The Story of Ibogaine

Long ago, lost in the history of tropical Africa, some villagers noticed a peculiar behavior among wild boars. They would jump around wildly and go into a frenzy after digging up and eating the roots of a certain plant. Naturally, these villagers were curious about the root and decided to try it themselves. The stimulant properties of the roots became well known. People found it useful to chew a small amount to combat fatigue and hunger. It was especially helpful to stay awake, sometimes for days, during lion hunts when it was understandably important to remain alert.

In higher doses, users discovered that the root caused an unusual state of dreaming without any loss of consciousness. It became a sacrament in religious rituals, particularly in Gabon and parts of Congo, where it is used by the Bwiti cult.

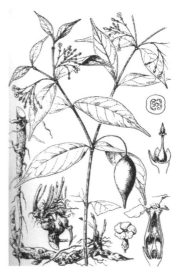

Iboga plant and its parts

The root is from a decorative shrub, *Tabernanthe iboga*, a member of the Dogbane (*Apocynaceae*) family. It is indigenous to the countries of equatorial Africa. The shrub produces a yellowish or pinkish white flower which yields a small, oval yellowish-orange fruit—about the size of an olive with an edible sweet pulp. Although the plant has other uses, it is cultivated widely for the bark from the root, which contains the stimulating substance.

The earliest documented reference to the use of Iboga occurred in 1864, when Griffon de Bellay brought specimens to Europe. A sample of the plant was displayed at the Paris Exposition in 1867. The psychoactive principle, ibogaine, was isolated in 1901.

The bark from the roots, especially the smaller ones, may contain up to six percent ibogaine. The bark is rasped from the roots and eaten directly, or dried and pounded into a powder to make tea.

After a dose of about 150 milligrams of the powdered root bark, the user might experience an increased sense of colors, similar to the effects of mescaline. With 300 milligrams, there is a slight nausea, dizziness, and a lack of muscular control or coordination. At one gram, there are hallucinations, which can last for days. The elimination half-life—the time it takes for half of the ibogaine to leave the body—is about 38 hours, suggesting that some effects can persist for a week or longer with a large dose.[1]

Ibogaine is unusual in that it has a variety of effects depending on the dose taken, and by its very long lasting action. It may act as a powerful stimulant, enabling the user to maintain high physical exertion without fatigue over a long period. The body seems lighter, and levitation—a feeling of floating—is often experienced. Spectrums or rainbow-like effects are seen in surrounding objects, and there is a distortion in the sense of time, so that a moment may seem like hours.

In addition to its hallucinogenic properties, ibogaine causes stimulation and tremors. Intoxication usually interferes with motor activity so that users often sit gazing intently into space, and eventually collapse. During this almost comatose period, their "shadow" (soul) is believed to have left the body to wander with the ancestors in the land of the dead.

To see Bwiti, they say, it is necessary to "break open the head"—by taking up to 100,000 times the stimulant dose.

Given the history of Iboga as a ritual hallucinogen in Africa, it is surprising that this plant was declared a Schedule I substance in the United States, where it is virtually unknown and certainly has never been shown to be a drug of abuse. How did this come about? The answer lies in the classification of ibogaine as a hallucinogenic substance by the World Health Assembly in

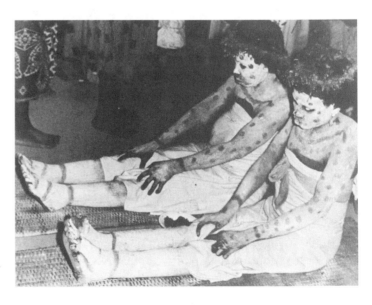

Initiates in the Bwiti cult, using Iboga to see the spirits of their ancestors

May 1967. Since ibogaine has a chemical structure similar to LSD (the ibogaine molecule contains the indole ring characteristic of many hallucinogens, see *Chapter 6*), the United States Federal Government classified ibogaine among substances analogous to LSD, and therefore made it illegal. Unlike LSD, however, ibogaine was never a recreational drug and it also shows promise as an anti-addictive medication. As research progresses, ibogaine may be rescheduled and marketed as a pharmaceutical.

ANTI-ADDICTION POTENTIAL

Soon after its discovery, Europeans began to experiment with ibogaine and found that it was effective in curing addiction to opiates, cocaine, alcohol, amphetamines, and nicotine. Self-help groups claimed that ibogaine reduces withdrawal symptoms and helps addicts stay away from other drugs. Some addicts claim that even a single dose has reduced drug cravings for periods up to six months.

Ibogaine was synthesized for use in research as an anti-addiction medication, and sold under the trade name Endabuse. Laboratory studies were carried out with animals to examine the interaction of ibogaine with addictive drugs of abuse. When rats were allowed to dose themselves with morphine and cocaine, they dosed themselves much less when they were given either natural ibogaine or its breakdown metabolite, noribogaine. The same effect was seen, to a lesser extent, in animals addicted to alcohol and nicotine.[2]

Although ibogaine is virtually unknown in the United States, the possibility that the drug might be of value in curing other drug addictions has created interest. One of the first to explore this use was Howard Lotsof, a non-scientist businessman who discovered that he and his friends stopped abusing drugs after experimenting with ibogaine. In the 1960s, he founded a New York corporation, NDA International, Inc., to market Endabuse. He went on to develop a formal detoxification program and took out several patents, beginning in 1985 with his "Rapid method for interrupting the narcotic addiction syndrome." In this program, one gram of ibogaine hydrochloride is taken by mouth, with effects lasting for about 30 hours. Following just this single treatment, it is claimed that the addict will no longer want to take heroin and show no perceptible signs of physical withdrawal.[3] Despite skepticism about this claim, the National Institute on Drug Abuse (NIDA) has added ibogaine to the list of drugs that show promise as a treatment for drug dependency.

Who Is Using Ibogaine?

The use of ibogaine is largely limited to native people in western and central Africa, particularly in the Bwiti cult of Gabon. This cult is widespread and may include both males and females, or separate groups of male (Bwiti) and female (Mbiri) participants. The cult is part of a movement back to traditional African religious beliefs, in reaction to the missionary spread of Christianity and Islam. Their customs, rituals, and beliefs transcend national boundaries, and serve to unify tribes in Congo and Gabon. The cult has been growing in its number of converts and in social acceptability.

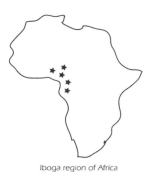

Iboga region of Africa

To enter the Bwiti cult, an initiate needs to establish contact with deceased ancestors, and to have a vision in which they see the spirit, Bwiti. Two to three teaspoons of the powdered dried bark are taken by women and three to five teaspoons by men. This amount provides hours of stimulation, leading to ceremonial drumming and dancing. To see Bwiti, however, initiates have to take considerably more—as much as a kilogram of powder.

Outside Africa, ibogaine is rarely found and its use is limited to research as a possible anti-addiction medication.

Chemical Characteristics

Ibogaine is an indole alkaloid similar in its chemical structure to other hallucinogens such as LSD and mescaline.

Both ibogaine and its metabolite noribogaine appear to decrease extracellular levels of dopamine in the nucleus accumbens of the brain. Ibogaine also blocks the dopamine released by morphine, cocaine, and nicotine. Since dopamine is considered to be responsible for addictive feelings, it is possible that ibogaine reduces addiction by blocking the action of the addictive drugs.

Ibogaine and noribogaine bind to kappa opioid and N-methyl-D-aspartate (NMDA) receptors and to serotonin uptake sites. Ibogaine also binds to sigma-2 and nicotinic receptors. It is likely that binding to the kappa opioid site removes the physical symptoms of withdrawal from opiates, binding to the NMDA receptors causes the decrease in craving for opiates, binding to the serotonin receptors decreases craving for alcohol, and binding to the nicotinic receptors decreases craving for nicotine. A versatile drug indeed!

It is also likely that yet other receptors, or combinations of receptors, may affect the interaction of ibogaine with different drugs of abuse.[4]

EFFECTS

The effects of ibogaine are felt about 15 to 20 minutes after ingestion. A buzzing sound is often heard, perhaps in waves, and the skin may feel numb. After 25 to 30 minutes, objects appear to vibrate. There may be nausea. After about an hour, the first visions appear. Then peak intoxication follows, lasting two to four hours, during which the user can experience difficulty walking, dizziness, pain with bright lights, and out-of-body sensations. There may also be tremors, abnormal breathing, spasms in the legs, and seizures. Some users have diarrhea, teary eyes, salivation, and a runny nose. Then the visions and numbness suddenly disappear, and for the next five to eight hours, the user is in a high-energy state, seeing flashes of lightning. This continues for about 20 hours, and ends when the user may go into a trance in which little physical activity is possible, or simply fall into an exhausted sleep.

Withdrawal Signs

There is no documented withdrawal syndrome.

Long-term Health Problems

Ibogaine may have long-lasting effects because it is stored in fat tissue and released slowly as noribogaine. Animal studies show that ibogaine destroys Purkinje cells in the cerebellum of the brain. Every rat treated with ibogaine had clear evidence of Purkinje cell degeneration, particularly in the intermediate and lateral cerebellum, as well as the vermis. Purkinje cells in lobules 5 and 6 were especially susceptible. These cells affect the muscle action of the head and upper extremities, and probably account for the tremor and incoordination often seen.[5]

It is not known how much of this effect in rats is present in humans. Perhaps because this drug has only recently been studied, there are no documented long-term health problems in humans.

What To Do If There Is An Overdose

Ibogaine appears to be safe even in amounts that greatly exceed the normal dose.[6] The greatest danger is in the paralysis that accompanies very high doses, but this is not properly considered an overdose, and resolves without adverse effects. There are unsubstantiated reports that excessive amounts of iboga ingestion have resulted in seizures, paralysis, and death by respiratory arrest.

Physical signs of overdose   Seizures
Paralysis
Respiratory arrest

Mental signs of overdose   Delirium

The major concern is probably anxiety and apprehension from the long-lasting effects. An overdose should be managed by support in a manner similar to the treatment of hallucinogens (see *LSD*). For suspected overdose, atropine has been used to suppress all signs of ibogaine intoxication.

LSD

LSD, lysergic acid diethylamide, is the most potent and highly studied hallucinogen known.

The Basic Facts

Type of drug	*Hallucinogen*
How taken	*Ingested, contact*
Duration of effect	*6 to 10 hours*
Physical danger	*None*
Addiction potential	*None*

Other Names

LSD-25	*acid, Alice, angel tears (liquid), angels in a sky, animal, backbreakers (LSD and strychnine), barrels, Bart Simpsons, battery acid, beast, big D, black sunshine, black tabs, blotter, blue acid, blue barrels, blue chairs, blue cheers, blue fly, blue heavens, blue microdot, blue mist, blue moons, blue vials, chinese dragons, windowpane*
LSD-49	*illusion*
LSD and PCP	*black acid, black star*

Acid: The Story of LSD

On the pleasant morning of April 16, 1943, Dr. Albert Hofmann worked as usual in his laboratory at Sandoz, a large pharmaceutical company in Basel, Switzerland. Five years earlier, he had been intrigued by the properties of ergot, a mold that grew on rye, and had synthesized many of its unique chemicals. Now, acting on a hunch, he turned his attention once again to a particular compound. It was the 25th in a series of combinations of lysergic acid and diethylamide, and he had called it LSD-25, from the initials for the German *LyserSaüre Diäthylamid*. As he prepared a fresh batch, a tiny amount of the liquid spilled on his bare hands. The rest of the day changed history.

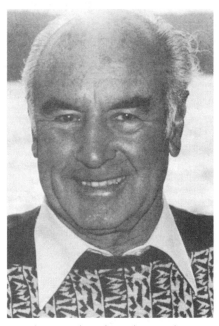

As the meticulous scientist wrote in his laboratory notebook, he soon began to feel odd. He suspected that he might have been poisoned by the lysergic acid, but he decided to keep working and let the sensation pass. The strange feeling grew and he sat back, alone in his laboratory, to watch a visual spectacle unfold of test tubes come alive and the walls pulsate and shimmer. Clearly, he was in no shape to work and decided to go home. He got on his bicycle and managed to ride home, wondering if he had lost his mind as the narrow lane seemed to stretch to infinity. A few hours later, his acid trip was over but the era of the modern hallucinogens had begun.

Little further notice of LSD was taken until 1947, when Werner Stoll, the son of Hofmann's superior, broadcast news of the discovery in an article entitled, "A New Hallucinatory Agent, Active in Very Small Amounts." Within two years, Sandoz began to market it under the trade name Delysid. Large quantities were brought to the United States and psychiatrists and the military began to explore its uses. By the end of the 1950s

"As I lay in a dazed condition with my eyes closed there surged up a succession of fantastic, rapidly changing imagery of a striking reality and depth, alternating with a vivid, kaleidoscopic play of colors."—Dr. Albert Hofmann, discoverer of LSD[1]

more than 500 scientific articles had appeared on LSD, increasing to 2,000 articles by the mid-1960s as it was studied for everything from mental illness to pain management (see *Chapter 2: Hallucinogens*).

 "Though LSD has had amazingly bad press, there seems to be no doubt of its immense and growing value."—Bill Wilson, founder of Alcoholics Anonymous [2]

If LSD had been discovered at any other time in history, it is unlikely that it would have had so great an impact. Three significant social developments generated interest in this new drug. The first was the Cold War between the United States and the Soviet Union, leading to a search for new chemical warfare weapons, no matter how unusual or far-fetched. The second was the development of psychopharmacology in the 1950s, when drugs began to replace traditional "talk therapy" and keen interest developed in any drug that might relieve mental illness. Finally, the baby boom generation born between 1946 and 1963 was one of the most adventurous and experimental populations in history and eagerly sought out the potential of mind-altering drugs. In the 1960s, LSD became the definitive hallucinogen, the most prominent of a new class of drugs that—unlike all other illegal drugs at the time—was not addictive, caused no physical injury, and did not involve organized crime.

The Beatles song Lucy in the Sky with Diamonds is believed to be a thinly disguised reference to the hallucinations of LSD.

Hallucinogens were not a threat to the person, but to society. They became a tool of social disorganization, and to a large part of the population, they were considered more dangerous than heroin.

The tremendous influence of LSD on art, music, and modern society— and the backlash from drug control operations—was a complete surprise to its discoverer, who later referred to it somewhat fondly as "my problem child."

Who Is Using LSD?

LSD use reached a peak in the 1960s, went through a steady decline, and has recently become popular once again, particularly among teenagers throughout the United States.

Since 1975, the National Household Survey on Drug Abuse has surveyed about 17,000 high-school seniors nationwide to determine trends and to measure attitudes and beliefs about drug abuse. Between 1975 and 1997, the lowest use of LSD was by the class of 1986, when 7.2 percent of highschool seniors reported using LSD at least once in their lives. This rate has steadily increased since then.[3] It is estimated that over 15 million Americans have used it at least once.

LSD is quite easily obtained in most highschools. In 1997, 51 percent of seniors said it would have been easy for them to get LSD if they had wanted it. Despite the ready availability, 80 percent of highschool seniors disapproved of people trying LSD, and 93 percent disapproved of people taking LSD regularly.

LSD use by students [4]

	8th Graders	10th Graders	12th Graders
Ever Used	4.7%	9.5%	13.6%
Used in Past Year	3.2%	6.7%	8.4%
Used in Past Month	1.5%	2.8%	3.1%

The Drug Enforcement Administration reports that the strength of LSD samples has declined in recent years, from the 100 to 200 microgram dose that was common in the 1960s and 1970s, to 20 to 80 micrograms currently. At these lower doses, LSD is likely to cause only a mild stimulation rather than a truly mind-altering experience.

LSD is available in various forms, including tablets, capsules, liquid, and as liquid absorbed onto a piece of paper ("blotter") or gelatin ("windowpane"). It is odorless, colorless, and may have a slightly bitter taste.

The manufacture of LSD is a complex process and involves the use of hydrazine, diethylamine, trifluoracetic acid, sulfur trioxide, and phosgene—most of which are either flammable, explosive, or extremely toxic to the eyes, lungs, and skin. The synthesis also requires a number of chemicals that are regulated and very difficult to obtain. These chemicals—especially ergotamine, ergonovine, and lysergic acid—are smuggled into the U.S. by European suppliers. Illicit labs may use a variety of methods to generate the necessary precursor chemicals. Some cultivate their own ergot-infested rye and use essentially the same method originally employed by Hofmann. Two hundred pounds of ergot will yield a pound of lysergic acid amides—enough for millions of doses of LSD. Newer sources of ergot alkaloids include plants such as the "Sleepy Grass" (*Stipa robusta*) of the desert American West. Because LSD manufacture is so difficult, it is estimated that fewer than ten underground laboratories, located in northern California, are responsible for the manufacture of the majority of all LSD sold in the United States.

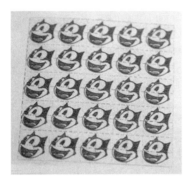

LSD blotter paper printed with cartoon designs

Nearly all retail sales of LSD are in the blotter paper form. The LSD is diluted in ethyl alcohol, and the blotter paper is dipped into the solution. Generally, the blotter paper is perforated into small squares called "tickets" and is stamped with pictures, designs, or characters as a trademark of the distributor. A "sheet" of blotter paper usually contains 100 perforated squares, and a "book" contains 1,000 squares.

LSD begins to degrade when exposed to sunlight or placed on paper. For this reason, LSD is sold in bulk as a liquid and then placed on blotter paper shortly before it reaches the consumer.

Pure LSD?

Since LSD is active in extremely small quantities, it is difficult to add or substitute another substance and still present it as a sheet of blotter paper or gelatin. These preparations are likely to be pure.

On the other hand, LSD sold as a pill, capsule, powder, or liquid could contain any number of other substances. A dose of 25 micrograms in a 500 milligram pill works out to one part LSD mixed in with 20,000 parts of some other substance, leaving plenty of opportunity for adulteration with other chemicals.

 "The synthesis of LSD is not a task to be undertaken lightly by the novice wannabe drug chemist."—Practical LSD Manufacture [5]

Current laboratory analyses show that only about 50 percent of the drug samples that are thought to be LSD prove to be actual LSD. Most of the adulterants are PCP or methamphetamine. Strychnine, easily obtained as rat poison, is also a common adulterant. It causes jitteriness and muscle cramps in small doses, which some users mistake for the effects of LSD. It is likely that any LSD sold as a pill contains adulterants.

Chemical Characteristics

LSD is the most powerful psychoactive substance known, 100 times stronger than psilocybin and 2,000 times more potent than mescaline. As little as a 25 microgram dose of LSD is enough to produce effects. To appreciate this small amount, consider that an average postage stamp weighs 60,000 micrograms, equal to 2,400 doses of LSD.[6] An amount of the weight of a copper penny would produce 112,000 doses; two gallons of LSD would be enough to intoxicate the entire population of the United States.

LSD is usually taken by mouth, although a recent trend in highschools is dropping the tiny blotter paper under an eyelid to be absorbed through the mucous membrane.

Twenty minutes to an hour after being swallowed, there is a dry or metallic taste in the mouth. This is often followed by sensations such as a slight chill, a vague sense of anxiety or physical unease, exhilaration and restlessness, tightness in muscles of the face and throat, queasy stomach, tingling in the extremities, and drowsiness. There may be a rapid pulse, dilated pupils, flushed face, and elevations in temperature or blood pressure.

The next state is more subjective. The senses are jangled and bombarded as colors appear more vivid, sounds are louder, and every sensation increases in intensity. Colors begin to shimmer and vibrate while depth perception is confused. Objects seem to become alive. Synesthesia (a sensory cross-over effect in which one kind of sensation is converted into another) may occur in which music may be seen and colors heard. There may be a complete loss of the sense of time. The boundary between body and space may be lost, so that the user feels dissolved into the environment or universe.

> "Reason and rationality take a back seat to the undifferentiated stimuli and subconscious material that come bubbling to the surface."[7]

The effects of LSD are unpredictable. They depend not only on the amount taken, but also on the user's personality, mood, expectations, and the physical or social environment. The rapidly changing imagery and moods, and especially the sense of depersonalization, can cause anxiety or panic. Some LSD users experience terrifying thoughts. They may have a fear of losing control, of permanent insanity or death.

The experience of a hallucinogenic drug has always reminded people of going on a mental journey—there is that same sense of leaving the familiar, known environment and going to a place that is foreign and unpredictable. Most injuries and a few fatalities have occurred when users found themselves overwhelmed by delusions and were injured either by accident or by intent. There are several reports of suicides of people on LSD. It is not certain what role LSD played in these deaths, but it is clear that the drug is not helpful to someone already suffering from mental illness.

For most users, it takes at least 20 micrograms to produce a noticeable effect. With a dose of 75 to 125 micrograms, the amount usually taken, LSD can emphasize internal phenomena. A heavy dose, 200 to 500 micrograms, tends to intensify rather than lengthen the experience. After 500 micrograms, there is a saturation beyond which an increase in dose makes little difference. For such a tiny amount of drug, it is remarkable that the concentration in the brain is lower than anywhere else in the body—only about 0.01 percent of the dose reaches the brain, and then only stays for about 15 minutes before it is metabolized and removed.

 The greatest mind-altering effects peak at about three hours, long after the drug itself has disappeared from the brain.

Like most hallucinogenic drugs, LSD produces its effects by over-whelming the serotonin neurotransmitter receptors in the brain. LSD, mescaline, DMT, and DOM all bind to the specific form of serotonin (hydroxy-tryptamine), known as 5-HT_2 receptors in the locus ceruleus and cortex of the brain. LSD differs from the others by binding to the 5-HT_{1A} receptors as well, which may give it some of its unique characteristics. Most of the effects of LSD are due to the inhibition of serotonin by binding to these receptors. The result is an increased and unregulated firing of sensory neurons, leading to the phenomenon of hallucinations.

In the 1990s, a newer variant of LSD was developed. LSD-49, sold with the street name "illusion," produces more visual distortions but is otherwise similar to LSD-25.

Withdrawal Signs

LSD is not toxic in the biological sense, and there is no sign of withdrawal from the drug. Rapid tolerance develops to repeated use. It requires up to one week without the drug for the user to experience a full effect again.

LSD is not addictive. Most users voluntarily decrease or stop its use over time, when the disagreeable sensations outweigh the novelty of the experience.

Long-term Health Problems

In the 1960s, there was a highly publicized concern that LSD causes chromosome damage. Animal studies have shown no adverse effects from LSD use, and the concern about chromosomal or other injury has been found to be false.

Although most users experience no long-term effects from LSD, four chronic reactions have been described:

- prolonged psychotic reactions, similar to schizophrenia
- worsening of pre-existing psychiatric illnesses
- severe depression
- flashbacks

It is unclear how much of the first three are caused by LSD. Like all psychoactive drugs, including alcohol, LSD will exacerbate any other mental health problems.

FLASHBACKS

The term "flashback" is given to brief episodes, usually just a few seconds, in which aspects of previous hallucinogenic drug use are unexpectedly re-experienced. The typical flashback is a sudden sense of the same perceptual distortions the user experienced during the drug trip. Sometimes the physical and emotional sense comes back as well. The sensation never lasts long and disappears spontaneously.

Flashbacks were first reported in the 1960s with the use of LSD.[8] They eventually were found to occur with almost all hallucinogens, including MDMA, PCP, and marijuana.[9] Flashbacks have been reported weeks or even months after taking the last dose.[10] Over time, flashbacks tend to decrease in frequency, duration, and intensity, as long as no further hallucinogens are taken.[11] Flashbacks occurring more than a year after the original drug experience suggest that a deeper type of mental illness may be present.[12]

There is no predictable association of flashbacks with the amount or frequency of the LSD taken. Some one-time users have experienced a flashback while others who have taken LSD hundreds of times deny it, and doubt that it even exists. Surveys have shown that 30 to 60 percent of heavy users—those who have taken 20 to 80 trips—have experienced flashbacks in one form or another.

Flashbacks can cause considerable anxiety, especially if the original drug experience was a bad one. The feeling can be triggered by stress, exercise, extreme fatigue, a situation reminiscent of the original drug experience, or for no apparent reason at all. The use of other drugs such as marijuana and alcohol can also trigger a flashback. Antidepressant medications such as Prozac are particularly likely to cause it. Not knowing when another flashback may occur can be quite unsettling. Treatment of disturbing flashbacks is simply a matter of alleviating anxiety with reassurance that the effects will gradually disappear.[13]

A newer psychiatric term for this condition is post-hallucinogen perceptual disorder (PHPD). Some psychologists use the term as a more formal-sounding phrase for flashback, while others believe that it is a distinct disorder with a much longer and more worrisome course. People suffering from PHPD describe it to be like "living in a bubble under water," with a continuous, uncomfortable distortion in perception, resulting in chronic anxiety, phobias, and depression.

What To Do If There Is An Overdose

If an excessive dose of LSD is taken, most users will suffer a temporary mental incapacitation but recover without harm. Others may undergo a very frightening experience that results in acute anxiety. Actual psychotic reactions are unusual, occurring in perhaps one to three percent of cases.

There is no specific antidote for LSD and no simple way to remove the drug from the body. The best treatment is to isolate the user in a quiet, dimly lit room, without the coming and going of strangers. The user is often frightened and paranoid. Someone whom the user trusts should stay and offer continual reassurance that the experience is not harmful and will soon end. The user should not be left alone, even for a few minutes, since the time distortion of LSD can make it seem like an eternity of abandonment.

 It may be necessary to repeat over and over such phrases as "it is only a drug," "you are not going crazy," "it will soon be over and you will feel normal."

The user should not be asked questions since this can provoke a flood of anxiety in a person struggling to maintain logical thought.

If anxiety is overwhelming, or the user falls into a panic, a sedative may be given, such as Valium, chloral hydrate, or sodium pentothal.

Physical signs of overdose usually imply that the LSD was mixed with other, more harmful drugs.

Physical signs of overdose

Fever
Rapid pulse
High blood pressure
Enlarged pupils
Hyperactivity
Drooling
Blank stare
Jerky eye movements
Muscle rigidity
Difficulty walking

Mental signs of overdose

Anxiety
Panic
Paranoia
Depersonalization
Mutism
Amnesia
Pressured speech

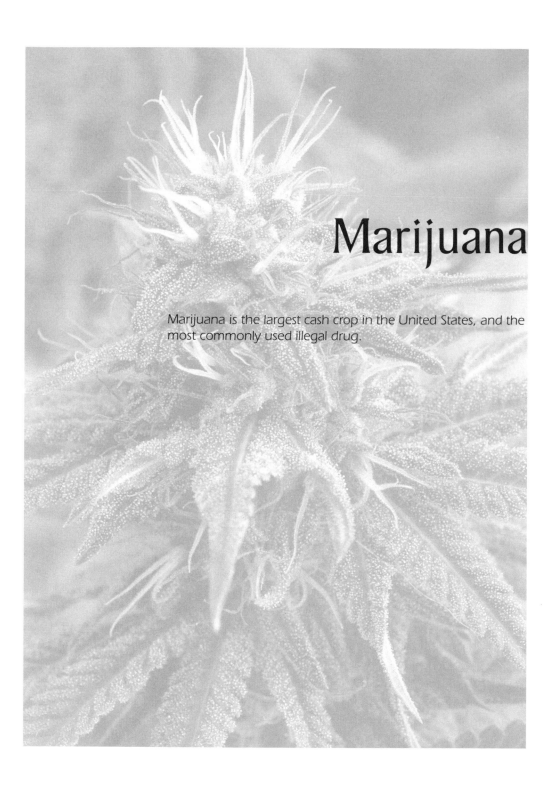

Marijuana

Marijuana is the largest cash crop in the United States, and the most commonly used illegal drug.

The Basic Facts

Type of drug	*Hallucinogen*
How taken	*Ingested, smoked*
Duration of effect	*2 to 8 hours*
Physical danger	*Low*
Addiction potential	*Low*

Other Names

Marijuana	*Acupulco Gold, African black, African bush, African woodbine airplane, Alice B. Toklas (brownie), amp joint (mixed with other narcotics), Angola, ashes, atshitshi, Aunt Mary, B (amount to fill a matchbox), B-40 (cigar filled with marijuana and dipped in malt liquor), baby, baby bhang, bale, bambalacha, bammer (weak marijuana), bar, Barbara Jean, bash, BC budd (from British Columbia), Belyando spruce, binky, black Bart, black gold, black gungi (from India), black gunion, black Maria, black Mo, black moat (mixed with honey), blanket, block, blue sage, blunt, Bob, bomber, boo, boom, bowl, broccoli, burnie, burning logs, can, canamo, canappa, cheeba, chronic, ganja, grass, herb, joint, Mary Jane, pakalolo, pot, reefer, weed, 420*
Marijuana and crack	*buda, chewies, cocktail, grimmie*
Marijuana and heroin	*atom bomb*
Marijuana and PCP	*ace, amp, fry, happy sticks, sherm, superweed, wet sticks*
Sinsemilla	*bud*
Hashish	*Alamout black hash (with belladonna), black ganja, black powder (ground into a powder), blond, charas, hash, kif, nup, shish, tar*
Hashish and opium	*black hash, black Russian, soles*
Hash oil	*green dragon, oil, shish oil*
Dronabinol	*Marinol*
Nabilone	*Cesamet*

Up in Smoke: The Story of Marijuana

Marijuana refers to the leaves and flowering tops of the cannabis plants, *Cannabis sativa* and *Cannabis indica*. These are probably not truly separate species, but variants of a single Cannabis species that originated in Asia and is now found throughout the world. *C. sativa*, the more common of the two, grows quickly and can reach a height of up to 15 feet. From seed to maturity takes three to five months outdoors, and as little as 60 days when grown indoors under ideal heat and light conditions. Historically, cannabis was grown to produce hemp for clothing, rope, paper, and other materials (see *Chapter 2: Marijuana*). The shorter variant, *C. indica*, has been cultivated around the world for the psychoactive properties of its resins. It reaches about four feet in height and is more bushy in appearance. Dried cannabis has a distinctive smell that varies according to the strain, with some having a strong pine or mint fragrance and others a skunk odor.

Archeological evidence shows that marijuana was used in China 12,000 years ago and then spread to the Middle East, North Africa, and Europe.[1] During the centuries of European conquest and colonization, its use extended to almost every country. In the United States, marijuana has a long history both as a medicinal tonic and as a recreational drug. Medical use reached a peak in the 19th century and then almost disappeared with the development of new medications. It is now again attracting interest as a remedy for people suffering from HIV, cancer, multiple sclerosis, and many other illnesses.

Until the 1960s, recreational use was largely confined to ethnic communities, artists and musicians. A survey in 1960 showed that only about three percent of population aged 18 to 25 had used marijuana. By 1970, this had increased to 40 percent

Marijuana is the flowering tops and leaves of the cannabis plant. These plants are often manicured to encourage more growth. Hashish is the resin exuded by the leaves to protect them from the sun's rays.[2]

and by 1980 to 70 percent, and marijuana had become widely regarded as a safe and non-addictive alternative to alcohol. It can now be considered mainstream—it is the most popular illegal drug in the United States and used throughout the country in every stratum of society.

 Marijuana is America's number one cash crop, with earnings estimated at $32 billion per year.

Home grown marijuana supplies only about one third of domestic consumption. The majority, 55 percent, is imported from Mexico, about 98 percent by vehicle.

JOINTS AND BLUNTS

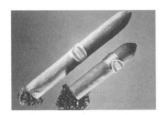

Blunts: cigars filled with marijuana

The most common way of using marijuana is by smoking it, either in a pipe or in a thinly rolled cigarette commonly referred to as a joint. These can easily fall apart and the smoke may be harsh, so many users empty a sturdy type of cigar or cigarette of its tobacco and replace it with marijuana. The result is known as a blunt, more stable than a cigarette and with a fragrant cigar smoke that helps mask the sweet smell of the marijuana.

ACAPULCO GOLD AND MAUI WOWIE

Much like tobacco, marijuana varies in potency depending on the type of plant, the way it is harvested, and the after-harvest processing. Marijuana grown in the United States was once considered inferior because of a low concentration of THC (delta-9-tetrahydrocannabinol, the major psychoactive ingredient). The best marijuana came from tropical areas such as Mexico and Hawaii—it was particularly popular in the tourist resorts of Acapulco and Maui. Acapulco Gold became a synonym for quality marijuana, no matter where it was grown.

 "Pot" probably comes from *potiguaya*, Mexican slang for marijuana.

By the 1980s, high penalties for importing drugs drove up the market value for potent marijuana and domestic suppliers responded by improving cultivation. In areas such as the Mendocino region of northern California, advancements in plant selection and cultivation resulted in highly potent products. In 1974, the average THC content of confiscated marijuana was less than one percent. By 1994 this had increased to five percent. Raids on outdoor growers encouraged suppliers to move their crops indoors, using specialized fluorescent grow lights. Indoor cultivation allowed year-round growing as well as much greater control over the crop and yet higher quality. Marijuana is now grown in this way throughout the United States and Canada.

"In buying grass, there are four things to remember: First, you don't want to get caught; second, you don't want to get bad grass; third, you don't want to overpay; and we can't remember the fourth."
—A Child's Garden of Grass [3]

Medium-grade marijuana is made from the dried flowering tops of female cannabis plants raised with, and fertilized by, male plants. Fertilization limits the psychoactive potency of the resulting marijuana because the female flower secretes THC-containing resin only until it is fertilized by male plants. After fertilization, the flower no longer needs the protective resin and it begins to produce seed.

When mature, marijuana appears as a green leafy bush that has a significant odor. The most distinctive feature is the shape of the serrated leaf, which may be wide or narrow and has three, five, seven, or a higher odd number of blades. The plant is harvested, ideally, when the resin glands begin to lose their luster and show a brown discoloration.

SINSEMILLA

In India, where marijuana has been popular since pre-historic times, potency was increased by selecting only small leaves and bracts of inflorescence from female plants. This preparation, called Ganja, was sometimes bundled together on a skewer, and more recently has been known as Thai Sticks. In California, selection was improved another step when the female plants were raised in isolation from male plants. The resulting marijuana is called sinsemilla, from the Spanish *sin semilla*, meaning without seeds.

Sinsemilla now accounts for about 85 percent of U.S. production. When these "buds" are harvested and dried, the concentration of THC can easily reach 10 percent, with some samples reaching up to 17 percent. In 1993, a new miniature hybrid variety was developed in the Netherlands. Called "skunk" on account of its odor, it is reputed to have a THC content as high as 30 percent. [4]

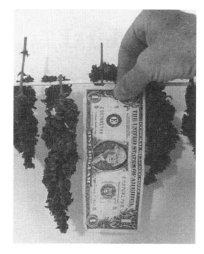
Sinsemilla buds, after harvesting

Indoor cultivation now accounts for the majority of home-grown marijuana, for many reasons: indoor cultivation allows year-round growth, the illegal operation can be more easily hidden, and the ability to precisely control the growing environment can produce a far higher quality product. During indoor growth, the amount of CO_2 can be increased in the closed environment of the growing area to speed up the rate at which plants will grow. Some operations use hydroponics, a fast and efficient method in which the plants are grown in a container of water and rocks with dissolved nutrients rather than in soil. Indoor cultivation has become quite sophisticated with Internet sites, specialty magazines, and even large supply shops catering to the needs of illicit farmers.

HASHISH

Hashish is the dried resin from flower tops and commonly contains up to 10 percent and as high as 20 percent THC. The purest form of hashish is virtually 100 percent resin. Most hashish, however, is not pure resin and contains varying amounts of other fibrous plant material. It is a dark-colored gummy ball that is rather hard, but not brittle.

Cheap labor is essential to produce hashish, as it takes an enormous number of man-hours to process. The resin is gathered in the summer months by hand-rubbing cannabis plants and forming little beads of the gooey material. When properly rubbed, the plant lives on and continues to produce resin until the seasonal rains bring an end to harvesting. After collection, the resin is compressed into a variety of forms, such as balls, cakes, or cookie-like sheets.[5] Pieces are then broken off, placed in pipes and smoked.

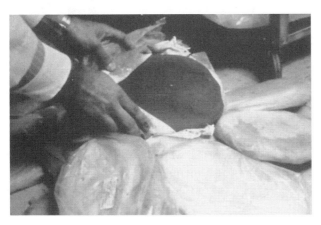

Hashish was developed in the Middle East and became popular throughout Northern Africa and Europe. Most hashish is smuggled into the United States from Pakistan, Nepal, Afghanistan, and Lebanon. Perhaps because of the need to import hashish, and the increased potency of sinsemilla, hashish has not become as popular in the United States as it is in other countries.

Large cakes of hashish for sale in Afghanistan

HASH OIL

Hash oil is made by boiling hash or marijuana in a solvent such as alcohol, gasoline, or kerosene, which absorbs THC. The sediment is then removed by filtering, resulting in a thick liquid that varies in odor and ranges in color from clear to yellow, dark brown, or black, depending on the process. Hash oil typically contains about 15 to 30 percent THC, with reports as high as 70 percent. A drop or two on a tobacco cigarette is as potent as a single marijuana joint.[6]

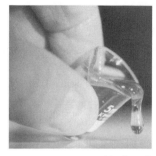
Hash oil

Most hash oil is imported from Jamaica and the Middle East. Because hash oil is light sensitive, it is normally packaged in dark colored glass vials.

SUPERWEED

Marijuana joints may be sprinkled with PCP or crack cocaine, or dipped in formaldehyde (embalming fluid), to obtain a more intense hallucinogenic or stimulating experience. This practice is common in the eastern United States.

MEDICAL MARIJUANA

Marijuana was used in ancient India and China as medication for a large number of ailments. Its medical use continued in Europe and the Americas until the 20th century. Between 1840 and 1900, European and American medical journals published hundreds of articles on the therapeutic use of marijuana, frequently referred to as cannabis or Indian hemp. It was recommended as an appetite stimulant, muscle relaxant, analgesic, hypnotic, and anticonvulsant. As late as 1913, the leading American medical authority Sir William Osler recommended it as the preferred remedy for migraine. There were 28 different preparations for sale in the United States, including pills, tablets, and elixirs. All were taken off the market after the Marijuana Tax Act (see *Chapter 3*).

By the early years of the 20th century, its use as a medication had begun to decline because of the uncertain potency of the preparations, the lack of a form that could be injected, and because newer, synthetic drugs such as aspirin and barbiturates became available. Concern was developing over the non-medical use of marijuana, particularly in western states, where it was considered to be a Mexican drug. Subtle hostility toward Mexican immigrants, who were thought to contribute to the labor surplus during the widespread unemployment of the Depression, was transferred to open hostility to marijuana (see *Chapter 2*).

Just as the prohibition of alcohol was finally achieved with the anti-German sentiment of the First World War, the prohibition against marijuana succeeded only when western state governments used anti-Mexican bigotry to make the drug illegal. The Federal Government, however, was not convinced. Rather than make it illegal outright, the United States Congress passed the Marihuana Tax Act of 1937, stipulating that any interstate transport of marijuana required a tax stamp from the Government. These stamps were rarely issued, however, and marijuana was removed from the U.S. Pharmacopoeia and became effectively illegal. In 1970, it was added to the list of Schedule I Controlled Substances, indicating that it had a high potential for abuse and no accepted medical use.

A number of physicians remained convinced that marijuana could be a valuable medication for certain illnesses. They argued that it should be moved to Schedule II, allowing its use as a prescription medication, while still otherwise illegal. In 1986, the U.S. Drug Enforcement Administration agreed to hold public hearings on the issue. In the following two years, a large number of physicians and patients testified to the safety and efficacy of marijuana, particularly in the treatment of AIDS, a new epidemic. In 1988, Francis L. Young, the administrative law judge of the DEA, acknowledged the medical potential of marijuana and ordered that it be moved to Schedule II. The order was overruled by the DEA.

 "Marijuana is one of the safest therapeutically active substances known to man"—Judge Francis Young [7]

Despite the Federal Government's adherence to the illegality of marijuana, 36 individual states have passed laws allowing medical use, and 10 have established formal research programs to evaluate marijuana as an investigational new drug (IND). Public sympathy with terminally ill patients persuaded the FDA to approve a number of physicians' requests for an Individual Treatment IND, also commonly referred to as a Compassionate IND. The application process is discouragingly complex, however, and with the legal status uncertain, most physicians are reluctant to risk losing their medical licenses if they prescribe marijuana.

 "When I started intravenous chemotherapy, absolutely nothing worked at all … Marijuana worked like a charm … was the greatest boost I received in all my year of treatment, and surely had a most important effect upon my eventual cure."—Stephen Jay Gould, Harvard Professor [8]

Many physicians continue to recommend marijuana informally to their patients. The most common uses are to alleviate the nausea and vomiting caused by cancer chemotherapy, and to help stimulate the appetite for HIV patients suffering from the wasting syndrome. Marijuana is also used to lower intraocular pressure in glaucoma, to prevent muscle spasms and seizures, and to alleviate phantom limb pain, menstrual cramps, and many other types of chronic pain—including Sir Osler's remedy for migraines.[9]

 "One of marihuana's greatest advantages as a medicine is its remarkable safety. It has little effect on major physiological functions. There is no known case of a lethal overdose."—American Medical Association, 1995 [10]

MARINOL: A MEDICAL SUBSTITUTE

While marijuana remains illegal, the major psychoactive constituent, THC, has been available for medical use since 1985. Dronabinol is synthetic THC and is marketed in capsule form under the brand name Marinol. In theory, dronabinol should be as effective as marijuana in relieving cancer pain and nausea. In practice, both patients and physicians disagree. A research program in New Mexico that allocated either marijuana or synthetic THC to 260 cancer patients found marijuana clearly superior in controlling nausea and vomiting—indeed, marijuana was even more effective than chlorpromazine, one of the most potent anti-vomiting agents.[11]

Why is dronabinol less effective than marijuana? The likely answer is that marijuana is a complex substance with many constituents other than THC. These other chemicals may have properties that contribute both individually and in combination to the overall effect. Cannabidiol, for example, is a component of marijuana that is not present in Marinol. Taken alone, cannabidiol has been shown to relieve anxiety. It is likely that the combination of THC with cannabidiol makes a more effective antinauseant than either drug alone.

Nabilone is a synthetic analog of THC that has been found to prevent vomiting after chemotherapy. Animal studies have shown nabilone to be a remarkably safe drug even after very intensive and prolonged use.[12]

THE DEBATE CONTINUES

When the Marihuana Tax Act of 1937 was passed, effectively making marijuana illegal, the American Medical Association was one of the few organizations that protested. Physicians now tend to be quiet on the matter, although many believe that there may be some legitimate medical uses and that the danger has been exaggerated. In a 1990 survey, 44 percent of cancer specialists said they had recommended that their patients smoke marijuana for the relief of nausea caused by chemotherapy.[13]

Perhaps the majority of physicians are concerned about the long-term effects of marijuana abuse but feel that this concern should not prevent its availability to those who might be helped by it. In 1999 the Institute of Medicine published a comprehensive review of marijuana. Their report concluded that marijuana has significant medical potential in the relief of nausea, pain, and appetite stimulation.[14]

"At present, the greatest danger in medical use of marihuana is its illegality, which imposes much anxiety and expense on suffering people, forces them to bargain with illicit drug dealers, and exposes them to the threat of criminal prosecution."—American Medical Association, 1995 [15]

Physicians opposed to the use of marijuana are more concerned about the practical and moral implications of giving credence to a widely abused substance. Those who recommend its medical use, they say, are simply using marijuana as a wedge to open the door for recreational use.[16] There is little doubt that allowing easy medical access would increase the overall use of marijuana, but whether this increase should be reason enough to disallow medical use is a matter of continuing debate.

Who Is Using Marijuana?

According to National Household Survey on Drug Abuse, there are currently 9,800,000 users of marijuana. Almost 20 million people have used marijuana at least once in the past year, about 5 million of them once a week or more. One third of all adult Americans have tried the drug. These are remarkable statistics given that simple possession of marijuana can destroy the career of many professionals or bring a lengthy prison sentence.

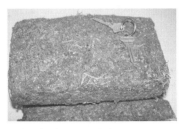

A brick of processed marijuana smuggled into the U.S.

The administration of President Clinton was widely viewed as a return to the more permissive attitude of President Carter, away from the hard-line approach of the Reagan and Bush administrations. However, the number of recent arrests for marijuana does not indicate a more lenient policy. During Clinton's time in office, about three million Americans were arrested for marijuana offenses. The 1997 total was the highest ever recorded by the FBI, with 695,200 people arrested for marijuana possession, double the number of arrests recorded in 1993.

In the United States, one marijuana smoker is arrested every 45 seconds, about 700,000 per year.[17]

 78% of high school students report that marijuana is used, sold, and kept at their schools.[18]

GOING DUTCH

In the rest of the world, attitudes to marijuana range from open tolerance to severe penalties including death. Of the industrialized countries, the most liberal is the Netherlands.

The Netherlands has pioneered an approach that attempts to control drug abuse while avoiding the criminality associated with the use of illegal drugs. Marijuana and hashish are technically illegal, but about 4,000 coffee shops are permitted to sell up to five grams (previously 30 grams, or about one ounce) to anyone over 16 years of age. Most of the marijuana consumed in the Netherlands is grown domestically indoors.[19] The lack of major smuggling operations, and ready availability of marijuana, has brought the price down and been effective in removing most of the criminal element.

Although smoking marijuana is certainly popular in the Netherlands and other countries that have removed criminal penalties, the worry that this might encourage users to progress to other drugs such as cocaine and heroin has not been borne out. In fact, the percentage of the population who use marijuana or other drugs in the Netherlands is much lower than in the United States.

 28   percentage of 10th grade students who have used marijuana in Holland
41   percentage of 10th grade students who have used marijuana in the United States [20]

 "I have never smoked marijuana. Why should I? I see people all day come in here to buy it. After they smoke, they look stupid."
—*Amsterdam marijuana shop employee* [21]

MEDICAL USE

In California, Proposition 215, the Compassionate Use Act of 1996, allows patients or defined caregivers to possess or grow marijuana for medical treatment so long as it is prescribed by a physician. Some physicians who favor legalization are happy to recommend it for almost all ailments and, in any case, complaints of nausea or pain are largely subjective and difficult to deny. In Arizona,

Proposition 200, the Drug, Medicalization, Prevention, and Control Act of 1996 went even further by giving physicians the right to prescribe other Schedule I drugs such as LSD for medical purposes.

There is a fine line between recreational and medical use of marijuana. If smoking marijuana to control pain or nausea is considered medicine, what about smoking it for anxiety or depression? What if an artist or musician uses marijuana to relax, or for inspiration? While the recreational use of marijuana goes through cycles of popularity, the purported medical use is steadily gaining.

NORML

In 1981, a group of people lobbying for the decriminalization of marijuana formed the National Organization for the Reform of Marijuana Laws.[22] The ultimate goal of NORML and The NORML Foundation is to permit the legal use of marijuana by adults in a private setting. Rather than favoring the open use of marijuana, NORML believes that the federal prohibition should be abolished and each state should determine to what extent it will allow the use of marijuana. In this way, various hypotheses of the outcome of liberalized use can be tested.[23]

Chemical Characteristics

Cannabis was previously believed to be a genus of plants with different species: *Cannabis sativa*, *Cannabis indica*, and *Cannabis ruderalis*. These are now generally considered to be variants of a single species. All variants contain the 61 compounds, called cannabinoids, that are found in no other plants. One of these, delta-9-tetrahydrocannabinol (THC), is considered to be the major psychoactive constituent, although the other cannabinoids have also been shown to be biologically active. The amount of THC varies among strains, among individual plants, within the plant itself, and during the plant's life cycle. The genetic quality of the seed is the single most important factor in determining the plant's ultimate THC potency.[24] It also is affected by the method of cultivation.[25] The highest concentration is in the tight group of buds, or cola, in the flowering tops, in which THC averages about seven percent of the total weight.

As the cannabis plant matures, the balance changes of the many chemicals. In the young plant, cannabidiolic acid (CBDA) predominates. It is converted to cannabidiol (CBD), which is then converted to THC as the plant begins to flower. Not all of the CBD is converted to THC, and the final amount determines the potency of the marijuana.

If the plant is not harvested when it flowers, it continues to mature and the THC is converted into cannabinol (CBN). The result is a type of marijuana with a heavier, more sedating effect.[26] A female plant that is not pollinated will continue to develop resin laden flowers rather than divert its energies into generating seeds, producing the highly potent sinsemilla. If it is pollinated, the seeds change their appearance as the plant becomes more mature.

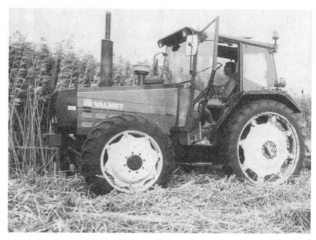

Legal hemp harvest—will this become a common sight?

Small, yellowish seeds suggest that the plant was cut early, before full maturity, while round and dark seeds indicate that the plant was harvested when the resin and THC content were at a peak.

 Cannabis contains 421 chemicals in 18 different chemical classes. Among these are 61 cannabinoids which are found in no other plants. Burning marijuana during smoking creates hundreds of additional compounds. The effect of most of these, alone or in combination, is not fully understood.

EFFECTS

The psychoactive parts of marijuana—the cannabinoids, including THC—are not water-soluble and therefore cannot be injected, but have to be smoked or ingested.

Until the mid-20th century, marijuana was usually taken by swallowing a baked preparation or an elixir, but now smoking is by far the most common method. About 30 percent of the THC in smoked marijuana is destroyed by pyrolysis. Another 20 to 40 percent is lost in side-stream smoke. Despite these losses, smoking is still the most effective method of using the drug, partly because the heat of combustion converts much of the delta-6 isomer of THC into the more powerfully psychoactive delta-1 form.

The effects of smoking marijuana begin in a few minutes, peak at 15 to 45 minutes, and then gradually diminish over two to six hours. Typically, the effects include euphoria, relaxed inhibitions, increased appetite, and disorientation. There may also be dry mouth and throat, dizziness, and increased visual and auditory awareness. Concentration, learning, perception, and fine muscle skills are somewhat impaired. Although the initial high may be gone within hours, some of the effects of marijuana on mental and physical functioning may be quite subtle and last for days. Studies of experienced pilots in a flight simulator showed a deficiency up to 24 hours later.[27]

"I now became unable to fix my attention on anything and I had the most irresistible desire to laugh. Everything seemed so ridiculously funny; even circumstances of a serious nature were productive of mirth."
—Dr. C.R. Marshall, medical marijuana researcher, 1897 [28]

Ingesting a cannabis extract such as hashish produces an onset of effects in about 30 minutes, which then last about three to five hours. The absorption is variable, depending on many factors.

Marijuana must be heated to be absorbed by the stomach. Simply eating marijuana, such as eating cannabis leaves in a salad, will produce little or no effect. In order for marijuana to contain THC in its free form, it needs to be subjected to intense heat or some other process which decarboxylates the acid precursor. This is usually done by boiling it in tea or heating in an oven, such as the popular "hash brownies."

MARIJUANA AND THE BRAIN

The action of marijuana in the brain has only recently become known. In 1992, researchers at the Hebrew University in Jerusalem discovered a nerve receptor that is specific for cannabinoids. This led to a search for a natural cannabinoid in the brain to match these receptors. When the researchers found it, they named it anandamide, from *ananda*, a Sanskrit word meaning bliss. A second naturally occurring cannabinoid, a derivative of arachidonic acid, 2-arachidonylglycerol (2-AG), has since been found in the brains of humans and animals. 2-AG is now considered to be the major natural cannabinoid.

The greatest concentration of cannabinoid receptors is located in the cerebellum, the basal ganglia, and the hippocampus. The hippocampus is believed to be active in forming new memories. It has long been known that marijuana interferes with memory, especially the ability to learn new information. Studies on rats showed that THC suppressed the activity of the hippocampal cells, hindering their ability to store new memories but not to recall earlier information. After the THC was eliminated, the hippocampal function returned to normal, without evidence of permanent changes or injury to the neurons. These findings suggest that marijuana may have a temporary effect on learning or memory, but this effect is not permanent.

Marijuana receptors are much more common in the brain than are opiate receptors. However, there are no marijuana receptors in the brain stem, which controls basic vital functions such as breathing, and this is why marijuana overdose is not lethal.

Drug testing

The standard drug test for marijuana employs immunoassay or gas chromatography/mass spectroscopy (GC/MS) to test urine for 11-nor-delta-9-tetrahydrocannabinol-9-carbolylic acid (THC-COOH). The Government-established cutoff value is 15 ng/mL.[29] This level indicates that the user was exposed to a very significant amount of marijuana—more than would be possible by only inhaling the smoke from other users.

 In the 1998 Winter Olympics, snowboarding gold medal winner Ross Rebagliati of Canada was disqualified because of a positive marijuana test. He argued that it was due to others smoking around him—and was allowed to keep his medal. This excuse is no longer permitted.

Cannabinoids are readily absorbed from the lungs and the gastro-intestinal tract. They enter the circulation and are stored and accumulate in fatty tissue, and then gradually excreted from the body. The half-life of THC has been estimated at anywhere from 18 to 48 hours. A person who smokes marijuana for the first time may test positive for one to three days at the 15 ng/mL cutoff. Because THC accumulates, a frequent marijuana user can test positive for more than four weeks after the last use.[30] Although THC is stored in fat, reducing body fat has not been shown to alter the rate at which THC-COOH is stored or excreted.[31]

If the drug test is positive for marijuana, the only legitimate excuse is either the use of dronabinol or, if allowed, the use of medically prescribed marijuana.

Withdrawal Signs

Most marijuana users—even those with long-term, heavy use—experience no withdrawal when they stop.[32] Some people have reported generally mild symptoms, including insomnia, hyperactivity, decreased appetite, nausea, diarrhea, restlessness, irritability, depression, anxiety, salivation, sweating, and tremors. There may also be a slight increase in heart rate, blood pressure, and body temperature.

If there are any symptoms at all, they usually occur within a day of withdrawal, peak in about two to four days, and then resolve within a week or two.

REVERSE TOLERANCE

An odd feature of marijuana is that many, perhaps most, people don't even get high the first few times they use marijuana. It seems that the user has to learn how to appreciate or perceive the psychoactive effects of the drug. This is the opposite of most other drugs, where users build up a tolerance to the effects. People who smoke a lot of marijuana are so familiar with the feeling that they respond to even fake marijuana cigarettes.

Long-term Health Problems

The main concern with the long-term use of marijuana is the effect of smoking on the lungs. Cannabis smoke has as much tar, carbon monoxide, cyanide and other toxic material as tobacco smoke. The two most potent cancer-causing agents in tobacco smoke, benzanthrene and benzpyrene, are present in even higher amounts in marijuana smoke. Because marijuana smokers tend to inhale more deeply, they absorb about five times as much carbon monoxide and tar than tobacco smokers.

Heavy marijuana smokers may eventually acquire the same health problems as tobacco smokers, including bronchitis, emphysema and bronchial asthma.[33] Marijuana has less effect on the heart than tobacco, but smoking marijuana does increase the heart rate by about 20 to 30 beats per minute.

Overall, the combination of heavy tobacco use and marijuana is far worse than each individually.

Holding it in
The typical marijuana smoker takes a puff and holds it in the lungs as long as possible. Research has shown that this practice, "toking," makes no difference in the amount of drug absorbed—it is just folklore.[34]

MARIJUANA AND THE IMMUNE SYSTEM

Marijuana has been reported to weaken the immune system. This may be a concern to people using medical marijuana to improve appetite and decrease nausea for cancer or HIV, both of which hurt the immune system. However, clinical research has not found that marijuana is hazardous on this account.

People with immune deficiencies should be concerned about contamination of marijuana with *Aspergillus* spores, which can cause the fungal infection aspergillosis. Baking the marijuana at 150° C (300° F) for 15 minutes will destroy the fungal spores, but not degrade the THC content.

OTHER HEALTH PROBLEMS

Lengthy use of marijuana has been reported to cause an impairment of memory, schizophrenia, and other mental illnesses. In the 1960s, there were claims that marijuana brought about a vaguely defined form of mental deficiency, which came to be called the "amotivational syndrome."[35] Further investigation found that there was no such syndrome and that the earlier findings were due to other social phenomena.[36]

Marijuana has been associated with a variety of other health problems, such as erectile dysfunction, decreased sperm counts and the development of breast tissue in men, and irregular menstrual cycles in women. Most of these reports were anecdotal, or from poorly done studies. More recent research has not found these effects.

On balance, even with long-term use, marijuana appears to be a remarkably safe and nontoxic substance.

IS MARIJUANA ADDICTIVE?

Marijuana does not cause a physical dependence. There is an active debate, however, about whether marijuana should be considered to cause psychological dependence. For reasons that are not clear, some users do develop the compulsive behavior that is characteristic of addiction, although to a much smaller degree than with other addictive drugs.

 "The smoking of cannabis, even long term, is not harmful to health."
—*The Lancet, 1995* [37]

What To Do If There Is An Overdose

Marijuana is considered a relatively safe drug. It does not directly cause significant harm to the body, and there is no known case of a lethal overdose. Research using animals shows that it is necessary to take about 40,000 times the normal amount to cause a lethal dose. By comparison, fatalities can be caused by five to ten times the intoxicating dose of alcohol, and as little as three times the normal dose of barbiturates or GHB. Most users simply stop smoking marijuana when they feel they have had enough. Overdoses are usually due to eating marijuana or hashish, when absorption can continue for hours and overwhelm the user.

If too much marijuana has been eaten, vomiting may be induced or a cathartic given to flush out the gastrointestinal tract. Otherwise, the user is expected to recover in hours without the need for medical care.

Physical signs of overdose   Racing pulse
                                   Low blood pressure

Mental signs of overdose   Unresponsive stupor

MDMA

MDMA, methylene-dioxy-methamphetamine, is more commonly known as Ecstasy. With chemical features of mescaline and the amphetamines, it is most often used to enhance intimacy and social openness.

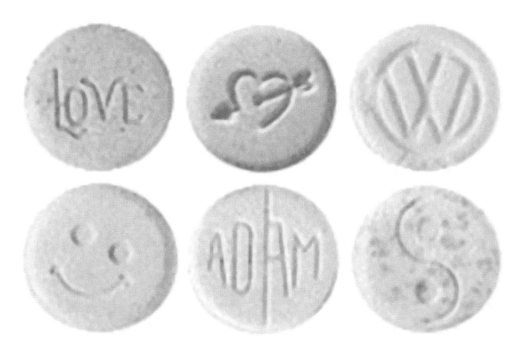

The Basic Facts

Type of drug	*Stimulant*
How taken	*Ingested, snorted, injected*
Duration of effect	*3 to 6 hours*
Physical danger	*Moderate*
Addiction potential	*None*

Other Names

2C-B	*bees, bromo, nexus, spectrum, venus*
DOM	*STP*
MDEA	*Eve*
MDMA	*Adam, baby slits, bean, booty juice, candy flip (with LSD), chocolate chips, clarity, E, ecstasy, essence, love drug, M, rave, roll, X, XTC*
PMA	*Death*

Adam, Eve, and Ecstasy: The Story of MDMA

FROM AMPHETAMINES TO MDA

Following the discovery of amphetamines a century ago, drug companies were eager to create other variants of these stimulants and explore their effects. MDA, methylenedioxyamphetamine, synthesized in 1910, was the first and simplest member of the new drug cluster. It is chemically very similar to the natural drug ephedrine.

On Christmas Eve, 1913, the German pharmaceutical company Merck took out a patent for another form of MDA, building on to methamphetamine rather than amphetamine. The new drug, MDMA, was thought to have potential as an appetite suppressant. Animal tests were not impressive in this regard, however, and it was never tested on humans.

MDMA was all but forgotten until 1953, when the U.S. Army Office of Strategic Services (OSS, which later became the CIA) began to explore psychoactive drugs as "non-conventional agents" for use in warfare and interrogation. MDMA, labeled EA-1475, was one of the Experimental Agents tested in Project MK-Ultra at the Chemical Warfare Service in Edgewood, Maryland. The Army did not find it of much use. In comparison to other chemical weapons, MDMA was found to be too weak to be of any interest, and it was once again passed over.

EMPATHY AGENT

In 1965, a biochemist working at Dow Chemical Company, Alexander T. Shulgin, synthesized MDMA. Dr. Shulgin was fascinated by psychoactive substances, and explored and synthesized hundreds of them. In 1978, Shulgin published the first scientific article on the effects of MDMA on humans, noting that the drug caused people to open up socially, turning timid users into garrulous talkers. It seemed to reverse any social deficiency. MDMA, he said, "could be all things to all people."

Shulgin recommended MDMA to Dr. Leo Zoff, a psychiatrist who began to use it in therapy. MDMA

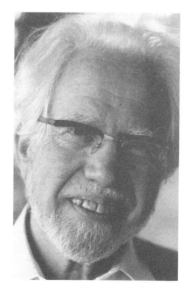

Dr. Alexander T. Shulgin popularized MDMA

was found to be particularly useful in marriage counseling, helping couples achieve insight and mutual understanding of their problems. It seemed to break through hardened defenses and promote trust and honesty.

 "I love the world and the world loves me."—MDMA therapy client

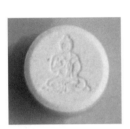

Word spread among psychotherapists of a new pill that created empathy. They began to take it themselves, alone or often together with their patients. An early enthusiast, Dr. George Greer, reported that the drug "enabled people to communicate ideas, beliefs, opinions, and memories that may have long been repressed in them." Ralph Metzner, Dean of the California Institute of Integral Studies, was particularly enthusiastic about the potential of this "empathy drug." At a 1983 conference at the University of California at Santa Barbara, he proposed the name "empathogen" to describe MDMA and related drugs. On the street, it was more commonly known by a partial re-arrangement of the letters MDMA to ADAM, making it easier to say and perhaps giving it a biblical hint of mysticism.

The real marketing coup occurred when one distributor decided to call it Ecstasy, resulting in an enormous boost in popularity. As Ecstasy, MDMA quickly spread from psychologists to college students and then to the general recreational drug market. By 1976, clandestine labs in California were producing 10,000 doses per month, rising to 30,000 in 1984 and 50,000 in 1985.

 The man who first named it "Ecstasy" told me that he chose the name because it would sell better than calling it "Empathy"—*Bruce Eisner, Ecstasy: The MDMA Story* [1]

The FDA has never approved MDMA for any purpose. When the drug was tested for safety, it was found to destroy brain cells in animals. Concern about these toxic effects, and the widely proliferating abuse, led the DEA to use its emergency powers to put MDMA on Schedule I, temporarily in July 1985, and then permanently on November 13, 1986, as a drug with high abuse potential and no acceptable medical use.[2]

DESIGNER DRUGS

MDMA was never manufactured for sale by a pharmaceutical company. As such, it joined a growing number of drugs that originally had been developed as pharmaceuticals but found to have insufficient medical use, and then diverted by others for recreational use (see *Chapter 6: Designer Drugs*). These are usually variations of approved medications. Since they have no accepted medical use, they are manufactured only in illicit operations. Some were made experimentally, or even accidentally, by amateur chemists trying to produce another mind-altering substance and circumvent existing drug laws.

 The cult leader Bhagwan Shree Rajneesh set up 600 communes worldwide. His followers slipped MDMA into the drinks of rich "sanyassins" to encourage donations.[3]

The result is an increasing number of new drugs. Most of these are simply called by their chemical acronym (see *Chapter 6: The Amphetamine Family*). For example, in MDMA, changing the *methyl* group to an *ethyl* group creates MDEA, a drug which is reported to have the same effects as MDMA but without the "rush" and many of the side effects such as jaw clenching, sweating, and withdrawal fatigue. Once the drug achieves some popularity, street names pop up. For example, MDEA became known as Eve (as a take-off on ADAM, no doubt).

A number of these new drugs were derived from myristicin, a psychoactive constituent of the aromatic oils of nutmeg and mace (see *Chapter 7: Nutmeg*). MMDA and other variants were discovered by Shulgin experimenting with myristicin. The irrepressible biochemist also synthesized DOM, 150 times more potent than mescaline and producing an intense experience of depersonalization described as "witness consciousness." In January 1967, 5,000 tablets of this substance, renamed STP (for Serenity, Tranquility, and Peace), were distributed free at the first "Human Be-in" in San Francisco. The result was disastrous as the users were unprepared for the powerful experience.

"Hundreds of people experienced hallucinatory episodes lasting three days, many ending up in the Emergency Departments of various Bay Area hospitals wondering if they would ever come down."[4]

The inventive Dr. Shulgin went on to synthesize DOB, DOET, and over 200 other new mind-altering substances, very few of which ever achieved popular use.

Designer drugs each have their own features. Some, like 2C-B, produce a visual experience and are reported to be very useful to recover repressed traumatic memories. Others, like MBDB, are less visual and promote a quiet sense of insight with the user less inclined to talk.

ALPHABET (AND CHEMICAL) SOUP

Most amphetamines and their derivatives are simple drugs that are relatively easy to manufacture, even in a rudimentary home laboratory. The drugs differ from one another in their potency, speed of onset, duration of action and their capacity to modify mood with or without producing overt hallucinations.[5] Because of their relation to the well-known drug mescaline, the potency of these new variants is often described in mescaline units.

Very few of these drugs are in popular use, and some are very toxic. PMA, for example, was often passed off as MDA between 1972 and 1973, but caused a dangerous rise in blood pressure and temperature and could result in convulsions. The drug caused a number of deaths in the U.S., and ten fatalities in Australia before it passed out of use. In 2000, it resurfaced in Canada labeled as Ecstasy. When two young men in Toronto died after taking it, Health Canada declared PMA one of the most dangerous hallucinogens in the world.

Some of the amphetamine designer drugs, their common acronyms, and potency relative to mescaline include:

Chemical	Common name	Mescaline units of potency
3,4-methylenedioxyphenyl-2-butanamine	BDB	?
4-bromo-2,5-dimethoxyphenethylamine	2C-B (Bromo, Venus)	8
4-bromo-2,5-dimethoxyamphetamine	DMA	6
2,5- dimethoxy-4-amylamphetamine	DOAM	10
4-bromo-2,5-dimethoxymethamphetamine	DOB	150
2,5- dimethoxy-4-butylamphetamine	DOBU	36
2,5-dimethoxy-4-ethylamphetamine	DOET	100
2,5- dimethoxy-4-methylamphetamine	DOM (STP)	80
2,5- dimethoxy-4-propylamphetamine	DOPR	80
N-hydroxy-3,4-methylenedioxyamphetamine	MDA	3
5-methoxy-3,4-methylenedioxyamphetamine	5-methoxy-MDA	3
N-ethyl-3,4-methylenedioxyamphetamine	MDEA (Eve)	4
3, 4-methylenedioxymethamphetamine	MDMA (Ecstasy)	4
N-methyl-3,4-methylenedioxyamphetamine	MDM	4
3-methoxy-4,5-methylenedioxyamphetamine	MMDA	3
N-ethylamphetamine	NEA	?
para-4-methoxyamphetamine	PMA (Death)	6
3,4,5-trimethoxyamphetamine	TMA	2
2,4,5-trimethoxyamphetamine	TMA-2	20
2,3,4-trimethoxyamphetamine	TMA-3	< 2
2,3,5-trimethoxyamphetamine	TMA-4	4
2,3,6-trimethoxyamphetamine	TMA-5	10
2,4,6-trimethoxyamphetamine	TMA-6	10

2C-B

Dr. Shulgin first synthesized 2C-B in 1974 while exploring variants of DOB. He tried it himself on June 25, 1975, described it as "beautifully active," and went on to recommend it as a psychedelic drug. When MDMA became illegal in 1985, 2C-B was marketed as a legal MDMA substitute. In 1993, 2C-B was placed on Schedule I in the United States, and by 1999 it was illegal in most of the world.

 DEADLY 'ECSTASY' TURNS UP IN CANADIAN NIGHTCLUBS
TORONTO—A deadly street drug disguised as "ecstasy" has surfaced at dance clubs around Ontario, prompting police to issue a warning ...
—Toronto Globe and Mail, Oct 14, 2000

2C-B continues to be sold as Ecstasy, but is more often sought by users for its unique effects, which are described as pleasurable energy, heightened bodily awareness, or a "sense of being in the body." Many users claim enhancement of both sexual interest and sexual pleasure, and may combine it with MDMA.[6] Others say it causes an unpleasant "buzzing" and find the increased bodily sensations very disagreeable.

On an empty stomach, a standard dose of 10 to 40 milligrams will have an effect in about an hour; this can be much longer depending on the type and amount of food taken. The small pills, which sometimes contain just five milligrams, can also be crushed into a powder and snorted for a shorter experience and quicker onset, but this is reportedly quite painful.

When taken by mouth, the effects of 2C-B last about four to six hours, followed by a gradual resolution of about two to four hours. At first, there is a sense of anticipation or anxiety. This is followed by a wide variety of perceptual changes, including visual patterns and movement with shifting colors. There is a sense of mental stimulation, new perspectives, feelings of insight, and emotional shifts ranging from happiness to anxiety and confusion. Overall, the effects are more subtle than other hallucinogens such as LSD or psilocybin, and those who like the drug say that it gives them a chance to reflect on their thoughts.

Most users report little or no after effects. However, many who try 2C-B find it intensely disagreeable. Diarrhea, cramping and gas are common, and some have complained of allergic-type reactions with coughing and runny nose. Some users feel anxious or have frightening thoughts and visions, though less so than with LSD.

Illicit 2C-B is often sold along with MDMA at raves and parties, as "Venus," "Bromo," "Spectrum," and by other names. Prices average $10 to

$35 per dose, with bulk prices at $100 to $500 per gram. Because it is a relatively unusual drug, confiscated drug samples show that it is generally pure and uncontaminated. Most use is by an exclusive and knowledgeable group.

Who Is Using MDMA?

By the late 1980s, MDMA became very popular among college students. A study at Stanford University in 1987 reported that 39 percent of the undergraduates had tried MDMA. Their use tended to be experimental—it was part of the college experience, especially for psychology or social science students. Once they had explored the effects, most students lost interest and disliked the longer lasting side effects.

"Desirable effects begin to change with each successive dose: freshmen love it, sophomores like it, juniors are ambivalent, and seniors afraid of it."[7]

From the universities, MDMA spread into the highschools and then into the dancehalls. Currently, 8.2 percent of U.S. highschool seniors say they have taken it, up from 5.8 percent in 1997.[8] Between 1998 and 1999, use rose 33% among 10th graders, and 56% among 12th graders.

Most MDMA users do not take it often, but there are some whose use borders on addiction. Some binge on it, in the same way that they would on amphetamines or cocaine, despite the rapid tolerance to the drug.

MDMA is especially popular at raves; along with GHB, it has become the drug of choice at these dances. Sometimes MDMA is combined with LSD, called "candyflipping," for a more intense experience.

"E makes shirtless, disgusting men, a club with broken bathrooms, a deejay that plays crap and vomiting into a trash can the best night of your life."
—Adrienne, a Midwestern woman and frequent MDMA user[9]

According to the United Nations Office for Drug Control and Crime Prevention (ODCCP), about 90 percent of the worldwide supply of MDMA is produced in illicit laboratories in the Netherlands and Belgium, and then trafficked internationally by Israeli organized-crime groups. Wholesale prices at the source are $.50 to $2.00 per tablet, which increase to $20 to $45 retail in the United States. One kilo of MDMA powder is enough for 10,000 tablets.

Most of the smuggled MDMA comes through New York. The traffickers usually employ couriers who pose as tourists to carry the powder or pills across borders. In 2000, customs officers seized 9.3 million tablets of MDMA, a huge increase over 1999 of 3.5 million, but this is only a small fraction of the imports. The DEA estimates that more than two million pills are smuggled from Europe into the United States each week.[10]

IS THAT PILL ECSTASY?

The manufacture of MDMA is not difficult, with several possible methods of synthesis. MDMA generally appears as a white crystalline substance, usually pressed into a small pill. About half of the tablet is MDMA and the rest filler. A brownish tint to the powder or tablets indicates that synthesis was incomplete. Although manufacture is relatively simple, sales of the precursor materials are monitored by the DEA. If these inexpensive materials can be obtained, there is plenty of profit for MDMA dealers.

 With manufacturing costs of less than a penny per tablet, MDMA is far more profitable than heroin.

Because MDMA is produced in illegal, unprofessional laboratories, it is rarely pure. The amount of actual MDMA in a capsule or tablet can vary from 50 up to 200 or 300 milligrams—or none at all.[11] Many other substances have been found in pills sold as MDMA, including amphetamine, ephedrine, caffeine, ketamine,[12] methamphetamine, acetaminophen, MDA, MDEA,[13] PMA, or dextromethorphan. In Switzerland, a large confiscation of Ecstasy tablets turned out to be 2C-B.[14]

DanceSafe is a pro-rave organization based in Berkeley, California. Largely funded by Microsoft millionaire Bob Wallace, the purpose of DanceSafe is to test MDMA pills for purity. DanceSafe sets up tables at raves and invites users to submit their pills for testing. A sliver of the pill is shaved off and a drop of solution poured onto it. The solution turns black when exposed to MDMA. In the rave samples tested by DanceSafe, up to 40 percent have been found to be fake. The most common substitutes were aspirin, caffeine, and over-the-counter cough remedies such as dextromethorphan. Fake Ecstasy may have 130 milligrams of dextromethorphan—13 times the amount included in cough suppressants such as Robitussin and enough to cause serious side effects such as blurred vision, vomiting, hallucinations and psychosis.[15] Like PMA, another toxic amphetamine sold as MDMA, dextromethorphan inhibits sweating and can easily cause heatstroke.

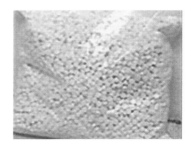

Confiscated bag of smuggled MDMA pills

Chemical Characteristics

MDMA increases the brain levels of serotonin, dopamine, and norepinephrine. Like all amphetamines, MDMA causes neurons that release these neuro-transmitters to actively dump them into the synapse space and block their re-uptake, flooding the synapse with the neurotransmitter.

Unlike the other amphetamines, MDMA releases much more serotonin than dopamine or norepinephrine. The result is less direct stimulation (an effect of norepinephrine) or addiction (a characteristic of dopamine), but more perceptual and mood effects (the serotonin).

MDMA is most potent if taken on an empty stomach. Effects are also reportedly diminished by alcohol or marijuana, and may be intensified to a dangerous level if taken together with cocaine.

EFFECTS

MDMA seems to cause effects that are a combination of the stimulation of amphetamines and the altered perception of hallucinogens. In laboratory studies, animals that were trained to recognize amphetamines also recognized MDMA. However, animals trained to recognize LSD or hallucinogens equally recognized MDMA. This similarity of a drug to both amphetamines and hallucinogens is very unusual.[16]

The primary influence is an elevated mood state with a feeling of euphoria, intimacy, and closeness to others. The positive feelings that people report are probably due to the release of serotonin. In this way, MDMA has effects similar to those of the popular anti-depressants and a number of weight-loss medications.

Typical effects[17]

Lower doses (40 to 80 mg)
☺ heightened interpersonal feeling toward others
☺ high self-esteem and confidence
☺ general state of euphoria
☺ intensified senses of touch and taste
☺ intensified colors
☺ feeling of "personal insight" into one's self

Higher doses (120 mg)
☹ panic
☹ depression
☹ confusion
☹ anxiety

The side effects of MDMA include loss of appetite, rapid heart rate, jaw tension, teeth grinding, dilated pupils, and sweating. About ten percent of users have transitory nausea, jitteriness, and a rise in blood pressure. Too much stimulation—especially when combined with intense physical exercise, heat, and dehydration (common at raves)—can cause a "head rush," a period up to three minutes in which dancers blank out all sights and sounds. More alarming is an increase in sudden deaths among MDMA users, particularly in Europe where such lethal reactions have been frequent. In October 1993, the Department of Medicine and Pharmacology at Sheffield University in Britain put out an explanation of the "sudden death syndrome." They discovered that about 1 in 12 individuals lacks the enzyme cytochrome P450-246, needed to metabolize MDMA. Without this enzyme, the person is susceptible to a fatal reaction to the drug.

The effects of MDEA are very similar to MDMA, while MDA acts more like a hallucinogen. The effects of NEXUS, BDB and other designer drugs have not been as well studied. In chickens, the administration of pure NEXUS causes a rigid, penguin-like posture. BDB causes a bursting-forward movement, an effect similar to the effects of LSD and harmine, a drug found in many natural hallucinogens.[18]

ECSTASY AND SEX

MDMA is reported to cause impotence in men, although some users say the opposite—they can sustain erection but not have an orgasm.

Many people say that MDMA decreases sexual interest at the peak of intoxication, but also that this effect wears off quickly and is followed by a high desire for sex. Together with increased social openness and lowered inhibition, the drug seems to make sexual activity with strangers more common. A study showed that after taking MDMA, men are 2.8 times more likely to have unprotected sex.

NERVE DESTRUCTION

MDMA is also different from the amphetamines in the way that it releases these neurotransmitters: it destroys the nerve terminal.[19] All amphetamines can be toxic to neurons in high doses, but MDMA, MDA, and the other variants appear to do this even in normal doses. Animal studies show a considerable destruction of serotonin nerve terminals after a single dose of MDMA or MDA.[20] Moderate doses produce damage to the end of the nerve terminal, but the overall serotonin system is still functional, so that the normally bushy nerve ending has a "pruned back" appearance under the microscope.[21]

Large doses destroy the nerve completely and permanently eliminate its ability to release serotonin.

Some evidence shows that MDMA may be safe in small quantities or if combined with fluoxetine (Prozac). Research on rats shows that neurotoxicity is prevented when MDMA is taken together with fluoxetine, perhaps because the nerve damage occurs when toxic substances are taken up into the serotonin nerve axon. Fluoxetine prevents this uptake. To achieve this protection in humans, it is suggested that the user take 40 milligrams of fluoxetine (twice the normal adult dose) about three hours after taking MDMA.

Withdrawal Signs

MDMA produces a rapid tolerance so that repeated use within a short time leads to the loss of desired effects. The positive feelings in mood, self-image, and empathy are followed by a rebound of the opposite feelings, leaving the user tired, uncaring, and miserable. If taken again within a few days, it can cause an *increase* in stress and many of the problems of amphetamine overdose.

TERRIBLE TUESDAYS

Coming down off a weekend rave, the aftermath of MDMA can feel like a bad hangover that some users refer to as the Terrible Tuesdays. Common symptoms include muscular aches, abdominal pain, chills, tremors, voracious hunger, anxiety, prolonged sleep, lack of energy, exhaustion, deep depression, and suicidal feelings.

In a clinical study of MDMA withdrawal, 29 volunteers were given pure MDMA. All 29 reported uncomfortable symptoms: 28 lost their appetite, 23 had extreme fatigue, 22 had teeth grinding or clenched jaws, 11 had insomnia, 9 had nausea, 8 had muscle aches or stiffness, and 3 had difficulty walking. Most of the volunteers reported sweating, rapid heart rate, and high blood pressure. These effects lasted from a few hours to a few days.

Long-term Health Problems

Frequent use of MDMA leads to a development of tolerance for the positive effects and a worsening of negative effects. Many of the long-term effects are similar to those of frequent amphetamine use. Some users have complained of panic attacks and paranoid psychotic symptoms. The negative effects of MDMA usually resolve after a few days, but may last for months. Persons with psychiatric illnesses are particularly susceptible to these effects, and even a single dose can cause long-term problems.

Monkeys show abnormal patterns of serotonin-producing neurons up to seven years after treatment with MDMA.[22] In people who have taken MDMA 20 times or more, analysis of the spinal fluid shows a depletion of serotonin metabolites, indicating a long-term disruption in normal brain functioning.

Brain damage

The MDMA destruction of serotonin nerve terminals is usually unnoticeable since the brain has billions of neurons with very complex interactions. Nevertheless, a study at Johns Hopkins showed that people who frequently used MDMA had impaired memory on standardized tests. There is evidence that suggests a long-term, potentially irreversible effect of MDMA on the human brain. As people age and experience a normal decline in brain functioning, this damage may begin to show up in diminished brain activity.

What To Do If There Is An Overdose

MDMA causes an overload of serotonin, not only in the brain but in the body as well. In fact, 90 percent of the serotonin in the body is outside the brain, most of it in the gut and in mast cells of the blood.[23] Stimulation of these cells helps cause an increase in body temperature. Overheating the body is worsened by vigorous physical activity and crowding. The combination has caused extremely high body temperatures in MDMA users, up to 110° Fahrenheit (43.3° C), which is enough to cook the brain.

The natural method used in the body to stabilize the effects of MDMA is by the enzyme monoamine oxidase (MAO). Some drugs and prescription medications inhibit this enzyme. If a user is taking MAO-inhibiting substances along with MDMA, there can be a serious or fatal reaction. MAO-inhibiting medications include Nardil (phenelzine), Parnate (tranylcypromine), Marplan (isocarboxazid), Eldepryl (l-deprenyl), Aurorex or Manerix (moclobemide), and the AIDS drug Ritonavir.

Since the start of its popularity in the 1980s, MDMA has been the cause of dozens of deaths. Most of the fatalities occurred at raves, where users collapsed unconscious or in convulsions while dancing. By the time they were taken to a hospital, they had a burning fever, racing pulse, and plunging blood pressure. The damage to the blood and muscle proteins caused the critical conditions of disseminated intravascular coagulation, rhabdomyolysis, and rapid kidney failure. Despite intensive care treatment, these people died within 2 to 60 hours.[24]

Many of the stimulant effects of MDMA are intensified by dehydration. Rave organizers are well aware of this, and profit by selling expensive drinks to the over-heated and thirsty dancers. Those who are unwilling to pay the high prices may end up paying in a different way. One MDMA user in Britain reacted to intense thirst by later drinking an enormous quantity of water, which caused a swelling of the brain and his death.

 About 14 MDMA pills make up a lethal dose. However, even a small amount of MDMA may be fatal in a susceptible person.

Anyone using MDMA who develops a fever or other physical signs of overdose should be taken to the Emergency Department immediately. They will be treated with rapid cooling measures and possibly with the antispasmodic drug dantrolene.

Physical signs of overdose

Fever
Rapid or irregular heart rate
Shallow breathing
High blood pressure
Dilated pupils
Blurred vision
Dry mouth
Profuse sweating
Teeth grinding
Tremors
Seizures
Stroke
Coma

Mental signs of overdose

Confusion
Agitation
Paranoia
Hallucinations

Methaqualone and Glutethimide

Methaqualone, more commonly known by its brand name Quaalude, is a central nervous system depressant. In the 1970s, it became a popular drug of abuse because it was considered an aphrodisiac. It was made illegal and removed from the market in 1983.

Glutethimide, sold as Doriden, is very similar to methaqualone. It was taken off the market in1986 and made illegal in 1991.

The Basic Facts

Type of drug	*Depressant*
How taken	*Ingested*
Duration of effect	*4 to 8 hours*
Physical danger	*Moderate*
Addiction potential	*Moderate*

Other Names

Methaqualone	*disco biscuits, love drug, ludes, Optimil, Parest, pillows, Q's, Quaalude, quacks, quads, soapers, Somnafac, sope, Sopor*
Methaqualone & antihistamine	*mandies, Mandrax*
Glutethimide	*Doriden, gofers, goofballs*
Glutethimide & codeine	*G&C, hits, loads, pancakes and syrup, sets, setups*

'Luding Out: The Story of Methaqualone and Glutethimide

By 1954, barbiturates were known to be addictive drugs with widespread abuse and responsible for many overdose fatalities. That year, glutethimide was introduced as a safer substitute for barbiturates. It was marketed under the brand name Doriden and became a popular prescription drug, with questionable use as a remedy for anxiety and insomnia.

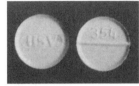

Although glutethimide was different from the barbiturates, it eventually proved to be even more addictive, with severe withdrawal symptoms. Doriden became a popular prescription remedy for anxiety and insomnia.

Glutethimide pills,
marketed as Doriden

In 1965, glutethimide was followed by methaqualone, a drug initially created in India in 1955 by researchers working on a cure for malaria.[1] Pharmaceutical companies in the United States noted the similarity of the two drugs. Several of them began to market methaqualone under the trade names Sopor, Parest, Optimil, and Mandrax. William H. Rorer, Inc., sold its methaqualone sleeping pills in units of 150 milligrams and 300 milligrams. It called them Quaaludes.

The pleasant, drunken states produced by these drugs made them highly sought after and created a strong black market demand. By the late 1960s, methaqualone had become very popular on college campuses. One study showed that 20,000 pills were consumed in a period of three weeks at Vassar, and a staggering 5,000 a day at Brooklyn College.[2] They were used so widely among young people camped out during the 1972 national political conventions that Flamingo Park in Miami Beach became known as "Quaalude Alley."

By then, Quaaludes and wine were a favored combination at college parties. "Luding out" was a way of dealing with any kind of stress. Quaalude also gained a reputation as the Love Drug because it lowered inhibition and enhanced the desire for sex. At Ohio State University, football players routinely took the drug while winding down from a game, and jars of the pills were available at fraternities. In New York, at least 15 nightclubs catered to "full-time, flat-out luders." The clubs were known as juice bars because in most of them the only drink available was fruit juice—convenient because many of the customers were underage.

 "I liked sopers because they made you feel drunk without a hangover."
—Ohio State college student, 1970s [3]

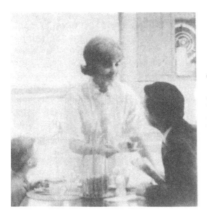

That "good morning" feeling... thanks to

∗

glutethimide

Worries about addiction and overdose first came from overseas. By the mid-1960s, half of all drug abusers in Japanese hospitals were addicted to Quaaludes. In 1962, the first death from an overdose was reported in Germany. The United States was not far behind. In 1974, 88 people died from methaqualone overdose, and in the following 12-month period, 5,500 people were taken to Emergency Departments for Quaalude use or withdrawal. When Broward County, Florida, began routine urine testing of intoxicated drivers in 1980, it found that 82 percent of them were on Quaaludes.

Methaqualone and glutethimide had been developed as a safer alternative to barbiturates. It became apparent, however, that they were equally addictive, overdoses were more difficult to treat, and fatalities were even more likely.

The turning point came in 1977 with two celebrity deaths. Freddie Prinze, star of the popular TV series *Chico and the Man*, was addicted to Quaaludes. In 1977, he took a dozen of the pills and shot himself. He was just 23 years old.

On August 16 of the same year, Elvis Presley was dead at age 42. He had increasingly depended on an elaborate schedule of drugs to get him through his days of publicity appearances, filming, recording, performing, and to help control his ballooning weight.

Five years later, John Belushi, part of the early Saturday Night Live crew and star of *The Blues Brothers*, took Quaaludes to try to relieve the anxiety and restlessness from his fatal cocaine habit. He was dead at age 33.

The rampant use of methaqualone in the United States, along with the many deaths from overdose, led to the end of pharmaceutical marketing in 1983. In 1984, it was declared a Schedule I Controlled Substance, indicating that it had a high abuse potential and no acceptable medical use. The last legal production in the world ceased in 1988.

Glutethimide continued to be prescribed for the short-term relief of insomnia and was a frequently stolen medication. After a surge of overdoses and deaths, it too was made illegal. In 1991, glutethimide was declared a Schedule II drug,[4] with very restricted medical use.

Who Is Using Methaqualone & Glutethimide?

Both methaqualone and glutethimide were originally prescribed primarily for anxiety, with other applications as a sedative, sleeping pill, and anticonvulsant. Because of their limited efficacy, and because so many of the pills were diverted for abuse, these drugs are no longer available by prescription in the United States.

Methaqualone and glutethimide are difficult to manufacture in clandestine laboratories. Both drugs are now much less common. They are rarely detected in workplace drug testing programs, and most drug testing laboratories stopped offering the tests in the late 1990s.

Many who try to make methaqualone illicitly end up producing mecloqualone or quinazolinone.[5] These related drugs are similar in effect to methaqualone and are often sold as Quaaludes. Most of this supply is from Mexico. Other reputed methaqualone sold on the street is likely to consist of Valium, PCP, or antihistamines.

In northwestern Pennsylvania, illegal glutethimide is often sold together with codeine as a "set." Nine deaths were reported due to this combination in a recent two-year period.[6]

Chemical Characteristics

Methaqualone and glutethimide are central nervous system depressants similar in action to the barbiturates. They cause slurred speech, disorientation, and drunken behavior without the odor of alcohol. High doses can cause fatigue, dizziness, sluggishness, numbness, delirium, seizures, and coma.

Like alcohol, both of these drugs initially create a slight sense of stimulation. The user feels more lively, friendly, and more confident in social settings. It is easier to approach others and to be

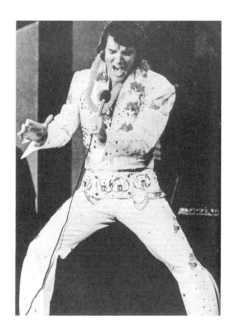

Elvis Presley's body contained Quaalude, Valium, and codeine in large concentrations, with trace amounts of chlorpheniramine, Demerol, morphine, pentobarbital, phenobarbital, and butabarbital. In the last two years of his life, he had been prescribed 19,000 doses of narcotics, stimulants, sedatives, and anti-depressants.

approached by them. Like alcohol, there is a sense of relaxation and lack of inhibition.

Along with the improved mood come muscle and visual disturbances, with a false perception of depth and distance. In the 60s, people would laugh at "wallbangers" who stumbled and bumped into walls. There may also be difficulty coordinating movement, with twitching and jerking—a condition of ataxia which users called "taxiing"—along with jumpy back-and-forth eye movements and sensations of tingling and prickling in the fingertips, lips, and tongue. Heavy users have intense sweating, and skin sores with blisters, rashes, and purple spotting from the bursting of fine blood vessels. This can also occur in the stomach and eyes, causing serious injury.

A common impurity of illicit methaqualone is ortho-toluidine, which can cause necrotizing cystitis, a bladder disease with the tissues appearing punched full of holes. Symptoms are nausea, vomiting, and blood in the urine. Another common impurity is methylene-dianaline, which causes severe liver damage.

The chemical name of methaqualone is 2-methyl-3-0-tolyl-4(3H)-quinazolinone. Most of the pills sold as "ludes" have anywhere from 0 to 500 milligrams of this substance, with the remainder consisting of contaminants or other drugs such as Valium or common antihistamines.[7]

The elimination half-life of both methaqualone and glutethimide is 10 to 42 hours, and they can be detected in the urine for about three days after use.

Withdrawal Signs

Most sedative drugs produce both addiction and physical withdrawal symptoms if they are taken regularly for more than a month or two. Withdrawal from frequent use of methaqualone and glutethimide typically results in anxiety and insomnia, and may be accompanied by tremors, sweating, fever, spastic blinking, anxiety, agitation, hallucinations, disorientation, and shock. Extreme withdrawal may result in delirium, convulsions, and possibly death.

In Australia, a case of glutethimide withdrawal produced persistent nausea, anxiety, sleep disturbance, and two generalized seizures resulting in a broken back and thigh. Intestinal paralysis occurred on the fifth day after withdrawal. Even three weeks later, the patient still required anti-seizure medication.[8]

Most addicts recover after a period of irritability, headaches, restlessness and insomnia. Many have nausea and stomach cramps. Symptoms usually begin one to three days after stopping the drug, and last for a few days.

The most worrisome feature of withdrawal from these drugs is a slowed throat reflex, so that the user may choke while vomiting. During medically supervised withdrawal, there is usually a gradual detoxification program, with daily doses decreased every one to three days until the addict is drug-free.

Long-term Health Problems

Tolerance to both methaqualone and glutethimide develops quickly. After just four days of use, the drugs have much less effect to calm, relax, or remove inhibitions. Within two weeks, the user no longer gets any benefit as a sleeping pill.

Long-term health problems are similar to those of the barbiturates: continual drowsiness and sluggishness, shortened memory and attention span, loss of coordination and awareness, emotional instability, rashes, nausea, anxiety and nervousness, involuntary eye movements, staggered gait, slurred speech, and trembling hands. These symptoms are worse in women, who get longer and stronger side-effects because the drug is stored in the fatty tissues of the body. The negative effects are also worse in people over age 30, who have a gradual decrease in their ability to metabolize the drugs.

What To Do If There Is An Overdose

Methaqualone and glutethimide are most dangerous if they are taken together with other sedative drugs such as alcohol. The combination can easily depress the central nervous system to the point of coma. If the brain is starved of oxygen for more than a few minutes, permanent damage may occur. In this case, the user may never recover.

With high doses of these drugs, breathing may be slowed to the point of coma or death. The heart rate, blood pressure, and muscle tone also decrease, and the user has less response to pain or loud noises. Eventually, the lungs may fill with fluid and the kidneys fail.

A mild overdose may resolve without the need for special medical care. If the user has any difficulty breathing or cannot be aroused, hospitalization is necessary. There, the person will probably be treated with a benzodiazepine, such as Valium, and perhaps an anticonvulsant medication such as phenobarbital.

Physical signs of overdose[9] Slurred speech
Jerky eye movement
Dry mouth
Flushed skin
Slow breathing
Low blood pressure
Difficulty walking
Seizures

Mental signs of overdose Confusion
Drowsiness
Delirium
Unresponsive coma

Opiates

"Among the remedies which it has pleased the Almighty God to give to man to relieve his sufferings, none is so universal and so efficacious as opium."
—*Thomas Sydenham, M.D., 1680*

Opiates are depressant drugs derived from the opium poppy plant, including morphine, codeine, and heroin. Opioids are synthetic drugs that have opiate-like activity but are not derived from opium.

Of the 178 drugs that are illegal in the United States, 122 are opiates or opioids. For convenience here, the term opiate is used for all of these drugs.

The Basic Facts

Type of drug	*Depressant*
How taken	*Ingested, smoked, snorted, injected*
Duration of effect	*2 to 6 hours*
Physical danger	*High*
Addiction potential	*High*

Other Names

Anileridine	*Leritene*
Codeine	*Number 3s, Number 4s,*
Fentanyl*	*Apache, China girl, China town, friend, goodfellas, Sublimaze*
Heroin	*AIP (from Afghanistan, Iran, and Pakistan), antifreeze, aries, Aunt Hazel, bad bundle (inferior quality), ballot, big bag, big daddy, big H, big Harry, blanco, bonita, boy, bozo, brick gum, brown sugar, caballo, carga, carne, China White, garbage, globo, H, hard stuff, Harry, horse, junk, mierda, Persian, Rufus, shit, skag, smack, stoffa, white stuff*
Heroin (Mexican tar)	*ball, black pearl, black stuff, chapapote, chiva, chocolate, goma, gomero, gum, gumball, Mexican mud, pedazo, tar, tootsie roll*
Heroin & amphetamine/cocaine	*speedball*
Heroin & crack	*hot rocks*
Heroin & freebase cocaine	*chasing and basing*
Hydrocodone	*Anexsia, Hycodan, Hycomine, Lortab, Lorcet, Tussionex, Tylox, Vicodin*
Hydromorphone	*Dilaudid, Dillies, drugstore heroin*
Ketobimidone	*Ketogin*
LAAM	*Lam, ORLAAM*
Meperidine*	*Demerol*
Methadone	*Amidone, Dolophine, juice*
Morphine	*M, Miss Emma, morph, Roxanol, MS-Contin, MSIR, Murphy*
Opium	*Ah-pen-yen, auntie, Auntie Emma, big O, black, black pill, hop, laudanum, O, op, Pantopon, Paragoric, poppy*
Oxycodone	*OC, oxy, OxyContin, Percocet, Percodan, percs*
Propoxyphene	*Darvocet, Darvon, pink ladies, pumpkin seeds, Wygesicc*
Tilidine and naloxone	*Valoron*

(*Illegally manufactured fentanyl and meperidine may also be called China White)

The First Narcotics: The Story of Opiates

The poppy flower *Papaver somniferum* (from the Greek *papaver*, "poppy," and Latin *somniferum*, "to induce sleep") was cultivated in the Mediterranean region as early as 5000 BC. It matures in about 90 days and grows to a height of about four feet. After maturity, the flower petals fall, leaving the one- to three-inch wide green seed pod. When cut, the walls of this seed pod will ooze a milky fluid. For thousands of years, this fluid was scraped by hand and dried to a gummy substance known as opium.

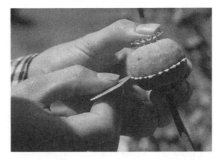

Opium oozing out of the cut poppy pod. There are 250 species of poppies, but only 2 of these produce opium.

The cultivation of opium poppies spread throughout Asia and North Africa where, from ancient times until the present, opium has been used to numb the body and mind (see *Chapter 2: Opium*). Opiate drugs eventually became popular throughout the world both for their medicinal value and for recreational use. Today, the many derivatives of opium are among the most addictive drugs known.

 Narcotics, from the Greek word meaning "to numb," refers specifically to opiates. The word is now often used to mean any illegal drug.

OPIUM

Raw opium is made by collecting the sap from the poppy to produce a brown, tarry substance. This material may be dried and rolled into a ball (gum opium), or crushed to a powder (powder opium). The process of collecting gum opium from poppies is very labor intensive. A more modern and efficient method uses machines to harvest the entire mature plant and cut it to poppy straw, which is dried and processed to a fine brownish powder. Most opium powder is produced this way, on specially licensed farms on contract to pharmaceutical companies.

Each year, more than 600 tons of opium powder are legally imported into the United States for legitimate medical use.[1] This powder is then refined to produce opiate medications. Opium and opiates that are imported illegally are usually already refined into their final form.

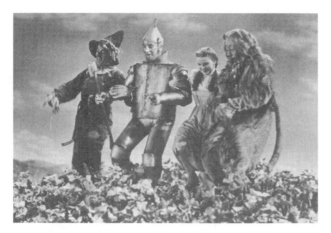

The Yellow Brick Road ... Walking through fields of cut poppies can be intoxicating.[2]

Poppies are grown in Australia, Turkey, France and Spain for the production of poppy straw. Farmers plant crops in spring or fall. Brightly colored flowers appear about three months later. After fertilization, the petals drop from the flower and expose the seed pod, a bulb about the size of a walnut. Opium is produced in the root system and distributed to all parts of the plant, but the majority collects in the thin wall of the seed pod. When the pod is cut, the milky white opium slowly bleeds from the incision, changing color to brown as it dries. This gummy material is scraped off and collected the following day. Pods may be incised up to five or six times before the opium is depleted.

The majority of opium is further refined into other drugs. When opium itself is used, it is typically smoked, but it can also be taken by mouth, usually by dissolving it in water or an alcoholic beverage. The taste is described as like that of bitter licorice.

Until the early 1900s, crude opium was a common medicine in the United States. Now, opium for pain relief has largely been replaced by other narcotics. Tincture of opium with alcohol (laudanum) or camphor (paragoric) is still prescribed for diarrhea and abdominal cramps.

Most medical opium is broken down into its alkaloid constituents. Over 40 pharmacologically active alkaloids have been identified in opium powder. The 3 most common of these are morphine (constituting from 4 to 20 percent of dried opium), codeine (1 to 5 percent), and thebaine (less than 1 percent).

Thebaine has no psychoactive properties and is not a drug of abuse. It is, however, widely employed in the manufacture of semi-synthetic opioids.

MORPHINE

Morphine is the primary constituent of opium and the first pure drug ever extracted from a plant. When raw opium was dissolved in hot water, adding lime brought morphine to the surface as a white suspension while the other solids settled to the bottom. It was discovered that there is a wide range of morphine

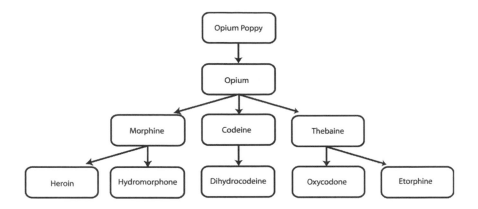

The Opiate Family

concentration in the natural plant. Now, commercial opium is standardized to contain ten percent morphine.

Morphine is one of the most effective drugs known for the relief of pain and remains the standard against which new pain-relieving medications are measured. It also has a number of medical applications beyond pain relief, with important use in emergency medicine. Morphine is available in oral solutions (Roxanol), sustained-release tablets (MS-Contin), suppositories, and injectable preparations. The injectable form can be given subcutaneously, intramuscularly, and intravenously.

Despite this very widespread use, especially in medicine, most of the morphine derived from opium is not used directly but converted into codeine and other opiates.

CODEINE

Codeine was isolated from opium soon after the discovery of morphine. However, most codeine used in the United States is not refined from opium but synthesized from morphine.

Codeine produces less analgesia, sedation, and respiratory depression than morphine. It also has good absorption if taken by mouth—unlike morphine, which is largely inactivated by the liver if taken as an oral preparation. Codeine is usually marketed in tablets or liquid, either alone or in combination with acetaminophen (for example, Tylenol #3) and other medications. This versatile drug is a particularly effective cough suppressant. It is by far the most commonly used narcotic in the world.

HEROIN

Heroin, diacetylmorphine, was discovered in 1874 by combining morphine and acetic acid (vinegar). Commercial production began in 1898. This new narcotic was synthesized from morphine in a search for a pain reliever that was less addictive. Its discoverers could not have been more wrong. Within a few years, it became apparent that heroin was being widely abused. Heroin was restricted in the Harrison Narcotic Act of 1914, the first significant control of drugs by the Federal Government, and made completely illegal in 1926. Today, heroin continues to be one of the major drugs of abuse in the United States and the world.

The illegal production of heroin begins when a farmer sells gum opium to a nearby processor. This material is then placed in boiling water, stirred into a mixture, and lime added to leach out the morphine as calcium morphenate. This is filtered out and ammonium chloride is added, causing the morphine base to settle to the bottom. Activated charcoal and hydrochloric acid are then added to produce morphine hydrochloride, which is dried and pressed into bricks for shipment to a heroin lab. The dried morphine base is often called heroin #1. It can be smoked, but is usually made into heroin #2. First, the morphine base is pulverized and mixed with acetic anhydride. Water and activated charcoal and then sodium bicarbonate are added, causing the heroin base to settle out. The mixture is filtered and the heroin base dried, producing heroin #2. This crude heroin is treated with hydrochloric acid to produce heroin hydrochloride, for final sale.

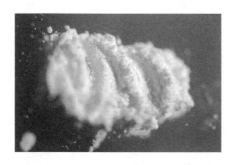

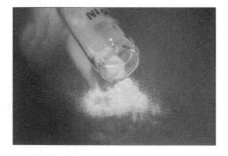

In the 1980s, a form of heroin from Mexico known as tar heroin became widely available in the western portion of the United States and today accounts for about five percent of America's heroin consumption. Tar heroin is produced by mobile labs near the poppy fields in Mexico. The color varies from brown to black and the consistency from that of sticky roofing tar to a solid coal-like substance. Most tar heroin samples have a vinegary smell, and have a purity of 20 to 80 percent. Due to its sticky consistency, tar heroin is often packaged in plastic or aluminum foil. It is usually dissolved in water and injected.

The DEA conducts a Heroin Signature Program to chemically analyze and identify batches of seized heroin to determine their source. In 1997, South American heroin accounted for 75 percent of all heroin seized in the United States, with another 14 percent from Mexico. Both are smuggled across the Mexican border by organized crime syndicates. Colombia produces about six metric tons of heroin each year, and almost all of it eventually finds its way to the U.S. market.

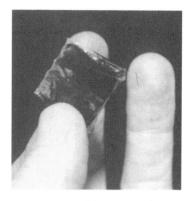

Mexican tar heroin

Heroin is usually injected, snorted, or smoked. When injected into a vein, the onset of euphoria occurs in seven to ten seconds. Intramuscular injection is slower, taking about five to eight minutes, and snorting is slower yet, taking about ten to fifteen minutes, and does not produce as intense a "rush" as the other methods. Despite the slower onset, many users now prefer to snort or smoke heroin because of concern about injection-related illnesses.

Medically Used and Abused Opiate Derivatives

Prescription opiates are very widely abused. They may be obtained in a number of ways: by fraud, theft, and smuggled sources, and by legitimate or forged prescriptions. Their abuse is actually much more extensive than abuse of illegally manufactured drugs such as heroin. Following are some of the most widely abused prescription opiates.

HYDROCODONE

Hydrocodone is a cough and pain medication, classified as a Schedule II narcotic in its pure form. It is an analog of codeine, but about six times more potent. The prescribed dose of five to ten milligrams is equivalent to 60 milligrams of oral morphine. As the sale and production of this drug has increased, so has the potential for the drug to be diverted for illicit use. Hydrocodone (found in Lortab, Vicodin, and many other medications) is one of the most common prescription drug addictions.

White and brown heroin

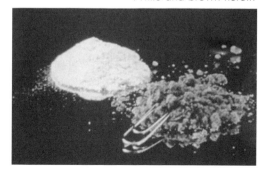

HYDROMORPHONE

Hydromorphone (Dilaudid) is marketed in both tablet and injectable forms. It is a very potent pain-relief agent, with an effect five to six times as strong as morphine and three times as strong as heroin. Because of its high addiction potential, it is not often prescribed. Most hydromorphone is obtained by fraudulent prescriptions or theft. The tablets are often dissolved and injected as a substitute for heroin.

There are really two types of opiate abuse:
- ☒   *illegally manufactured drugs*
- ☒   *diverted prescription drugs*

While most people are concerned about illegal drugs, prescription drug abuse is actually far more common.

KETOBIMIDONE

Commonly abused in Europe, ketobimidone is similar to morphine. It is less popular in the United States.

OXYCODONE

Oxycodone (e.g., OxyContin, Percodan, Percocet) was introduced in 1995 as a long-lasting pain killer. Synthesized from thebaine, it is more potent then codeine but less so than morphine.

Oxycodone is a commonly abused prescription drug, second only to hydrocodone. Users smash the pills and snort the powder, or dissolve the tablets in water, filter out the insoluble material, and then inject the drug intravenously. The result is a high that is claimed to be as strong as that of heroin.

In some rural towns, OxyContin has overtaken cocaine and marijuana as a recreational drug. In 2000, communities in eastern Kentucky reported 59 deaths from overdose, and Maine reported 35 fatalities due to the drug. [3]

THEBAINE

Thebaine was named after the ancient Egyptian city of Thebes, where inscriptions describing opium were found. It is chemically similar to both morphine and codeine, but stimulates rather than depresses the central nervous system. Thebaine is not used directly in medicine. It is converted into a number of other drugs such as codeine, hydrocodone, oxycodone, oxymorphone, nalbuphine, naloxone, naltrexone and buprenorphine.

TILIDINE

Tilidine is a pain reliever similar to dextropropoxyphene. It is about one tenth as potent as morphine and half as potent as meperidine.[4] Toxic doses of tilidine can cause coma, convulsions, and respiratory arrest.[5] To prevent abuse and overdose, tilidine is not sold separately but is marketed in a form combined with naloxone, an opiate antagonist.

Opioids: Synthetic Narcotics

Properly speaking, opiates are derived directly or indirectly from the opium poppy.[6] Opioids, on the other hand, are produced entirely in the laboratory. These products are chemically similar to the opiates, and include both pharmaceutical variations and accidental byproducts of the illegal manufacture of other opioids.

ANILERIDINE

Anileridine has a chemical structure similar to meperidine, but it is much more potent. Several people have died from overdose of this alternative to Demerol.[7]

ETORPHINE

This extraordinarily potent opioid was discovered in 1960 in an Edinburgh lab when the morning tea was accidentally stirred with a glass rod used in an experiment. It knocked the unsuspecting scientists into a coma. Once they recovered, they analyzed the new compound and found it to be 10,000 times as strong as morphine.

 Etorphine is the key ingredient in "Immobilizer," used in dart guns to stun elephants and rhinos.

Etorphine is not used medically. A scratch of a contaminated needle may kill a person, and two milliliters will knock unconscious a full-grown rhino.

FENTANYL

Fentanyl is about 100 times more potent than morphine. It was first synthesized in Belgium in the 1950s and later marketed as an intravenous anesthetic under the trade name of Sublimaze. Fentanyl was followed by two variants: alfentanil (Alfenta), an ultra-short acting analgesic, and sufentanil (Sufenta), a powerful pain-relief agent for use in heart surgery.

The effects of other fentanyl-type drugs are indistinguishable from those of heroin, but hundreds of times more potent.[8] The result is a very high potential for abuse. Fentanyls are most commonly injected but, like heroin, they may also be smoked or snorted. The first illicit use of fentanyl was in the mid-1970s when anesthesiologists and other medical personnel who had access to the drug succumbed to the temptation to use it themselves.

Medical fentanyl is tightly controlled. Clandestine laboratories have tried to manufacture it, with mixed success, resulting in a number of chemical analogs of fentanyl from improper manufacturing and the occasional production of very toxic by-products. These fentanyl analogs are potent and dangerous drugs with poorly known effects. All of them are illegal. They include:

Acetyl-alpha-methylfentanyl
Alpha-methylfentanyl
Alpha-methylthiofentanyl
Benzylfentanyl
Beta-hydroxyfentanyl
Beta-hydroxy-3-methylfentanyl
Carfentanil
3-Methylfentanyl
3-Methylthiofentanyl
Para-fluorofentanyl
Remifentanil
Thenylfentanyl
Thiofentanyl

LAAM

LAAM, levo-alpha-acetyl-methadol, is a close relative to methadone, approved in 1993 for use as a maintenance drug for narcotic addicts. Like methadone, LAAM has a very long duration of action, from 48 to 72 hours.

LAAM appears to be as effective as methadone in clinical studies,[9] but it may not always be appreciated by addicts who prefer methadone because of its "rush-like" effect.[10] In one study designed to test LAAM, the addicts refused to take it because it could not be sold or manipulated like methadone.[11] More recent studies have shown LAAM to lead to a more stable and consistent recovery.[12]

Adverse reactions to LAAM are similar to those of methadone, and include arrhythmias, flu-like symptoms, abdominal cramps, diarrhea, and muscle aches.

MEPERIDINE

Commonly known as pethidine or by its brand name, Demerol, meperidine was developed in the 1930s as a synthetic narcotic similar to morphine, but available for use either orally or by injection. Meperidine is most often used for the relief of moderate to severe pain, particularly in obstetrics and after surgery. It is relatively safe, but can cause convulsions in high doses.

Like other medicines with a high abuse potential, the distribution of meperidine is tightly controlled. Clandestine laboratories have tried to manufacture it and have inadvertently developed several chemical analogs of the drug. The effects of these analogs are not well known and have resulted in many deaths from overdose. Meperidine analogs include:

Hydroxypethidine
MPPP (1-methyl-4-phenyl-4-propionoxypiperidine)
PEPAP (1-[-2-phenethyl]-4-phenyl-4-acetoxypiperidine)
Pethidine-intermediate-A (4-cyano-1-methyl-4-phenylpiperidine)
Pethidine-intermediate-B
Pethidine-intermediate-C
Trimeperidine

In one notorious case, a by-product was developed that caused a severe form of Parkinson's Disease (see *Chapter 6: Designer Drugs*).

METHADONE

Methadone was invented as a substitute for morphine by German scientists during the Second World War, when morphine was in very short supply. Although methadone is chemically different from morphine, its effects are similar, making it a useful drug for severe pain. Methadone has a much longer effect than morphine or heroin, lasting up to 24 hours, and is less likely to cause addiction.

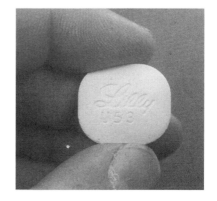

In 1947, the pharmaceutical company Eli Lilly began to manufacture methadone in the United States as the pain-relief drug Dolophine. It continues to be used for this purpose, especially for severe and chronic pain in cancer patients, but now the most common use of methadone is as a maintenance drug for narcotic addicts. In theory, addicts on methadone are better able to tolerate withdrawal from their addiction. Unfortunately, many of these addicts simply add methadone to their other narcotic habits, or even sell methadone for illicit use by others. For this reason, methadone prescription programs are very tightly controlled under specific guidelines by The National Institute on Drug Abuse.[13] There are now about 115,000 patients in long-term methadone maintenance programs in the U.S., most of them in New York State, at a cost of about $4,000 per patient per year. Methadone is also used in short-term programs to detoxify heroin addicts, but most addicts who detox return to heroin use.[14]

Methadone is effective both orally and by injection, and is usually given once a day as a large pill or in a lemon or cherry-flavored liquid. Although tolerance and addiction may occur, withdrawal is milder than from morphine or heroin. The typical use of methadone involves an initial dose of 15 to 30 milligrams per day, which may be increased to 30 to 100 milligrams as needed. Like other opiates, methadone can cause respiratory depression, and many deaths have occurred from overdose.

PROPOXYPHENE

Propoxyphene, also known as dextropropoxyphene, is chemically similar to methadone, but is less potent and shorter-lasting. It was first marketed in 1957 under the trade name Darvon.

Propoxyphene has a pain-relieving strength about half that of codeine and about ten times stronger than aspirin. It is a very popular medication for mild to moderate pain: more than 100 tons are produced each year in the United States, with about 25 million prescriptions.

Bulk propoxyphene is a Schedule II controlled substance. High doses can cause respiratory depression. Since propoxyphene is readily available as a prescription drug, it is often abused and it is among the top ten drugs causing death from overdose.

OTHER ILLEGAL OPIOIDS

There are many variants of synthetic opioid drugs. These "designer drugs" are sometimes intentionally produced, but most are accidental by-products of attempts to manufacture potent opioids such as fentanyl or meperidine.[15] Illegal chemists tend not to be overly concerned about quality control: if their product sells, that is all that matters. Possible toxicity or brain injury to the user takes a low priority when their main worries are getting paid, avoiding attacks from other criminals, and keeping a step ahead of the police.

A number of synthetic opioid derivatives have been identified and declared illegal:

Acetorphine
Acetyldihydrocodeine
Allylprodine
Alphameprodine
Alphaprodine

Benzethidine
Benzylmorphine
Betacetylmethadol
Betameprodine
Betamethadol
Betaprodine
Bezitramide

Clonitazene
Cyprenorphine

Desomorphine
Dextromoramide
Diampromide
Diethylthiambutene
Difenoxin
Dihydrocodeine
Dihydromorphine
Dimenoxadol
Dimepheptanol
Dimethylthiambutene
Dioxaphetyl butyrate
Diphenoxylate
Dipipanone
Drotebanol

Ethylmethylthiambutene
Ethylmorphine
Etonitazene
Etorphine hydrochloride
Etoxeridine

Furethidine

Hydromorphinol

Isomethadone

Ketobemidone

Levomethorphan
Levomoramide
Levophenacylmorphan
Levorphanol

Metazocine
Methyldesorphine
Methyldihydromorphine
Metopon

Moramide-intermediate
Morpheridine
Myrophine

Nicocodeine
Nicomorphine
Noracymethadol
Norlevophanol
Normethadone
Normophine
Norpipanone

Oxymorphone

Phenadoxone
Phenampromide
Phenazocine
Phenomorphan
Phenoperidine
Pholcodine
Piminodine
Piritramide
Proheptazine
Properidine
Propiram

Racemethorphan
Racemoramide
Racemorphan

Thebacon

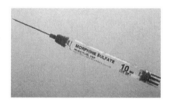

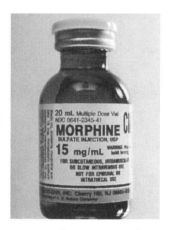

Morphine in various forms for medical use

Who Is Using Opiates?

Survey estimates show that 1,260,000 Americans abuse opiates every month. Approximately 2,450,000 Americans have tried heroin at least once in their lives, and from 300,000 to 800,000 are regular users.[16]

By far the greatest amount of opiate abuse occurs with prescription drugs. The extent of this consumption is shown by the legal production of opiates: in 1996, the United States used 1,225,600 pounds of opium , mostly for production of morphine, codeine, and other prescription opiates.[17]

 In Michigan, an 1878 survey found 7763 "opium eaters"—about 1 in 200 people. Results of a 1971 survey of narcotic addicts: about 1 in 200 people.

Of the illegal opiates, heroin is the most prominent. It has a cyclical popularity, going in and out of fashion for reasons that are not well understood. Until the 1980s, the most common way of using heroin was injecting it. In part because of worries of hepatitis or HIV and the fear and disgust associated with needles, heroin use declined. A decade later, heroin returned to popularity as a purer drug that could be snorted or smoked. Heroin is usually smoked by placing a small amount on aluminum foil and heating it from below by a match, called "chasing the dragon." Heroin also joined cocaine in a highly addictive combination that allowed the user to take more of both drugs (see *Cocaine*).

 A "speedball" is heroin laced with cocaine. It combines the stimulating high of cocaine with the pleasant, sleepy "rush" of heroin.

PURITY OF HEROIN

The medical supply of opiates comes from the poppy farms of Turkey, middle-eastern countries, Mexico and South America. Heroin is legally manufactured in England, with small amounts produced in France and Belgium. In the United States, imported opium and poppy straw is refined into prescription opiates. The U.S. does not legally manufacture heroin, but imports small amounts for highly restricted use in research and for terminally ill hospice patients.

Most of the illegal supply of heroin is produced in Southeast Asia, especially the "Golden Triangle" countries of Burma, Thailand, and Laos; with Burma (Myanmar) alone contributing about 60 percent of the total. Historically, opium was shipped from these countries to other locations, such as France, for processing into morphine and heroin. The notorious "French Connection" was composed

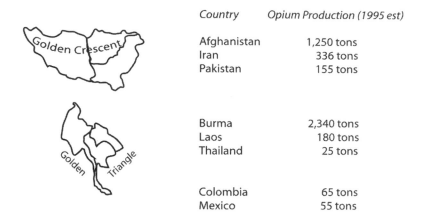

Country	Opium Production (1995 est)
Afghanistan	1,250 tons
Iran	336 tons
Pakistan	155 tons
Burma	2,340 tons
Laos	180 tons
Thailand	25 tons
Colombia	65 tons
Mexico	55 tons

of a cartel that dominated the opium trade from Turkey to the south of France, especially Marseilles, where the heroin labs were located. This monopoly resulted in high prices and very poor quality—in 1970, the street purity averaged just three percent. The cartel's domination of the trade led to a decrease in heroin use in the United States. In an irony of drug control politics, when the cartel was broken in the 1980s, heroin production was opened to farmers and dealers in Mexico, followed in the 1990s by the heavy hitters of the Colombian cocaine trade, resulting in much greater volume and distribution.

Some of the heroin from Southeast Asia is quite pure. For example, samples of "China White" have been tested up to 99 percent purity. "Persian Brown" from Iran, Afghanistan, Pakistan, and Turkey is about 90 percent pure. "Pink" heroin from India, Cambodia, and Malaysia or Sri Lanka is usually about 50 percent pure. By the time it gets to the street, the purity of illegal heroin varies widely but it has gradually increased over time. In the 1960s, street heroin might have contained from 1 to 10 percent actual heroin. Currently, the national average is about 35 percent pure, with some samples much higher.

Heroin is distributed in two basic forms: powder and tar. Powder is the traditional method of manufacture, and is very easily diluted with similar looking substances. Pure heroin appears as a white powder with a bitter taste. This form is rarely found on the illegal market. Illegal heroin has both natural impurities and cheaper additives, including sugar, starch, talcum powder, baking powder, powdered milk,

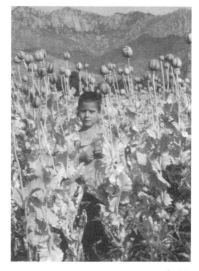

Opium poppy fields

or quinine, and anything that can give an extra kick to the product, including caffeine, amphetamines, PCP, and local anesthetics such as xylocaine. It can range in color from white to dark brown. Heroin products may also have small amounts of codeine, partly from impure processing from opium powder and partly because it is often deliberately added by dealers to increase volume. Codeine is much cheaper and more readily available than heroin. It can be purchased without a prescription in many countries, including Canada (for example, 222 and AC&C) and Mexico. In New Zealand, morphine and heroin are often made from legally available codeine preparations, in a simple process of codeine demethylation that uses pyridine hydrochloride to form a product called "homebake."

Killer quality
Any new sample of heroin is a gamble since it can range in purity from zero to 99 percent. If a user expects 5% purity and gets 50%, the overdose can be fatal.

In the 1980s, a cruder form of heroin from Mexico, "black tar," became popular in California. Although it has a naturally lower purity than refined powder heroin, it has a hard texture and is difficult to cut, with the result that it is unlikely to become further contaminated or diluted. Nonetheless, dealers try to extend their supply by putting tar heroin in an oven on low temperature to heat it until it becomes soft and gummy, and then knead other substances into it, such as starch, molasses, cocoa mix, coffee and brown sugar.

Heroin with a low purity must be injected to have a significant effect. Traditionally, users dissolved the powder or tar in a small amount of liquid in a spoon by heating it with a match, and then strained the solution through a tuft of cotton before injecting it. This method is a feeble attempt to purify the product and more often results in a host of illnesses and infections (see *Chapter 4: Intravenous Drug Use*).

Sophisticated users purify heroin by first dissolving it in hydrochloric acid (HCl). About a gram of heroin is placed in a small glass container, such as a test tube, and several drops of 28% HCl are added, followed by 5 ml of distilled water, and the mixture is shaken vigorously. Any particulate matter settles to the bottom, and the top solution is removed with a pipette or eyedropper. Ammonium hydroxide is then added, one drop at time, giving the solution a milky appearance. The solution is poured into 100 ml of ethyl ether, followed by the addition of baking soda to cause the mess to bubble in reaction. The final solution is dried, yielding a pure heroin powder that may be much smaller in volume.[18]

ANOTHER FORM OF CHINA WHITE

In 1979, an illegal California laboratory produced a variant of fentanyl later identified as alpha-methyl-fentanyl. They called it China White to convince users that it was the ultra-pure form of heroin. The new drug certainly was as potent as pure heroin—in fact, it was vastly more potent.[19] Over 100 deaths occurred from overdose before the word got out to avoid this new substance. Part of the risk of overdose was the wide range of potency in the samples, which varied as much as 300-fold.[20] In late 1983, an even more powerful analog appeared, 3-methyl-fentanyl, with an effective dose of less than 0.5 milligrams. In 1986, it spread to the east coast, where another 99 deaths were reported in the following two years.[21] It has since disappeared, awaiting the next unscrupulous manufacturer.

 The United States consumes 45 percent of the world's legal production of opium.

Chemical Characteristics

Opium alkaloids fall into two groups of chemicals: phenanthrenes and isoquinolines. The phenanthrenes are the psychoactive constituents, including morphine, codeine, and thebaine. Isoquinolines have no significant effects on the central nervous system, and are therefore not controlled substances, but have other useful medical properties (for example, as a medication for diarrhea).

Morphine was the first opiate molecule to be analyzed, and it is still the standard by which the others are measured. Heroin is made by combining morphine with acetic anhydride (for this reason, acetic anhydride is also a controlled substance). Heroin is not really a different drug from morphine. It is more potent than morphine because it is more soluble in fat, and therefore enters the brain faster. Once in the brain, however, it is converted back to morphine and has the same effects.

The psychoactive properties of the opiates have stimulated research into the functions of the brain, and led to some of the most significant discoveries of how nerve cells communicate. Scientists have long been intrigued by the concept of "euphoria." How can a drug produce this feeling? And how are drug effects different from the natural euphoria that comes from romantic love, strenuous physical activity, or religious practices?

The answer came in the early 1970s, when the brain was discovered to have its own, self-created neurotransmitters that were similar to the opiates (see *Chapter 6*). Opiates mimic these endorphins—a term coined from endogenous morphine—by binding to the same receptors on the nerve cells. More and more types of these receptors have been discovered, and it is likely that the effects of drugs will be largely explained by their specific stimulation of these receptors.

Opiates cause euphoric feelings by attaching to mu (μ) opioid receptors at several distinct anatomical locations in the brain, including the ventral tegmentum, the nucleus accumbens, the medial frontal cortex, and especially the locus ceruleus. Opiates inhibit the activity of the locus ceruleus, a center for stimulating impulses and the "fight or flight" response, and therefore produce the dreamy contentment desired by its users. Unfortunately, long-term use of opiates causes adaptation to this inhibition so that the brain works much harder to send out its stimulating impulses. Sudden withdrawal of opiates results in an excess of neuronal excitement, bringing about the muscle spasms, dilated pupils, and the overall "flu-like" feeling of withdrawal. Clonidine has an inhibiting effect on the locus ceruleus and is often prescribed for the relief of these withdrawal symptoms.

EFFECTS

Taking a small amount of an opiate results in a short-lived feeling of euphoria leading to several hours of physical and mental relaxation. Many other effects may be present, varying with the user, the amount taken, and the type of drug. Although opiates differ widely in their action, most include the following signs and symptoms.

Physical effects include drowsiness, respiratory depression, constricted pupils, a dull facial appearance, ptosis (a drooping of the upper eyelid), nausea, vasodilation (the "flush and rush"), slurred speech, impaired attention, and impaired memory. Users often have a peculiar head-nodding behavior ("the nod") that seems to be somehow comforting to themselves.

Mental effects include mental dullness, impaired judgment, impaired social function, and overall confusion.

Opiates cause a release of histamine in the body, the same effect that occurs with allergies and some viral infections, causing a general itching and maybe a skin rash.

 Opiate users often complain of dry, itchy skin and may absentmindedly scratch themselves for hours.

Opiates affect almost every part of the body, including the heart, lungs, brain, eyes, voice box, muscles, reproductive system, excretory system, immune system, and cough and nausea centers. The muscles are relaxed: speech becomes slurred and slowed, the eyelids droop, and the head may begin to nod. It may become difficult to walk. The pupils of the eyes become pinpointed and do not react to light.

The reproductive abilities of both men and women are affected, with a decrease in sexual desire or total indifference. In women, the period is delayed, and in men, less testosterone is produced.

 Opiates take away both the desire and the disgust of sex with strangers. This is one reason—along with the need for money—why users are more susceptible to becoming prostitutes.

Opiates also affect the nausea and cough centers of the brain. Many heroin users vomit each time they take it, and even use this feature as reassurance to know they have taken good stuff. The action of opiates on suppressing the cough center in brain was one of the original reasons for their medical use, and continues to make codeine-based cough medicines among the most widely prescribed drugs.

TESTING FOR OPIATES

After ingestion, most opiates are rapidly absorbed and metabolized. Morphine, codeine, heroin, and their metabolites can be detected in urine up to four days after use.

When morphine is taken, either by mouth or by injection, about ten percent is excreted in the urine as morphine. The remainder is converted to conjugated forms of morphine, primarily morphine-3-glucuronide.

Codeine is metabolized primarily to codeine-6-glucuronide, a conjugated form. About 10 to 15 percent of codeine is demethylated, forming morphine and norcodeine, mainly in the form of conjugates. Therefore, after taking only codeine the urine can be positive for codeine, norcodeine, morphine, or all three. Codeine is rapidly cleared from the body, with an elimination half-life of approximately 3.3 hours.[22] Morphine takes somewhat longer, as long as four days.

Heroin is diacetylmorphine. After it enters the body, it is rapidly deacetylated to 6-acetylmorphine (6-AM), also called 6-monoacetylmorphine (6-MAM). This metabolite is specific for heroin and it always indicates heroin use. Heroin itself is rarely detected in urine. After a single dose of heroin, 6-AM may be detectable in urine for two to eight hours at concentrations generally ranging from 10 to 250 ng/mL.[23] 6-AM is stable in urine refrigerated for up to 10 days or frozen for up to 2 years. Heroin users have morphine in their urine, from the body's metabolism of heroin, and may also have codeine in their urine because heroin is often cut with codeine. Therefore, after heroin use, both morphine and codeine may be detected in urine.

Taking ...	shows up in urine as ...
Morphine	→ Morphine metabolites
	↘ Morphine
Codeine	↗ Norcodeine
	→ Codeine
	↘ Morphine
Heroin	↗ 6-AM
	→ (Codeine)
	↘ Morphine

The synthetic and semisynthetic opiates—for example, hydromorphone, hydrocodone, oxycodone, propoxyphene, methadone, meperidine, and fentanyl—do not metabolize to codeine, morphine or 6-AM. Taking any of these prescription drugs does not cause a positive result in testing for opiates.

POPPY SEED POSITIVE

Poppy seeds used in breads and pastries are from flowers similar to opium poppies. Eating as little as five grams, about one teaspoon, of poppy seeds can result in a positive test for opiates. The amount of actual morphine or codeine in poppy seeds is quite low, but some people say they can feel the effects. Eating a large quantity of poppy seeds can produce elated feelings, and is often done for this purpose in Eastern Europe.[24] Withdrawal symptoms from a "poppy seed habit" have even been observed.[25]

"It must have been those bagels"
There is no direct way to be sure whether a urine test positive for morphine or codeine is due to poppy seeds or to drugs.[26] Eating a single poppy seed bagel can result in a positive drug test for up to three days.[27]

Eating a normal amount of poppy seeds can result in peak urine morphine concentrations of more than 4,000 ng/mL and peak codeine concentrations of more than 2,000 ng/mL.[28] This is enough to test positive for morphine or codeine use. There is no direct way to determine whether positive urine test results are due to poppy seeds or to drug use. A common indirect test is to compare the amount of morphine to codeine: poppy seeds contain much more morphine than codeine, so the morphine-to-codeine ratio should be greater than 2:1.[29] If the ratio is less than 2:1, codeine use should be suspected.

Withdrawal Signs

Opiates are physically and psychologically addictive, with a withdrawal syndrome that is characterized by flu-like symptoms and a very uncomfortable experience. Symptoms usually peak at 24 to 72 hours after the last dose and then gradually subside and disappear within seven to ten days. Unlike other addictive drugs, such as barbiturates, opiate withdrawal is not life-threatening and generally resolves without the need for medication.

Withdrawal from opiates is not life-threatening—but it is an utterly miserable experience. You only feel like you are going to die.

The earliest signs of withdrawal are watery eyes, runny nose, yawning and sweating. The pupils become dilated and there is a loss of appetite with irritability, tremors, panic, muscle cramps and restless legs, nausea or vomiting, diarrhea, fever and chills, and insomnia. There may be a rapid pulse and goose-flesh (which is why abrupt withdrawal is called "cold turkey").

Withdrawal from opiates may cause uncontrollable diarrhea. This is because all opiates cause constipation. Indeed, the relief of diarrhea was one of the first historical uses of opiates, and even now it is one of the more common medicines in preparations such as diphenoxylate (Lomotil), used to alleviate loose bowel movements. When the body adapts to the constipating action of opium, withdrawal produces the opposite effect.

Withdrawal can also cause extreme insomnia. After three days without sleep, withdrawing addicts can be utterly exhausted and frustrated beyond their ability to cope.

Opiate effect and ...	the withdrawal symptom[30]
Numbness	becomes pain
Euphoria	becomes anxiety
Dryness of mouth	becomes sweating, runny nose
Constipation	becomes diarrhea
Slow pulse	becomes rapid pulse
Low blood pressure	becomes high blood pressure
Shallow breathing	becomes coughing
Pinpoint pupils	becomes dilated pupils
Sluggishness	becomes severe hyper-reflexes
Relaxed muscles	become muscle cramps

Some of these symptoms can be alleviated by the use of clonidine,[31] a prescription medication for the treatment of high blood pressure. Clonidine depresses the locus ceruleus in a manner similar to heroin, and greatly reduces anxiety. It is usually combined with a sleeping pill, such Librium, temazepam (Restoril), or alprazolam (Xanax). Imodium may be given for diarrhea and Tylenol for muscle aches.

"Clonidine alone will transform the nightmare of withdrawal into a bad dream."[32]

If flu-like symptoms were the worst of opiate withdrawal, the treatment of addiction would be relatively short and simple. Unfortunately, there is another symptom that is longer-lasting and much more difficult to deal with. The medical term for this is dysphoria, but it is best explained as "just feeling lousy." [33] Opiates cause the brain to experience euphoria. When this occurs on a regular basis, the brain no longer needs to produce its own endorphins to produce good feelings and down-regulates their production. The result is that withdrawal from opiates brings about a deficiency of these positive-mood endorphins until the brain once again resumes their production. Withdrawing opiate addicts simply feel miserable, and they know opiates will reverse this feeling. The physical craving may soon resolve, but the psychological desire can last for months or years, with the memory of a euphoria that normal life just doesn't seem to bring. This aspect of opiate addiction is very difficult to treat.

"The last of the codeine was running out. My nose and eyes began to run, sweat soaked through my clothes. Hot and cold flashes hit me as though a furnace door was swinging open and shut. I lay down on the bunk, too weak to move. My legs ached and twitched so that any position was intolerable, and I moved from one side to the other, sloshing about in my sweaty clothes."—William Burroughs, Junkie

TREATING OPIATE ADDICTION

Before 1914 in the United States, physicians treated patients addicted to opiates by simply giving them other opiates. In fact, physicians often caused addictions by treating almost all illnesses with narcotics. This practice ended in 1920, when the American Medical Association recommended a ban of this method of treatment. For the next 50 years, opiate addiction was treated instead by the criminal justice system: going cold turkey in jail. It was not very successful. The relapse rate for opiate addiction without medical care was estimated to be close to 100 percent.

The current standard method of treating opiate addiction is the use of methadone (or, more recently, LAAM). Methadone has a slow onset of action and a long effect. It therefore provides the same pleasant feeling but not the rush and the intense reward-cycle that is characteristic of addictive drugs. The purpose of methadone is to relieve the physical and psychological need for opiates, and wean users away from substances such as heroin. Methadone programs are most effective if they use a high dose, long-term regimen, with realistic goals coupled with social and psychological counseling. These programs have been shown to improve health, reduce criminal activity, and decrease the spread of HIV and other infections.[34]

Four common methods of opiate withdrawal

- cold turkey
- clonidine
- opioid substitution (e.g., methadone)
- antagonist therapy (rapid detox)

Naltrexone (Trexan) is another medication often used to prevent opiate addicts from relapsing. Naltrexone is an opiate antagonist. It binds to the μ-receptor in the brain and blocks the effects of opiates for about three days. If there is recent opiate use, naltrexone will cause immediate and severe withdrawal symptoms. This medication may be safely used after withdrawal is complete, and will discourage the user from resuming the use of opiates. It is therefore recommended as a long-term regimen for those who have difficulty staying clean.

Buprenorphine (Buprenex), is a newer, semi-synthetic narcotic derived from thebaine. It is a long-acting, mixed opioid agonist-antagonist with properties similar to either methadone or naltrexone, depending on the dose.[35] It also appears to be effective for detoxification and is being used in some maintenance programs.

Ultra-rapid detox

With all of the conventional methods—cold turkey or opiate substitution—opiate detoxification is a long, drawn-out process with plenty of chances for relapse. A new method developed in the last few years compresses the physical detoxification process into just a few hours. This is done by not only stopping opiate administration but also giving additional drugs that have an effect opposite to opiates. Normally, such an extreme action would be unbearably painful. For this "ultra-rapid detox," the addict is put into a deep sleep with a general anesthetic and the body is flooded with an opiate antagonist for four to six hours.

Although ultra-rapid detox is very effective in speeding up withdrawal, it is not a substitute for long-term addiction management, and former users will soon return to opiates if they have not addressed other aspects of addiction.

Long-term Health Problems

Opiate addiction in itself is minimally injurious to the body. With the exception of being chronically impotent and constipated, the typical user is able to function quite well and live a long and normal life. Throughout history, many people—including famous artists, writers, and countless others of great achievement—were life-long opiate addicts. From Benjamin Franklin to the rock musician Jerry Garcia of the Grateful Dead, even addiction for many decades was well tolerated and they eventually died from unrelated diseases.

It is the lifestyle of the addict, rather than the drug itself, which is dangerous. In a recent three-year heroin maintenance program in Switzerland, not a single heroin-related death occurred in over 1,000 patients.[36]

There are two major dangers of long-term opiate use, and both of these are largely due to the illegal status of these drugs. The first and greatest problem of all illegal drug use, and opiates in particular, is that these drugs have an unknown purity and potency. Every use is therefore a gamble with an unknown substance. The list of problems that can occur because of contaminated drugs is lengthy (see *Chapter 4: Drug Use Illnesses*).

Maternal support ...

With the needle still in his arm, Lenny Bruce died from an overdose of too-potent heroin. The famous comedian had been given the heroin by his mother.

The risk of illness from an illegal drug is radically increased when the drug is used intravenously. Human immunodeficiency virus (HIV) is a major concern of IV drug use. In many parts of the United States, the epidemic of HIV has shifted from sexual transmission to infection from dirty needles. In some cities, 80 percent of IV drug addicts are HIV-positive. Infection with the hepatitis B and C viruses is even more common, and may not appear for years or even decades after use. Tuberculosis has also dramatically increased among intravenous opiate users, particularly newer forms of tuberculosis that are resistant to antibiotics and extremely difficult to treat.

The second long-term danger of opiate use is addiction, specifically the criminal activities involved in the compulsive search for the drugs. It is estimated that more than 95 percent of opiate addicts commit crimes in order to support to their addiction—either to get drugs, or to get money to buy drugs. Theft is the most common offense, but other crimes range from prostitution to homicide. In 1993, more than one quarter of all inmates in state and federal prisons, and about 60 percent of those in federal penitentiaries, were imprisoned for drug offenses.

What To Do If There Is An Overdose

Like all popular drugs, opiate use goes in cycles. Following a decline in the 1970s and 80s, there has once again been an increase in use. From 1991 to 1995, the annual number of opiate overdoses reported by large hospitals rose from 36,000 to 76,000, and the annual number deaths from opiates increased from 2300 to 4000. According to the Drug Abuse Warning Network (DAWN), heroin is the second highest cause of deaths from illegal drugs, after barbiturates.

Opiates cause depression of the central nervous system. The user typically looks confused and falls easily into a stupor. The most dangerous feature of opiate drugs by far—and the usual cause of death—is the suppression of breathing, which can be fatal within minutes after an injection. If an overdose is suspected, the most important measure is to clear the airway and maintain respiration, and to prevent shock by keeping the patient warm and elevating the feet.

Physical signs of overdose[37]	Slow, shallow breathing
	Irregular heart beat
	Low blood pressure
	Slurred speech
	Difficulty walking
	Pinpoint pupils
	Clammy skin
	Seizures
Mental signs of overdose	Confusion
	Drowsiness
	Delirium
	Unresponsive coma

If there is difficulty breathing, the overdose patient should be taken immediately to the Emergency Department. The opiate antidote naloxone

(Narcan) will probably be given. Naloxone displaces the opiate molecules from their receptor sites in the brain within minutes, and can cause rapid withdrawal. If there is any chance that the patient took cocaine along with the opiate ("speedball"), naloxone should not be given because it increases the effect of cocaine and can result in an irregular heart beat.

River Phoenix, a young actor with great potential, died on Halloween, 1993, after taking a "speedball" combination of cocaine and heroin.

If the overdose is of methadone, the excess can be flushed out by making the urine more acidic. Giving Vitamin C, for example, will increase the rate of excretion by 5 to 22 percent,[38] which may be enough to manage the excessive dose.

PCP

PCP, phencyclidine, is an anesthetic drug with depressant, stimulant and hallucinatory effects. Its main function is to dissociate awareness from the body.

The Basic Facts

Type of drug	*Hallucinogen, stimulant*
How taken	*Ingested, smoked, snorted, injected*
Duration of effect	*8 hours*
Physical danger	*Moderate*
Addiction potential	*Low*

Other Names

PCP	*AD, amoeba, angel, angel dust, angel hair, angel mist, angel poke, animal tranquilizer, aurora borealis, black whack, blue madman, blue star, boat, busy bee, butt naked, Cadillac, cliffhanger, cyclones, dust, fresh, goon, gorilla biscuits, hog, jet fuel, loveboat, mellow yellow, monkey dust, peace, rocket fuel, scuffle, selma, sherman, shermies, sherm sticks, snorts, surfer, T, TAC, TIC, tranks, zombie dust*
PCP mixed with crack	*beam me up Scottie*
PCP mixed with marijuana	*ace, amp, CJ, crystal joints, fry, happy sticks, kay jay, killer weed, mint weed, supercools, superweed, wet sticks, whacky weed*
PCP mixed with heroin	*alien sex fiend*

Angel Dust: The Story of PCP

Phencyclidine (PCP) was first synthesized in 1926 at a time of great development of new drugs. It did not find a use until 1957, when the Parke-Davis company marketed it as a general anesthetic under the trade name Sernyl. Phencyclidine initially showed promise as a novel type of anesthetic that did not depress the central nervous system, paralyze the diaphragm, or limit breathing (see *Chapter 7: Ketamine*). Bad reactions soon began to be reported, however. Too many patients coming out of anesthesia complained of delirium, delusions, visual disturbances, and varying degrees of psychotic behavior. In 1965 Parke-Davis withdrew Sernyl from medical use, and then reintroduced it in 1967 as the veterinary drug, Sernylan (apparently, animals had fewer complaints of psychosis).

The same year of its advertisement as a veterinary anesthetic, recreational users discovered it. The drug showed up at San Francisco music festivals, billed as the "PeaCe Pill," which was shorted to PCP. Use spread quickly, at first from diverted veterinary supplies and then from illicit labs. In 1978, the commercial manufacture of phencyclidine was discontinued and it was made illegal as a Schedule II Controlled Substance.

PCP is one of the most complex psychoactive drugs, with many different effects depending on the amount taken and the characteristics of the user. In a normal dose, PCP typically causes drunken behavior with drowsiness, slurred speech, and poor coordination. There is an altered sense of time and distance. The user feels detached and removed from the environment and less sensitive to pain. Some people have a sense of strength and invulnerability. This feeling of being invincible—along with its pure white, powdery appearance—gave it the name "angel dust."

At higher doses, PCP can produce a completely dissociative state in which the user has a blank stare or jerky eye movements and is oblivious to the environment. There may be radical mood swings, visual distortions, and auditory hallucinations in which the person hears voices or commands. After recovery, the user often has no memory of the whole event.

Pills may be stamped with popular logos, such as this Pokemon character

There are countless stories of incredible feats performed by individuals under PCP. No medical evidence exists that PCP increases strength or any other ability. It can, however, cause a total loss of sensitivity to pain. This feature accounts for the stories of PCP-intoxicated people ignoring severe burns, running on two broken legs, pulling their own teeth, and other horrendous and seemingly superhuman accomplishments.

In some people, PCP causes extreme anxiety and a feeling of impending doom, or paranoia and violent hostility, leading to wild and risky behavior. For this reason, many people, especially law officers, believe PCP is the most dangerous of all drugs.

Who Is Using PCP?

Because of its extreme and unpredictable effects, PCP has never achieved the popularity of other recreational drugs. Drug surveys show that it accounts for about one percent of all positive drug tests, but it is difficult to estimate population use because many of these tests are laboratory proficiency testing samples. Actual use of PCP is probably quite limited, and mostly confined to groups such as motorcycle clubs and street gangs.

Almost all of the PCP now available in the United States is produced illegally. Pure PCP is a white, crystalline powder that is easily dissolved in water. The PCP that is available on the street often contains a number of impurities. It varies in color from tan to brown, and in consistency from powder to a gummy mass. It may be sold in tablets, capsules, powder or liquid. PCP is usually smoked, but may be swallowed, snorted, or injected intravenously. Many users smoke PCP after sprinkling the powder or liquid on tobacco, marijuana, or herbs such as parsley, mint, or oregano.

The illegal manufacture of PCP can produce other chemical analogues of PCP that are similar in effect. The first four of these substances have also been made illegal:[1]

PCE	N-ethyl-1-phenylcyclohexylamine
PCPy	1-phenylcyclohexyl-pyrrolidine
TCP	1-[1-(2-thienyl)-cyclohexyl]-piperidine
TCPy	1-[1-(2-thienyl)-cyclohexyl]-cyclohexyl-pyrrolidine
PCC	1-(1-piperidinyl)-cyclohexane-carbonitrile[3]
THP	N-[1-(thienyl)-cyclohexyl]-pyrrolidine
PCDEA	N,N-dimethyl-1-phenyl-cyclohexylamine

For such a complex drug, the manufacture is surprisingly simple. The ingredients are bromobenzene, cyclohexanone, ether, pentamethylene dibromide, phenylmagnesium bromide, piperidine, potassium cyanide, and sodium bisulfide. Most of these materials are readily available. The exception is piperidine, the most important of the ingredients. It is difficult to obtain by illicit chemists because distribution is controlled by Federal law. Piperidine is a clear liquid with an odor similar to pepper. It has industrial uses as a solvent, as an additive to certain fuels and oils, and in the production of rubber. To avoid illicit use, any quantity of piperidine that is purchased from chemical supply houses in excess of 500 grams must be reported to the DEA.

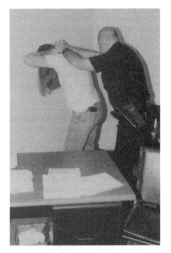

"So, in total, you have someone running around drunk, insensitive to pain, and very uninhibited. Is it any wonder that PCP-intoxicated people frequently find themselves in trouble with the law?"[2]

The synthesis of PCP is a two-step process. First, an intermediate product known as PCC is made. This is then converted into PCP. If all impurities and chemicals used in the manufacturing process are removed, the end product is an odorless, metallic or bitter-tasting white powder. However, poor manufacturing usually produces PCP that varies in color from tan to brown and has a strong odor.

Most illicit labs are controlled by inner-city gangs. They also distribute it, and are the majority of its consumers. By the time it gets to the end user, the drug is often diluted to 20 to 1, or even more.

PCP is typically sprinkled on cigarettes and smoked. Cigarettes or cigars with heavy, dark paper are preferred because they can conceal the liquid discoloration and do not fall apart after being soaked. The most popular brand of cigarettes for this purpose are Shermans, and PCP-laced cigarettes are often referred to as sherms, shermies, or sherm sticks.

Chemical Characteristics

The full chemical name of PCP is 1-1-phenylcyclohexyl piperidine hydrochloride. It produces its psychoactive effects by binding to glutamate and NMDA neurotransmitter receptors in the brain, and by stepping up the release of dopamine.

Glutamate is one of the most common neurotransmitters in the brain, and the major means of stimulation. When glutamate is blocked by PCP, the result is a feeling of disconnection from the body and environment.

When PCP binds to the NMDA (N-methyl-D-aspartic acid) channel, it impedes the flow of calcium ions into neurons. This prevents activation of the neurons and results in the loss of pain sensation.

PCP also releases dopamine, in a manner similar to the amphetamines. The amphetamine-like action is considered to be responsible for the agitation, stimulation, and addictive potential.

Intoxication begins several minutes after taking PCP. The peak experience usually lasts for four to six hours. Residual effects may last for days afterward; some heavy users can remain intoxicated for days, weeks, or even months after the last dose. PCP is well absorbed no matter how it is taken. It is highly fat-soluble and accumulates in fat tissue and in the brain.[4] Small doses, less than five milligrams, typically produce a drunken state with slurred speech, numbness and depression, which is then followed by a sense of stimulation. With a moderate dose, about ten milligrams, the effects become more difficult to predict, and include muscle rigidity, lack of coordination, agitated or combative behavior, distorted mental images, and hallucinations. These features, along with a loss of sensitivity to pain, account for the often bizarre behavior of PCP users.

TESTING FOR PCP

About ten percent of a dose of PCP is excreted in the urine unchanged. The rest is slowly released from fat tissue and excreted over weeks. A single dose of PCP may show up in urine for as long as two weeks. If use has been very extensive, a urine drug test may be positive for 30 days or more.[5]

There are no medications approved in the United States that contain PCP. Most accurate drug tests look for the major metabolite, 4-hydroxy-phencyclidine. Taking diphenhydramine (Benadryl) can cause a positive PCP urine test if one of the simpler tests is used. However, confirmatory testing with GC/MS (see *Chapter 5*) will be positive only if PCP was used.[6]

Chemically, PCP is a weak base. If the urine is acidified, the elimination rate is increased. Users can take vitamin C, vinegar, or acidic fruit juices such as cranberry juice to help rid the body of PCP.[7]

Withdrawal Signs

PCP users have not shown a distinct withdrawal syndrome, even after long-term use. However, many users have complained of depression, anxiety, irritability, excessive sleep, and craving for PCP.[8]

Long-term Health Problems

A single use of PCP can result in an abnormal psychiatric state that might persist for days, and some users suffer from perceptual disorders that last for years. Most of these are auditory and visual hallucinations such as "machinery voices" and after-images seen with moving objects.[9] Some PCP users have reported LSD-like flashbacks, especially with heavy use.

 Unlike other hallucinogens, PCP flashbacks are true chemical effects—caused by residual amounts of drug remaining in the body—and are not just psychological.

In animal testing, PCP and its analogues have been shown to cause spasms in the arteries of the brain.[10] It is not known what sort of temporary or permanent injury this may cause in humans.

What To Do If There Is An Overdose

PCP accounts for about three percent of all deaths from illegal drug use.[11]

The greatest concern is the possibility that the conscious user may slip into a coma, which can resolve in minutes or last as long as a week. Coma may develop spontaneously or after a period of bizarre or violent behavior. The comatose user may awaken briefly in an agitated or hostile state, and then fall back into the coma—a patient calm one minute may appear violent the next.

Anyone who has overdosed should be observed for at least 12 hours, by which time the symptoms generally resolve.

Overdose of PCP has been described as taking place in three stages:

The user is conscious, with largely psychological effects

 The user is poorly responsive, or responsive to pain only

 The user is comatose and unresponsive to pain

Physical signs of overdose[12]   Blank stare
Inability to speak
Pressured speech
Impulsive or violent behavior
Fever
Rapid pulse
High blood pressure
Hyperactivity
Drooling
Jerky eye movements
Muscle rigidity
Difficulty walking

Mental signs of overdose   Anxiety
Panic
Paranoia
Memory loss

Young children have become intoxicated by putting the butts of used PCP cigarettes into their mouths, or from inhaling the sidestream smoke. They may become lethargic, severely depressed, or have jerky eyes and difficulty walking.

There is no specific antidote for PCP.[13] For most users, the best therapy is a reassuring person who can talk them down in a quiet room. If the user is agitated, a benzodiazepine such as Valium may be given, or if extremely agitated or violent, haloperidol (Haldol) is often used. Neuroleptic medications that have strong anticholinergic actions (for example, Thorazine), should not be used since these contribute to the anticholinergic properties of PCP.

PCP excretion can be speeded up by making the urine more acidic. Care should be taken if multiple drugs are involved, because acidification will slow down the excretion of barbiturates and aspirin. Experimental work is now being done with anti-PCP monoclonal antibody binding fragments, which would provide a specific antidote.[14]

Peyote and Mescaline

Peyote is the top of a small cactus which grows in Texas and Mexico. It contains mescaline, a hallucinogen.

Peyote has been used for thousands of years as a medicine and as a religious sacrament. It continues to be used legally by the Native American Church.

The Basic Facts

Type of drug	*Hallucinogen*
How taken	*Ingested*
Duration of effect	*4 to 12 hours*
Physical danger	*None*
Addiction potential	*None*

Other Names

Peyote

britton, buttons, cactus, chief, dry whiskey, green whiskey, half moon, hikuri, hyatari, medicine (Native American Church), nubs, tops

Mescaline

beans, blue caps, mesc, mescap, mescy, mese, moon

Divine Cactus: The Story of Peyote and Mescaline

Peyote refers to the top, above-ground "button" of a small, spineless, flowering cactus, *Lophophora williamsii*. The buttons contain about one percent mescaline by dry weight, on average, with some samples having as high as six percent.

The peyote cactus grows mainly in a restricted area near the Rio Grande River in Texas and Mexico. In the United States, ranchers who own the land where wild peyote grows may allow harvesting of the cactus by licensed representatives of the Native American Church (NAC). Except for this unusual exemption, both peyote and mescaline are illegal Schedule I drugs under the Controlled Substances Act.

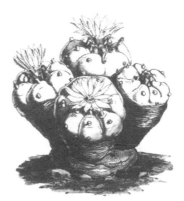

The earliest known illustration of peyote, 1847

The button of the peyote cactus is about one to four inches in diameter and grows on top of a turnip-like root. Peyote seeds germinate quickly, within three to seven days, but require two years or more to mature and flower. The top part of the plant may be harvested repeatedly, with several new buttons sprouting from the cut. Eventually, large clusters can be formed up to several feet wide. Some plants live for a hundred years or longer.

Peyote buttons are eaten fresh or are dried for later use. Most peyote is distributed as the hard, dried buttons. These may be steeped as a tea, ground into a powder, or simply chewed and swallowed. The buttons have an extremely noxious and bitter taste. Most users become nauseated and vomit if they take more than a small amount. To avoid the disagreeable taste, some users grind the buttons into a fine powder and take it encased in gelatin capsules. For those who are unable to swallow the material, peyote tea may be used as an enema by using a small bulb syringe to infuse it into the rectum. There are also reports of users smoking the powder, mixed with herbs or marijuana.

A normal dose of peyote is 4 to 12 buttons, taken by mouth. Mescaline and other alkaloids of peyote are efficiently absorbed. After about one hour, a number of disagreeable symptoms are experienced, including nausea, vomiting, dizziness, sweating, palpitations, and headache. Pupil dilation is common, making bright lights uncomfortable. Most people feel a generalized restlessness and discomfort, with an urge to urinate, tremors, or stomach cramps. This phase may last up to three hours, and is followed by a second phase characterized by euphoria, visual imagery and distortion of perception. The user may have a paradoxical sensation of simultaneous elation and depression. The greatest effect, however, is a sense of psychological insight and understanding. This effect is sought after for both religious and medicinal purposes. A gradual resolution follows over about ten hours, leaving the user fatigued but otherwise without residual effects.

VARIETIES OF HALLUCINOGENIC CACTI

Dozens of hallucinogenic cacti have been discovered in the Americas. Historically, three species were well-known in South America, while Indians in Central Mexico recognize over 15 other species for medicinal and ritual use.

The most prominent of the South American species is the San Pedro cactus, *Echinopsis pachanoi* (also designated *Trichocereus pachanoi*), which contains mescaline but in a lesser concentration than peyote. It is indigenous to Peru and Ecuador where it has been used for perhaps 3,000 years. Although it is reported to grow in the southwest United States as well, it has rarely been used in this country and is not illegal (see *Chapter 7: San Pedro*). A cousin of San Pedro, *Trichocereus peruvianus*, has a lighter blue color and three to four inch thorns. It is reported to have ten times the amount of mescaline content of San Pedro, or about the same as peyote.

In North America, the *Doña Ana* (or *Doñana*) cactus, *Coryphantha macromeris*, contains several psychoactive compounds, notably macro-merine, but apparently not mescaline. It is only about one-fifth as potent as peyote.[1]

Native Americans also refer to peyotillo, the "little peyote" (*Pelcyphora aselliformis*), which they used medicinally. It has very small amounts of mescaline, probably not enough for psychoactive effects,[2] but

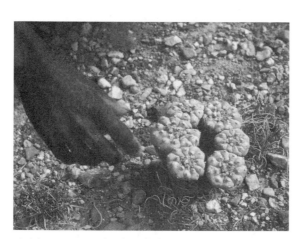

Wild peyote may be legally harvested only by a registered peyotero

many of the other alkaloids of peyote. In garden stores, it is sometimes called the "hatchet cactus" because of its oddly flattened tubercules.

Other cacti in traditional use include that named by the Huichol Indians *Tsuwiri* (*Ariocarpus retusus*) and *Sunami* (*Ariocarpus fissuratus*), "false peyote," which they believed to be more potent than peyote. They are known by other tribes as *chautle* or *chaute*, and commonly sold in gardening stores as "living rock." This cactus contains mostly hordenine, however, and not mescaline.

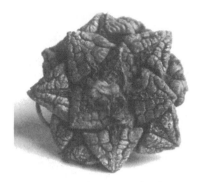

Living Rock cactus, also known as false peyote

THE FLESH OF GOD

Archeological evidence shows that peyote has been used in North America for over 10,000 years. Plant remains have been found in human sites dating to 8,500 BC, and the ancient Colima culture of 2,000 years ago has prolific art showing the use of peyote.

Peyote came to European attention when the Aztec civilization of central Mexico was conquered by Hernán Cortés in 1519. His appointed archbishop, Juan de Zumarraga, searched throughout the empire for information about their civilization and burned thousands of documents including a tremendous store of knowledge of plants and medicines.[3] The Franciscan friar Bernardino de Sahagún accompanied the conquistadors. Fortunately for historians, he was a better naturalist than missionary, and recognized the value of this information that was about to be lost. He worked tirelessly with Aztec physicians to record their medical practices, and after decades of effort produced the monumental *Historia general de las cosas de Nueva España* (*General History of Things of New Spain*). In this work, he described a cactus used by the Chichimecas, "which they call *péyotl*, and those who drank it took it in place of wine."[4] He went on to write that "it is like a food to the chichimecas, which supports them and gives them courage to fight and they have neither fear, nor thirst, nor hunger, and they say that it protects them from every danger."[5]

The new conquerors were not pleased to learn

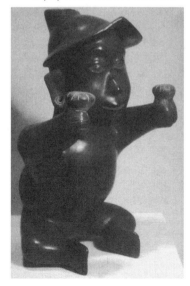

Statue of dwarf holding a pair of peyotes, Mexico, 200 BC

of a plant which gave courage and removed fear and hunger. In 1571, a harsh repression began of all traditional religious practices, and in 1620, the use of peyote was declared to be the work of the devil.[6] In the eyes of the government, peyote was as evil as murder and cannibalism and its use severely punished, sometimes by death.

The Mexican inquisition asked: "Have you murdered? Have you eaten the flesh of man? Have you eaten peyote?"[7]

Although peyote was repressed, it continued to be used secretly by healers and shamans, and more openly by remote tribes including the Yaqui, Cora, and Tepecano. Two tribes in particular, the Huichol and the Tarahumara, have carried the peyote tradition up to the present as a central, dominant feature of their culture.

The Huichol tribe now consists of about 25,000 people who live in the Sierra Madre Occidental mountain region of northwestern Mexico. Most of their sacred practices revolve around the use of peyote, which they hold as the physical manifestation of God. Peyote, they believe, "will give one heart" and greatly increases *Kupuri*, the energy force that creates life. Because the cactus does not grow in their territory, Huicholes travel hundreds of miles to the peyote fields each year in a ritualistic journey that involves prayer, abstinence, and celebration. Their annual pilgrimage is made at the end of the rainy season, in October or November. The pilgrimage is led by a Huichol shaman, the *mara'akame*, who is in contact with *Tatewari*, the grandfather-fire, also known as *Hikuri*, the Peyote-God. For the Huichol, peyote is much more than an intoxicant; it is a central feature of their lives. They pray to it, tell stories and dance to it, and use it for all types of illnesses, even childbirth, and rub the juices of fresh peyote into wounds to prevent infection and promote healing.

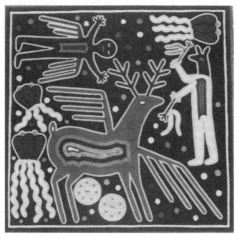

Brightly colored Huichol yarn paintings show their reverence for peyote.

The Tarahumara historically lived north of the Huichol in the Sierra Madre Occidental, but now many of the 50,000 members of the tribe have migrated to the hills and plains southwest of the city of Chihuahua. Tarahumaras are famous as great distance runners, delighting in 20 to 40 mile races over rugged mountain trails. Their races are not

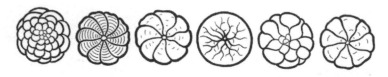

Variants of peyote are shown in the button patterns.

only for sport but also have religious meaning. Athletes carry only a little leather pouch containing peyote, which they use for endurance and to keep focused on the meditative spirit of the run.[8] While the outward ritual of their peyote use is different from the Huichol, they share the belief that peyote is the flesh of God.

The Huichol and other tribes recognize two forms of peyote, one larger, more potent and bitter than the other. The larger one is called Peyote of God, and the smaller one Peyote of the Goddess. Biologists consider them to be a single species, different only in age, since the buttons become increasingly potent as they grow older and larger.

Peyote is widely used in traditional Mexican folk medicine, even by those who do not participate in formal religious ceremonies. This use includes the treatment of arthritis, tuberculosis, influenza, intestinal disorders, diabetes, snake and scorpion bites, and datura poisoning. Because of excessive harvesting of the wild peyote, the Mexican Government has placed peyote on the endangered list of plants.

In 1967, the botanist H.H. Bravo found another species of peyote near Queretaro in northeastern Mexico, which he named *Lophoph-ora diffusa*. It has a yellow-green color, instead of the gray-green of *L. williamsii*, and is softer and ribless. It contains less mescaline and a different alkaloid mixture than *L. williamsii*, but is otherwise very similar to the untrained eye.

The United States law specifically identifies *Lophophora williamsii* and does not address the Mexican variant of peyote.

All other cacti which endogenously produce mescaline are not explicitly outlawed under Federal and state drug laws. However, manufacturing a controlled substance is a crime, and this includes extracting a controlled substance from a natural source. Therefore, use of these other cacti for drug purposes would be illegal.

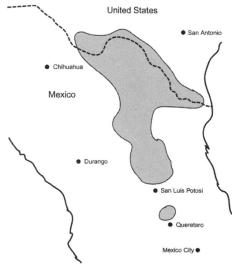

Peyote growing regions

MESCALINE

In 1887, Dr. Louis Lewin received a sample of dried peyote buttons in his laboratory in Germany. The sample was labeled "Mescale Button" because they were obtained from the Mescalero Apaches, a border tribe that adopted the peyote ritual from Native Mexicans. For the next nine years, the buttons were shelved until they came to the attention of Lewin's colleague, Arthur Heffter. In 1896, this meticulous scientist isolated many of the alkaloids found in the buttons, and ingested each one individually to examine its effects. When he discovered the psychoactive compound, he called it mescaline.[9] Peyote therefore became the first hallucinogenic plant to be chemically analyzed and its psychoactive agent identified.[10]

Mescaline was synthesized in 1919, but its manufacture is quite complex. It may be extracted from peyote by the use of sodium hydroxide, benzene, sulfuric acid and water, and then dried to form long needle-like crystals. Pure mescaline has a translucent white color and a very bitter taste. It is rarely seen on the illicit market.

Heffter's unwitting use of the term mescaline for a constituent of peyote has caused a lot of confusion in the study of psychoactive drugs, since mescal also refers to entirely different substances. Mescal is the name of a distilled liquor, similar to tequila. It comes from a Nahuatl (the language of the Aztecs) word referring to the fermented juice of the Agave cactus—probably from *me(tl)*, Agave (or maguey), and *(i)xcalli*, "something cooked."

Mescal also refers to a toxic and hallucinogenic bean from the Texas mountain laurel, *Sophora secundiflora*. However, Mescal beans contain cytisine and not mescaline. The bean probably got its name from confusion with peyote after reports of southwest Indians using a hallucinogenic button. The confusion is not surprising, since some Apaches and many other tribes actually did use the Mescal bean for intoxicating rituals.[11] Adding to the similarity, the tree is often found growing near peyote. Moreover, the Mescalero Apaches wear necklaces of Mescal beans in their peyote ceremonies (although they no longer eat the Mescal beans), and consider these beans sacred.

Peyote never became prominent outside Native American use. A few artists and writers noticed its mind-altering properties, but they were put off by its nauseating taste and subsequent vomiting, and the buttons did not become popular.

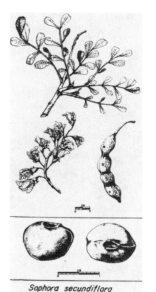

Sophora secundiflora

The Mescal bean is psychoactive but also very poisonous. It does not contain mescaline.

Pure mescaline, on the other hand, was clean and simple with a typical 500 mg dose equivalent to about a dozen peyote buttons, but without the noxious taste or effects. Word of the new drug spread among California intellectuals and many artists were intrigued.

 Allen Ginsburg wrote his most powerful poem, Howl, after a night on peyote walking the streets of San Francisco.

Aldous Huxley was already a famous writer when he moved to the Hollywood Hills of Los Angeles. On a May morning in 1953, he took 400 milligrams of mescaline and it changed his life. His account, published the following year as *The Doors of Perception*, is widely credited with inspiring the drug culture of the 1960s, and gave the name to a local rock band, The Doors.

 An early user of mescaline described a "furious succession" of visual images. Walt Disney was impressed by the description and hired him as the chief visualist for Fantasia.[12]

Synthetic mescaline is relatively difficult to make, however, and it was overtaken by other, more readily available hallucinogenic drugs such as LSD and psilocybin. Mescaline now has a very minor role as a popular hallucinogen.

NATIVE AMERICAN CHURCH

After the European colonization of North America, the health, culture, and social organization of Native Americans were all but destroyed. They were robbed of their lands and, under the Indian Religious Crime Code, even their religious practices were prohibited. By the mid-19th century, the great buffalo herds were gone and Indians were pushed onto reservations of the least-valued land. Most tribes were stricken with poverty and disease, and many were forbidden even to speak their own language.

In 1872, a Caddo-Delaware-French individual named John Wilson began a messianic movement called the Ghost Dance, to make white men vanish and bring back the buffalo. The white government misinterpreted the cult as an armed resistance movement and outlawed it, which led to a number of skirmishes. By 1890, the final pockets of resistance were crushed in the campaign that ended with the Wounded Knee massacre in South Dakota. After Wilson fled into seclusion, he learned of peyote from a Comanche medicine man and began to see salvation not as a process of armed struggle but accommodation to change.

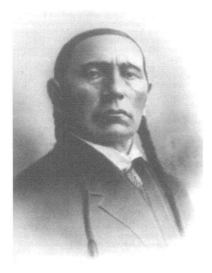

"The white man goes into his church house and talks about Jesus; the Indian goes into his tepee and talks to Jesus."—Commanche Chief Quanah Parker

James Mooney, anthropologist, proposed the Native American Church

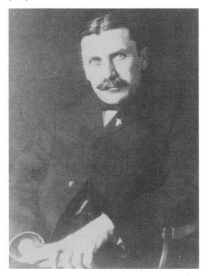

The chief of the Comanche at the time was Quanah Parker, a man of mixed Native and European ancestry. He fell deathly ill in 1884. When white medicine failed to help, he was taken to a Tarahumara *curandera* who cured him with peyote tea. The experience changed his life. He decided to turn away from violence and spread *peyotl* as a force to unify all tribes. Along with John Wilson, Mary Buffalo, Elk Hair, John Rave and many others who preached the use of peyote, he formed an amalgam of traditional Native and Christian beliefs with a set of moral instructions including abstinence from liquor, restraint in sexuality, matrimonial fidelity, and prohibitions against deceit, vengeance and violence. These teachings came to be known as the Peyote Road, and the leader of a ceremony as the Roadman.

In 1891, an anthropologist from the Smithsonian Institution named James Mooney was sent to the politically unstable region of the Oklahoma Territory to study Indian culture. He participated in Kiowa peyote ceremonies and became convinced that peyote could provide a way out of despondence, alcoholism and strife among Indians. Mooney called for a meeting of the Roadmen, and argued that they must band together to protect the use of peyote. He proposed the name Native American Church, partly to recognize the practice as a legitimate religion and partly as a cover for protection under the First and Fourteenth Amendments of the United States Constitution protecting religious freedom. In 1918, the Native American Church was incorporated in Oklahoma City.

The NAC preached resignation instead of resistance, accommodation to present realities rather than a return to paradise lost, and above all, personal responsibility for everything in one's life. It combined traditional Indian religious rituals—including chants, dances, and the sacred use of tobacco and eagle feathers—with Christian practices

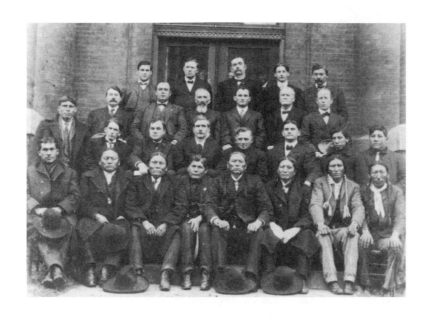

The founders of the NAC, 1918

such as the use of the Bible, sermons, baptism, and christening. Especially striking was the belief that peyote was the actual body of Christ, as in the Catholic Eucharist. Peyote ceremonies were not intended to displace Christian religion, but to complement them. Most NAC members continued to participate in services in a more traditional church. Ceremonies were held Saturday nights, both to accommodate the modern work week as well as to respect the Christian Sabbath.

The Peyote Road

Brotherly love	Members should be honest, truthful, friendly and helpful to one another.
Care of family	Married people should not engage in extra-marital affairs, and should cherish and care for one another, and their children. Money should be spent on the family as a whole, rather than selfishly.
Self-reliance	Members should work steadily and reliably at their jobs, and earn their own living.
Avoidance of alcohol	Peyote and alcohol don't mix.

By 1922, the NAC had grown to 13,000 members, largely in the plains states. It continued to expand throughout the United States and into Canada. At present, it is estimated that there are about 300,000 members, many combining it with membership of more orthodox Christian churches. The NAC remains a loose federation without universally recognized leaders, defined lines of authority, or well documented doctrines or rituals.

 "Peyote is like a Bible to us here. Peyote is our Bible. When I'm with this Herb sometimes it is like a book ... like turning the pages in a book."
—*Washo man* [13]

From the beginning, the peyote movement was held in suspicion by both white governments and other Indians. The Navajo were particularly opposed, since peyote had never been part of traditional Navajo culture. Later, Federal antagonism on other issues brought them into the pan-Indian movement, and the Navajoland NAC chapter is now one of the largest in the country.

The first legal case against peyote indicted three Kickapoos in Oklahoma in 1907; they were found guilty and fined. From 1917 to 1937, most western states passed laws against peyote, and nine bills banning it were introduced in Congress. Each of these was withdrawn or repealed after being challenged as an assault on religious freedom. By 1934, the Bureau of Indian Affairs refused further attempts to suppress the NAC. In 1960, Judge Yale McFate overturned the Arizona state law and sanctioned peyote use by Native Americans.

 What if He came back,
What if He came back as a plant?
—*A Peyote Song* [14]

The Drug Abuse Control Amendments of 1966, which outlawed hallucinogenic drugs, specifically exempted Indian peyote use from the regulation. The Comprehensive Drug Abuse Prevention and Control Act of 1970 followed suit, banning peyote as a Schedule I drug but providing a specific allowance, under section 21 CFR 1307.31 of the law, for the "nondrug use of peyote in bona fide religious ceremonies of the Native American Church."

Peyote therefore has a unique status as a hallucinogenic substance tolerated by Government and society so long as it is used only by Indians, but forbidden for others as a most dangerous drug.

WHY IS PEYOTE ILLEGAL?

The legal status of the religious use of peyote is very murky. Despite the apparently simple language in the Controlled Substances Act, further laws have been enacted with the purpose of clarifying who may and who may not use peyote. Their effect has been just the opposite, with further obfuscation.

It is clear, for example, that any Native American may engage in the ceremonial use of peyote under the Joint Resolution American Indian Religious Freedom Act of 1978, and the Native American Free Exercise of Religion Act of 1993. Other laws specifically allow peyote "when used by a bona fide religion as a sacrament."

> In 1975, Pope Paul VI gave a Papal Blessing to the Native American Church, Pine Ridge Reservation

It is not clear, however, what constitutes a "bona fide religion." May any group declare themselves to be a Native American Church? The NAC, neither in its charter nor in its current registry, defines the process of how a chapter of the church is incorporated, how members may join, who may be allowed to become a member, who may participate in ceremonies, or who may conduct ceremonies. In Utah, for example, there are five independent chapters of the NAC. Some do not recognize the others, and have even filed legal proceedings against them. The issue is further complicated because Utah State law does not include the Federal exemption of peyote for religious use; however, Indians can claim that tribal reservations are not state property, and therefore fall under Federal rather than state regulations.

Are non-Natives allowed to participate in a Native American ceremony? The federal law does not address this question. To forbid participation, in any other religion, would be considered discriminatory. For example, it would be thought absurd to allow only persons of Italian descent to participate in a Catholic mass. Yet several states have attempted to restrict the NAC to documented Indians. Texas requires a minimum of 25 percent Native American ancestry to participate in a ceremony. The Supreme Court of California has taken a relatively liberal view,[15] while the Supreme Court of Oregon has taken a very restrictive view. In a case that twice went to the Supreme Court of the United States, in 1988 and 1990, the use of peyote was forbidden for American Indian substance abuse counselors who were not American Indians themselves, even though they used it within the legitimate practice of the Native American Church.

Since most Native American Churches do not allow non-Native participation, an attempt was made by non-Natives to form analogous churches, including the Peyote Way Church of God, the Church of the Tree of Life, the Church of the Awakening, the Neo-American Church, and several others. All of these have been disallowed by the Court.

The case of the Peyote Way Church of God is particularly illustrative of the legal conundrums that come up between church and state. This church was incorporated in Arizona on May 11, 1979, by a group of non-Indians who held deep religious beliefs about peyote. The ruling against them, by Judge Maloney of the Fifth Circuit Court of Arizona in 1988, stated:

1.   There is a limited supply of the Holy Sacrament peyote, and all of it is needed for the Native American Church of North America.

2.   Federal and Texas State laws are not racist, they are political. Native American Church members belong to a sovereign nation.

"The Court therefore concludes that regardless of the sincerity of Peyote Way's members' beliefs in peyotism, the exemption provided the Native American Church cannot be expanded to include non-Native American Church use of peyote.
    "The Court further concludes that the overriding interest of Congress to control the use of narcotics and psychotropic drugs outweighs the interest of expanding an exemption that clearly was meant to be a grandfather clause."

In other words, the Court declared that the use of peyote is like owning a piece of property. The Native Americans were the first to claim it, and no one else should be allowed to do so.

At this time, peyote use is legal for Native Americans within the Native American Church, questionable for non-Natives in the NAC, and illegal otherwise.

 The Native American Church is the only case in which the Government curtails religious freedom on the basis of ancestry.

Why is peyote illegal at all? There is very little evidence of its abuse as a recreational drug, nor is it habit-forming. There is no record of illnesses or injuries due to the intoxicating aspects of peyote. Peyote is legal in Europe, and may be purchased over the counter, but very few people use it and peyote has never been considered to cause a drug problem. The legal status of peyote appears to stem from its history as an instrument of Native American empowerment and its association with other popular hallucinogenic plants.

In 1993, Congress attempted to liberalize this restriction with the Religious Freedom Restoration Act (RFRA), which stated that the "government

shall not substantially burden a person's exercise of religion."
The Act was hailed by some states but denounced by others
as an imposition on state drug control laws.

In 1997, the U.S. Supreme Court ruled that RFRA
was unconstitutional because it improperly infringed upon
the states' rights to control their own police power.[16] This
ruling was considered to effectively overturn RFRA.
However, a Superior Court decision in Guam[17] interpreted
the Supreme Court ruling more narrowly, stating that RFRA
still applied to the Federal Government.[18] Therefore, the
religious use of peyote on property under Federal jurisdiction
(including national parks) would still be protected under
RFRA. Other states provided RFRA-like exemptions:
Oregon, for example, now protects all religious users of peyote
so long as they use it "in a manner that is not dangerous to the
health of the user or others who are in the proximity of the
user."[19] Arizona, Colorado, and New Mexico passed similar laws.
California and New York, while not having specific statutory
exemptions, have court decisions on the books which recognize
a religious defense to peyote use.

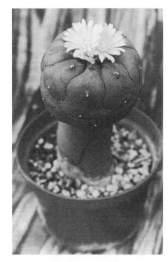

Peyote cactus for sale in Amsterdam

 "The uncontroverted evidence on the record [is] that peyote is not a narcotic substance and is not habit forming."
—*Supreme Court of North Dakota*

In 1997, the military declared that it will allow American Indian soldiers
to use peyote. The policy applies only to the 9,262 American Indians in the
military, 0.6 percent of its population. It also allows American Indians to answer
"No" when asked if they have ever used drugs.[20]

 "If they're using peyote in their religious practice, it's a sacrament, not a drug, just as sacramental wine is not considered a drug."
—*Air Force Maj. Monica Aloisio, Pentagon spokesperson*

The result is a curious and inconsistent patchwork of laws which allow
some people to use peyote, even at the highest level of responsibility in the
U.S. Armed Forces, while others may be punished for mere possession of the
plant with penalties equal to those for heroin and the most dangerous drugs.

Who Is Using Peyote And Mescaline?

Peyote is not commonly used as a recreational drug because it so bitter and nauseating. The vast majority of it is consumed by the Native American Church. There are 98 branches of this loosely organized church in 24 states and Canada. It is estimated that there are now about 300,000 members of the NAC, although neither membership nor attendance is well recorded. At a typical peyote ceremony, an average of 4 to 20 buttons may be consumed; therefore, a regular participant might use 500 buttons per year. The total annual consumption by the NAC is about 2 million buttons, with requests for up to 10 million limited by the supply. Almost all of this is as dried buttons (which may be steeped into a tea or ground into powder).

Virtually all peyote comes from the Rio Grande region of south Texas, particularly Starr County, much of which is owned by ranchers and oil companies. The State of Texas and the DEA license nine distributors to harvest peyote for the NAC. After they obtain a permit from the Texas Department of Public Safety, these *peyoteros* pay fees to enter private ranches and collect peyote by using machetes or a special short-handled shovel. In some areas, there may be as many as 60,000 peyote cacti growing per acre. The harvest takes place with a great deal of respect, and a prayer is said to each plant as its button is excised with care to avoid damaging the root. Once cut, it takes about three years for another button to grow. After being harvested, the buttons are sun-dried for about seven days, and packaged in bags of up to 1,000 to be sold for about 15 cents a piece.

Only wild peyote is harvested, as the Federal restrictions do not allow cultivation. Contrary to popular belief, however, peyote is easily cultivated (the author has even seen it grown indoors in The Netherlands). It takes about three years to grow peyote from seed to flowering plant. Growth can be speeded up by grafting a piece of peyote as small as a quarter inch on to the stalk of another, faster and more tolerant cactus such as San Pedro or Blue Myrtle (*Myrtillocactus geometrizan*), both of which are readily available in gardening stores.

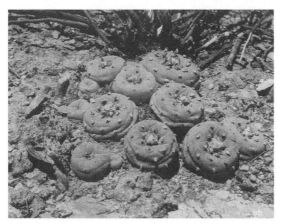

After harvesting, peyote often regrows in clusters

INSIDE AN NAC PEYOTE CEREMONY

Branches of the NAC have differing policies regarding permission to attend ceremonies. In Texas, for example, a NAC participant is expected to have at least 25 percent Native American ancestry. Many others allow any person, of any ancestry, to participate if that person is respectful of NAC beliefs and traditions. Most NAC branches have no formal policy and permit attendance based on the individual discretion of the Roadman.

A peyote ceremony is traditionally held at night and lasts for about 12 hours. Most tribes fast for a least a day before taking peyote and end the ceremony with a feast. In the course of the ritual, anywhere from 2 to 40 buttons may be eaten in a series of rounds during which all participate. The dry buttons may be eaten directly, chewed slowly to moisten and swallow the bitter substance, or drunk as a tea or powder slurry. Some ceremonies allow a drink of unsweetened grapefruit juice to neutralize the bitter taste; others allow no water or food to be taken, or, for that matter, any bathroom breaks. Ceremonies usually involve considerable vomiting by the participants.

The following was told by a young man who had been arrested for drug abuse. His exhausted parents had spent a lot of money on counseling and rehab programs to no avail, and in desperation sent him to a NAC ceremony:

"I was getting bombed every day, and twice ended up in the emergency room from GHB. When they told me about this place where they take peyote, I thought, what the hell, it might be fun— I'd tried just about every other drug already.

"We sat in a circle in the teepee, on the dirt floor with some blankets. Everyone was quiet. The medicine man was sitting behind a small altar with some eagle feathers and stuff. Burning sage, like incense. He talked for a while about sacred traditions, and then there was singing and drumming. After an hour, he gave each of us some peyote powder. It was the most disgusting stuff I've ever tasted. I could hardly gag it down. There was more singing and drumming, and the medicine man started talking again, but I had a hard time following. I started feeling really uncomfortable, sweating, just like, totally miserable. Somebody beside me was whispering into my ear, 'Listen to what he's saying. It's about you.' But I could hardly concentrate. Some people were crying or throwing up into a plastic bucket in the middle of the room. I grabbed it and puked and puked, right there in front of everybody.

"Then the medicine man turns to me and says in this dead-calm voice, 'What's going on with you?' That's when it happened. It all just came together. I realized what a total screw-up I'd been. I was just so sick of everything. Sick, pissed off, like FUCK YOU to the whole world. That's when I finally got it. I felt like I puked my whole life right into that bucket."

From that point on, he stopped using drugs. When asked about it a year later, he said, "I don't think it was really the peyote that made me change. It was just that I didn't know what I wanted, and the peyote helped me see it."

Throwing up, rather than attempting to hold it in, is encouraged as a purging of both physical and psychological ills.

Peyote ceremonies are complex rituals with considerable improvisation by the Roadman. They may involve prayer, singing, drumming, the burning of tobacco, cedar, sagebrush, and other materials, and occasionally dancing. Some ceremonies function in a way analogous to group psychological counseling, where personal problems are explored and resolved.[21] Other ceremonies may be conducted as a method of healing.[22]

MESCALINE USE

The NAC does not use mescaline or other drugs. Mescaline was a popular recreational hallucinogen during the 1960s and continues to have a small role in the American drug culture. It is a white crystalline powder, often sold as a pill. By far the majority of purported mescaline, however, is actually LSD and occasionally other substances. Controlled laboratory studies show that users cannot distinguish between mescaline, psilocybin, and LSD. Since LSD and psilocybin are easily obtained, but mescaline is difficult to synthesize, there is little demand for mescaline.

In a study done by PharmChem on 185 samples said to be mescaline, only 17 percent were found to contain mescaline. Of the remainder, 73 percent were LSD, or LSD mixed with PCP, and 7.6 percent contained no drug at all.

Chemical Characteristics

Of the more than 55 pharmacologically active substances found in peyote, mescaline is considered the most important and accounts for the main psychoactive effects. About one percent, or about 45 mg, of the dry weight of peyote is mescaline.[23] The action of the other constituents is not well known, but they may be very important in the overall effect and contribute to the efficacy of peyote in relieving alcohol and other drug addictions.

Mescaline (3,4,5-trimethoxy-phenethylamine) is an indole hallucinogen resembling the neurotransmitters dopamine and norepinephrine (see *Chapter 6*).[24] It has about 1/2000th the potency of LSD, and 1/20th the potency of psilocybin. Mescaline can be extracted from peyote, but almost all available mescaline is produced synthetically.[25] A 500 mg dose of mescaline is equivalent to about a dozen peyote buttons.

Alcoholism and other drug abuse are common among Native Americans, and peyote appears to be remarkably effective in resolving these addictions.[26]

The United States Public Health Service Hospital in Clinton, Oklahoma, has reported some success in a program at its alcoholism rehabilitation center using peyote in group sessions that resemble Alcoholics Anonymous.[27] The beneficial action of peyote in relieving alcohol or other addictions is poorly understood. It is possible that certain biochemical alkaloids found in the peyote cactus, and not just mescaline, are pharmacologically similar to the neuroamine-derived alkaloids formed in the brain during alcohol intoxication. By replacing the neurologic effects of alcohol, the alcoholic can more easily abstain.[28] The chemistry of this effect is not clear, but it does seem to work. Theoretically, peyote tolerance develops quickly and there should be little effect if it is taken for more than a day or so. The NAC, however, will encourage drug addicts to take peyote every day for weeks or even months, with the result that the addiction is often cured.

 "Peyote is not harmful ... It is a better antidote to alcohol than anything [the] American Medical Association, and the public health services have come up with."—Dr. Karl A. Menninger, renowned psychiatrist [29]

Withdrawal Signs

The principal after-effect of the use of peyote or mescaline is fatigue. Anxiety or mental depression have also been reported.[30] Withdrawal is otherwise uneventful.

A single dose of mescaline will cause tolerance within a day and diminish the effects of further doses for several days. Physical dependence does not occur.

Long-term Health Problems

There are no reports of long-term health problems from the use of peyote. A multigenerational study of extensive peyote use among Huichol Indians showed no evidence of illness or other adverse outcomes related to peyote even after decades of regular use.[31] Remarkably, peyote is also routinely used during pregnancy and childbirth; no averse outcomes have been reported.[32]

An extensive survey of the medical literature revealed just three cases of illness from peyote, due to botulism resulting from eating peyote that had been improperly preserved. All recovered spontaneously.[33]

 "We have seen almost no acute or chronic emotional disturbance arising from peyote use. ... approximately one bad reaction per 70,000 ingestions."—Dr. Robert Bergman, Director of U.S. Public Health Service, Navajo Reservation, Arizona [34]

What To Do If There Is An Overdose

It is almost impossible to overdose on peyote because the drug causes extreme nausea. Any excess will simply be vomited. Peyote is used by hundreds of thousands of members of the Native American Church, yet reports of bad experiences or health problems are very rare. A single death was reported of a man who had severe alcoholic liver disease, and died from bleeding into the stomach when he vomited.[35]

Very high doses of mescaline have been known to cause respiratory depression, low blood pressure, and a low heart rate. There is no record of fatalities, however.

Like other hallucinogens, mescaline can cause anxiety or panic in an unprepared user. A sedative medication such as Valium may be of value in this situation.[36] Overdose is not physically dangerous, and symptoms will resolve spontaneously within hours with comfort and reassurance.

Physical signs of overdose[37]

Vomiting
Low blood pressure
Respiratory depression
Difficulty walking

Mental signs of overdose

Anxiety
Panic

PART III

Self-help Resources

Notes and References

Index

Self-help Resources

DRUG IDENTIFICATION

Illegally obtained drugs always have questionable purity. There are two ways to find out about the contents of a drug sample. The first is visual identification. Several free services are listed here that show pictures of popular illegal drugs, and describe their contents. The second method is to send a sample of the drug to a laboratory for identification. Addresses for these services are listed below.

The California Department of Justice operates a free website that helps visual identification of drugs: www.stopdrugs.org/identification.html

Readi-TCID charges a small fee for drug identification: www.drugid.net

PharmChem is a private company that will conduct a confidential drug analysis for a small fee. Pharmchem may be contacted at: www.pharmchem.com

and at:

TEXAS DIVISION
7606 Pebble Dr.
Fort Worth, TX 76118
(817) 215-8800
Fax (817) 215-8863
(800) 967-8378

MEDSCREEN
1A Harbour Quay
100 Preston's Rd. UK
London, England E149PH
+44 171-712-8000
Fax +44 171-712-8001

Drug Identification: www.intrlink.net/smartchoices/drug.htm

Drug Identification and Influence Recognition: www.drugid.org

Project Inform Drug Identification Chart: www.thebody.com/pinf/idchart.html

FURTHER INFORMATION

There are several ways in which you can get further information about illegal drugs:

You can search the Internet for sites providing information about drugs. Some of the more reputable sites include:

www.onhealth.com
www.drugfreeamerica.org
www.nida.nih.gov
www.drugdigest.org

www.clubdrugs.org
www.healthfinder.gov
www.whitehousedrugpolicy.gov
www.lindesmith.org
www.publicagenda.org/issues/frontdoor.cfm?issue_type=illegal_drugs
http://usinfo.state.gov/topical/global/drugs
http://freeadvice.com/law/519us.htm
www.druglibrary.org
www.drugsense.org/lists
www.drugscope.org.uk

You can research the medical literature directly to learn more about drugs. Searching a medical database takes time and experience, but gives the information right from the source. Medline can be searched free at:

www.medmatrix.org/info/medlinetables.asp
www.ncbi.nlm.nih.gov/PubMed
www.igm.nlm.nih.gov

Other free academic medical information sites include:

www.emedicine.com
www.medmatrix.org/reg/login.asp
www.shef.ac.uk/uni/academic/R-Z/scharr/ir/netting.html
www.mwsearch.com
www.nthames-health.tymde.ac.uk/connect/journals.htm
www.pslgroup.com/dg/medjournals.htm
www.guidelines.gov
www.cma.ca/cpgs

Other sites provide drug information, but are not supported by universities, government, or health agencies. They are operated by people who have a special interest in drugs and often describe drugs or drug features that are less commonly known. However, some of these sites also contain misinformation.

Pro-drug orientation
www.theforbiddenfruit.com/books/books.htm
www.entheogen.com
www.erowid.org
www.norml.org
www.hofmann.org

Anti-drug orientation
www.teenchallenge.com
www.streetdrugs.org
www.druguse.com
www.trashed.co.uk
www.openhere.com/health1/substance-abuse/illegal-drugs

DRUG ABUSE PREVENTION AND TREATMENT COORDINATORS

You can get direct help and advice—and talk to a real person—at a number of State and Federal Government offices. A list of these providers follows. Since you have already paid for these services through your taxes, you should not hesitate to make use of them. All of these offices are there for your benefit.

Alabama
Head: Commissioner
Address: Dept of Mental Health
            and Mental Retardation
            RSA Union Building
            100 Union Street
            P.O. Box 3014 1 0
            Montgomery,
            Alabama 36130-1410
Phone: (334) 242-3961

Alaska
Head: Director
Address: Division of Alcoholism
            and Drug Abuse
            Department of Health
            and Social Services
            P.O. Box 11 0607
            Juneau, Alaska 99811-0607
Phone: (907) 465-2071

Arizona
Head: Manager
Address: Drug Abuse Section
            Department of Health Services
            Division of Behavioral Health Services
            2122 East Highland Street
            Phoenix, Arizona 85016
Phone: (602) 220-8999

Arkansas
Head: Director
Address: Office on Alcohol
            and Drug Abuse Prevention
            5800 West 10th Street, Suite 907
            Little Rock, Arkansas 72204
Phone: (501) 280-4500

California
Head: Director
Address: Department of Alcohol
            and Drug Programs
            1700 K Street
            Sacramento, California 95814
Phone: (916) 445-0934

Colorado
Head: Director
Address: Alcohol and Drug Abuse Division
            Department of Human Services
            4300 Cherry Creek Drive South
            Denver, Colorado 80222-1530
Phone: (303) 692-2930

Connecticut
Head: Executive Director
Address: Dept of Mental Health
            and Addiction Services
            Office of Substance Abuse
            410 Capitol Avenue,
            Mail Stop #14COM
            Hartford, Connecticut 06105
Phone: (860) 418-6832

Delaware
Head: Director
Address: Div. of Alcoholism,
            Drug Abuse & Mental Health
            1901 North DuPont Highway
            Newcastle, Delaware 19720
Phone: (302) 577-4660

District of Columbia
Head: Administrator
Address: Addiction, Prevention
            and Recovery Admin
            1300 First Street N. E.
            Washington, D. C. 20002
Phone: (202) 727-1765

Florida
Head: Director
Address: Substance Abuse
            & Mental Health Program Office
            1317 Winewood Boulevard
            Building 3, Room 102
            Tallahassee, Florida 32399-0700
Phone: (904) 488-0900

Georgia
Head: Deputy Director
Address: Alcohol and Drug Section
            Division of Mental Health
            Mental Retardation,
            and Substance Abuse
            Dept of Human Resources 4th Floor,
            Suite 550
            2 Peach Tree Street
            Atlanta, Georgia 30303
Phone: (404) 657-6407

Hawaii
Head: Division Chief
Address: Alcohol and Drug Abuse Division
            Department of Health
            1270 Queen Emma Street, Room 305
            Honolulu, Hawaii 96813
Phone: (808) 586-4007

Idaho
Head: Director
Address: Bureau of Mental Health
               and Substance Abuse
               Department of Health and Welfare
               P. O. Box 83720, 5th Floor
               Boise, Idaho 83720-0036
Phone: (208) 334-5935

Illinois
Head: Director
Address: Department of Alcoholism
               and Substance Abuse
               James R. Thompson Building
               100 West Randolph Street, Suite 5-600
               Chicago, Illinois 60601
Phone: (312) 814-3840

Indiana
Head: Deputy Commissioner
Address: Addiction Services
               FSSA/Division of Mental Health
               402 West Washington Street,
               Room W363
               Indianapolis, Indiana 46204-2739
Phone: (317) 232-7816

Iowa
Head: Director
Address: Iowa Department of Public Health
               Division of Substance Abuse
               and Health
               Lucas State Office Building,
               3rd Floor
               321 East 12th Street
               Des Moines, Iowa 50319
Phone: (515) 281-3641

Kansas
Head: Commissioner
Address: Alcohol and Drug Abuse Services
               300 S. W. Oakley,
               2nd Floor Biddle Building
               Topeka, Kansas 66606
Phone.   (913) 296-3925

Kentucky
Head: Division Director
Address: Substance Abuse Division
               275 East Main Street Frankfort,
               Kentucky 40621
Phone   (502) 564-2880

Louisiana
Head: Director
Address: Department of Health and Hospitals
               Alcohol and Drug Abuse Prevention Services
               Baton Rouge Area Substance Abuse Clinic
               1201 Capitol Access Road
               Baton Rouge, Louisiana 70802
Phone: (504) 342-9354

Maine
Head: Director
Address: Dept of Mental Health
               and Substance Abuse
               AMHI Complex,
               Marquardt Building, 3rd Floor
               159 State House Station
               Augusta, Maine 04333
Phone: (207) 1-87-2595

Maryland
Head: Director
Address: Alcohol and Drug Abuse Administration
               201 West Preston Street
               Baltimore, Maryland 21201
Phone: (301) 225-6910

Massachusetts
Head: Director
Address: Bureau of Substance Abuse Services
               250 Washington Street, 3rd Floor
               Boston,
               Massachusetts 02108-4619
Phone: (617) 727-8617

Michigan
Head: Administrator
Address: Department of Community Health
               Center for Substance Abuse Services
               P. O. Box 30206
               Lansing, Michigan 48909
Phone: (517) 335-8810

Minnesota
Head: Director
Address: Department of Human Services
               Chemical Dependency Division
               444 Lafayette Road
               St. Paul, Minnesota 55155
Phone: (612) 296-3991

Mississippi
Head: Director
Address: Division of Alcohol and Drug Abuse
               Department of Mental Health
               1101 Robert E. Lee Building
               239 North Lamar Street
               Jackson, Mississippi 39201
Phone: (601) 359-1288

Missouri
Head: Director
Address: Division of Alcohol and Drug Abuse
               Department of Mental Health
               P.O. Box 687
               Jefferson City, Missouri 65 102
Phone: (573) 751-4942

Montana
Head: Administrator
Address: Public Health and Human Services
           Alcohol and Drug Abuse Division
           P. O. Box 4210
           Helena, Montana 59620
Phone: (406) 444-3904

Nebraska
Head: Director
Address: Division of Drug and Alcohol Abuse
           Department of Public Institutions
           P.O. Box 94728
           Lincoln, Nebraska 68509
Phone: (402) 471-2851

Nevada
Head: Bureau Chief
Address: Bureau of Alcohol and Drug Abuse
           Dept of Employment
           Training Rehabilitation
           505 East Kina Street, Room 500
           Carson City, Nevada 89710
Phone: (702) 687-4790

New Hampshire
Head: Director
Address: Office of Alcoholism and
           Drug Abuse Prevention
           State Office Park,
           South 105 Pleasant Street
           Concord, New Hampshire 03301
Phone: (603) 271- 6100

New Jersey
Head: Commissioner
Address: Division of Addiction Services
           Department of Health
           and Senior Services, CN 362
           Trenton, New Jersey 08625
Phone: (609) 292-5760

New Mexico
Head: Director
Address: Department of Health Services
           Division of Substance Abuse
           P. O. Box 26110
           Santa Fe, New Mexico 87502
Phone   (505) 827-2601

New York
Head: Director
Address: Alcoholism and Substance
           Abuse Services
           1450 Western Avenue
           Albany, New York 12203
Phone: (518) 457-2061

North Carolina
Head: Deputy Director
Address: Alcohol and Drug Abuse Services
           Division of Mental Health
           and Substance Abuse
           325 North Salisbury Street
           Raleigh, North Carolina 27603
Phone: (919) 733-4670

North Dakota
Head: Director
Address: Division of Mental Health
           and Substance Abuse
           600 South 2nd Street, Suite IE
           Bismarck, North Dakota 58504
Phone: (701) 328-8920

Ohio
Head: Director
Address: Ohio Department of Alcohol
           and Drug Addiction
           280 North High Street, 12th Floor
           Columbus, Ohio 43215
Phone: (614) 466-7893

Oklahoma
Head: Commissioner
Address: Alcohol and Drug Programs
           Department of Mental Health
           and Substance Abuse
           1200 North East 13th
           P. O. Box 53277
           Capitol Station
           Oklahoma City,
           Oklahoma 73152-3277
Phone: (405) 522-3857

Oregon
Head: Assistant Director
Address: State Alcohol and
           Drug Programs Office
           1178 Chemeketa Street, N.E., #102
           Salem, Oregon 97310
Phone: (503) 945-9850

Pennsylvania
Head: Deputy Secretary
Address: Office of Drug
           and Alcohol Programs
           Department of Health
           Health and Welfare Building, 9th Floor
           P.O. Box 90
           Harrisburg, Pennsylvania 17108
Phone: (717) 783-8200

Rhode Island
Head: Assistant Director
Address: Division of Substance Abuse
            Department of Health Cannon Building,
            Room 105
            3 Capitol Hill
            Providence, Rhode Island 02908
Phone: (401) 277-4680

South Carolina
Head: Executive Director
Address: Department of Alcohol
            and Other Drug Abuse
            3700 Forest Drive,
            Suite 300 Columbia,
            South Carolina 29204
Phone: (803) 734-9520

South Dakota
Head: Director
Address: Division of Alcohol and Drug Abuse
            Hillsview Plaza
            500 East Capitol
            Pierre,
            South Dakota 57501-5070
Phone: (605) 773-3123

Tennessee
Head: Assistant Commissioner
Address: Bureau of Alcohol
            and Drug Abuse Services
            Tennessee Department of Health
            Cordell Hull Building, 3rd Floor
            Nashville, Tennessee 37247-4401
Phone: (615) 741 1-1921

Texas
Head: Executive Director
Address: Texas Commission on Alcohol
            and Drug Abuse
            9001 North Interstate Highway 35,
            Suite 105
            Austin, Texas 78753-5233
Phone: (512) 349-6600

Utah
Head.   Director
Address: Department of Human Services
            Division of Substance Abuse
            120 North 200 West, Room 201
            Salt Lake City, Utah 84103
Phone: (801) 538-3939

Vermont
Head: Director
Address: Office of Alcohol
            and Drug Abuse Programs
            108 Cherry Street
            Burlington, Vermont 05402
Phone: (802) 651-1550

Virginia
Head: Director
Address: Department of Mental Health
            and Substance Abuse
            Office of Substance Abuse
            Specialty Services
            P.O. Box 1797, 12th Floor
            Richmond, Virginia 23214
Phone: (804) 786-3906

Washington
Head: Director
Address: Division of Alcoholism
            and Substance Abuse
            Department of Social
            and Health Services
            Mail Stop 45330
            Olympia, Washington 98504-5330
Phone: (360) 438-8200

West Virginia
Head: Director
Address: Division of Alcohol
            and Drug Abuse
            State Capitol Complex,
            Building 3, Room 717
            Charleston, West Virginia 25305
Phone: (304) 558-0627

Wisconsin
Head: Director
Address: Department of Health
            and Family Services
            Division of Supportive Living
            Bureau of Substance Abuse Services
            P.O. Box 7851
            Madison, Wisconsin 53707-7851
Phone: (608) 266-2717

Wyoming
Head: Manager
Address: Div Behavioral Health Alcohol
            and Drug Abuse
            451 Hathaway Building, 4th Floor
            2300 Capitol Avenue
            Cheyenne, Wyoming 82002-0480
Phone: (307) 777-7094

DEA DIVISION OFFICES

Aviation Operations Center
2300 Horizon Road
Ft. Worth, TX 76177-5300
(1817) 837-0000

DEA Atlanta Division
75 Spring Street, S.W., Room 740
Atlanta, GA 30303
(404) 331-4401

DEA New England Division
50 Staniford Street, Suite 200
Boston, MA 02114
(617) 557-2100

DEA Caribbean Division
2432 Loiza Street
Santurce, PR 00913
(809) 253-4200

DEA Chicago Division
230 S. Dearborn Street, Suite 1200
Chicago, IL 60604
(312) 353-7875

DEA Dallas Division
1880 Regal Row
Dallas, TX 75235
(214) 767-7151

DEA Detroit Division
431 Howard Street
Detroit, MI 48226
(313) 234-4000

EPIC
11339 SSG Sims Street
El Paso, TX 79908-8098
(915) 564-2033

DEA Houston Division
333 West Loop North, Suite 300
Houston. TX 77024
(700) 527-9000

DEA Los Angeles Division
255 East Temple Street, 20th Floor
Los Angeles, CA 90012
(213) 894-2650

DEA Miami Division
8400 N.W. 53rd Street
Miami, FL 33166
(305) 590-4870

DEA New Orleans Division
3 Lakeway Center
3838 N. Causeway Blvd, Suite 1800
Metairie, LA 70002
(504) 840-1100

DEA New York Division
99 Tenth Avenue
New York, NY 10011
(212) 337-3900

DEA Newark Division
970 Broad Street, Room 806
Newark, NJ 07102
(201) 645-6060

DEA Philadelphia Division
600 Arch Street, Room 10224
Philadelphia, PA 19106
(215) 597-9530

DEA Phoenix Division
30 1 0 North 2nd Street, Suite 301
Phoenix, AZ 85012
(602) 664-5600

DEA Rocky Mountain Division
115 Inverness Drive, East
Englewood, CO 80112-5116
(303) 784-6300

DEA San Diego Division
4560 View Ridge Avenue
San Diego, CA 92123
(619) 616-4100

DEA San Francisco Division
450 Golden Gate Ave.
San Francisco, CA 94102
(415) 556-6771

DEA Seattle Division
220 West Mercer, Suite 300
Seattle, WA 98119
(206) 553-5443

DEA St. Louis Division
7911 Forsythe Boulevard, Suite 500
St. Louis, MO 63105
(314) 425-3241

DEA Washington, D. C. Division
400 Sixth Street, S.W., Room 2558
Washington, D.C. 20024
(202) 401-7834

NATIONAL GUARD COUNTERDRUG COORDINATORS

Alabama
Attn: Counterdrug Coordinator
Address: P. O. Box 3711
            Montgomery, AL 36109-0711
Phone: (334) 271-7473

Alaska
Attn: Counterdrug Coordinator
Address: P.O. Box 5800 Bldg 49000
            Ft. Richardson, AK 99505-5800
Phone: (907) 428-3617

Arizona
Attn: Counterdrug Coordinator
Address: 5636 E. McDowell Road
            Phoenix, AZ 85008-3495
Phone: (602) 267-2623

Arkansas
Attn: Counterdrug Coordinator
Address: Camp J.T. Robinson
            Attn: DPT-MS-CD
            North Little Rock, AR 72199-9600
Phone: (501) 212-5492

California
Attn: Counterdrug Coordinator
Address: 9800 Goethe Road
            Sacramento, CA 95826-9101
Phone: (916) 854-3889

Colorado
Attn: Counterdrug Coordinator
Address: 6868 S. Revere Pkwy
            Englewood, CO 80112-6703
Phone: (303) 397-3058

Connecticut
Attn: Counterdrug, Coordinator
Address: 360 Broad Street
            Hartford, CT 06105-3795
Phone: (860) 524-4980

Delaware
Attn: Counterdrug Coordinator
Address: First Regiment Road
            Wilmington, DE 19808-2191
Phone: (302) 326-7085

District of Columbia
Attn: Counterdrug Coordinator
Address: 2001 E. Capital, SE
            Washington, D.C. 20003-1719
Phone: (202) 433-5221

Florida
Attn: Counterdrug Coordinator
Address: P. O. Box 1008
            St. Augustine, FL 32085-1 008
Phone: (904) 823-0438

Georgia
Attn: Counterdrug Coordinator
Address: P. O. Box 672108
            Marietta. GA 30006-0036
Phone: (770) 919-3473

Guam
Attn: Counterdrug Coordinator
Address: 622 E. Harmon IND Park Rd.
            Tamuning, GU 96911-4421
Phone: 011 (671) 647-6019

Hawaii
Attn: Counterdrug Coordinator
Address: 3949 Diamond Head Road
            Honolulu, HI 96816-4495
Phone: (808) 737-9450

Idaho
Attn: Counterdrug Coordinator
Address: 4736 Kennedy, Bldg T-927
            Boise, ID 83705-8135
Phone: (208) 422-6044

Illinois
Attn: Counterdrug Coordinator
Address: 1301 N. MacArthur Blvd.
            Springfield, IL 62702-2399
Phone: (217) 785-3728

Indiana
Attn: Counterdrug Coordinator
Address: 2002 South Holt Road
            Indianapolis, IN 46241-0326
Phone: (317) 247-3516

Iowa
Attn: Counterdrug Coordinator
Address: 7700 NW Beaver Drive,
            Camp Dodge, P.O. Box 269101
            Johnston, IA 50131-4643
Phone: (515) 252-4606

Kansas
Attn: Counterdrug Coordinator
Address: 2302 Militia Drive
            Jefferson City, MO 65101-1203
Phone: (573) 526-9952

Kentucky
Attn: Counterdrug Coordinator
Address: I 00 Minuteman Parkway,
             Bldg 124 #1 05
             Frankfort, KY 40601-6188
Phone: (502) 564-6256

Louisiana
Attn: Counterdrug Coordinator
Address: Hq Bldg 35, Rm 251
             Jackson Barracks
             New Orleans, LA 70146-0330
Phone: (504) 278-8491

Maine
Attn: Counterdrug Coordinator
Address: Camp Keyes
             Augusta, ME 04333-0033
Phone: (207) 626-4316

Maryland
Attn: Counterdrug Coordinator
Address: 29th Division St., 5th Regiment Armory
             Baltimore, MD 21201-2288
Phone: (410) 576-6135

Massachusetts
Attn: Counterdrug Coordinator
Address: 25 Haverhill Road
             Reading, MA 01867-1999
Phone: (617) 994-0500

Michigan
Attn: Counterdrug Coordinator
Address: 2500 So. Washington Avenue
             Lansing, MI 48917-5101
Phone: (517) 483-5896

Minnesota
Attn: Counterdrug Coordinator
Address: 20 West 1211 Street
             St. Paul, MN 55155-2098
Phone: (612) 282-4147

Mississippi
Attn: Counterdrug Coordinator
Address: 144 Military Drive
             Jackson, MS 39208-8860
Phone: (601) 936-7670

Missouri
Attn: Counterdrug Coordinator
Address: P. O. Box 19012
             Topeka, KS 66615-0012
Phone: (913) 862-0001

Montana
Attn: Counterdrug Coordinator
Address: 1100 North Main, P. O. Box 4789
             Helena, MT 59604-478
Phone: (406) 444-6938

Nebraska
Attn: Counterdrug Coordinator
Address: 1300 Military Road
             Lincoln, NE 68508-1090
Phone: (402) 458-1132

Nevada
Attn: Counterdrug Coordinator
Address: 4600 Alpha Avenue, #8212
             Reno, NV 89506-1276
Phone: (702) 677-5233

New Hampshire
Attn: Counterdrug Coordinator
Address: State Military Reservation
             4 Pembroke Rd
             Concord, NH 03301-5652
Phone: (603) 288-8534

New Jersey
Attn: Counterdrug Coordinator
Address: 3650 Saylor Pond Road
             Fort Dix, NJ 08460-7600
Phone: (609) 562-0812

New Mexico
Attn: Counterdrug Coordinator
Address: P. O. Box 5610
             Albuquerque, NM 87185-5610
Phone: (505) 846-7152

New York
Attn: Counterdrug Coordinator
Address: 1 Air National Guard Road
             Scotia, NY 12302-9752
Phone: (518) 344-2056

North Carolina
Attn: Counterdrug Coordinator
Address: 4105 Reedy Creed Road
             Raleigh, NC 27607-6410
Phone: (919) 664-6322

North Dakota
Attn: Counterdrug Coordinator
Address: P. O. Box 5511,
             Fraine Barracks, Rd, #190
             Bismarck, ND 58502-5511
Phone: (710) 224-5269

Ohio
Attn: Counterdrug Coordinator
Address: 2825 W. Dublin Granville Road
             Columbus, OH 43235-2789
Phone: (614) 889-7146

Oklahoma
Attn: Counterdrug Coordinator
Address: 3501 Military Circle, NE
             Oklahoma City, OK 73111-4398
Phone: (405) 425-8688

Oregon
Attn: Counterdrug Coordinator
Address: 1921 Turner Road, SE
                 Salem, OR 97302-2099
Phone: (503) 945-3281

Pennsylvania
Attn: Counterdrug Coordinator
Address: Fort Indiantown Gap, Bldg 9-7
                 Annville, PA 17003-5002
Phone: (717) 861-8223

Puerto Rico
Attn: Counterdrug Coordinator
Address: G. P. O. Box 9023786
                 San Juan, PR 00902-3786
Phone: (787) 289-1677

Rhode Island
Attn: Counterdrug Coordinator
Address: Command Readiness Center
                 645 New London Avenue
                 Cranston, RI 02920-3097
Phone: (401) 457-4285

South Carolina
Attn: Counterdrug Coordinator
Address: 1 National Guard Road
                 Columbia, SC 29201-4766
Phone: (803) 806-1559

South Dakota
Attn: Counterdrug Coordinator
Address: 2823 West Main Street
                 Rapid City, SD 57702-8186
Phone: (605) 399-6723

Tennessee
Attn: Counterdrug Coordinator
Address: 3041 Sidco Drive
                 Nashville, TN 37204-1502
Phone: (615) 313-0648

Texas
Attn: Counterdrug Coordinator
Address: P. O. Box 5218, Bldg 10,
                 Camp Mabry
                 9001 North Interstate Highway 35,
                 Suite 105
                 Austin, Texas 78763-5218
Phone: (512) 465-5516

Utah
Attn: Counterdrug Coordinator
Address: 12953 Minuteman Drive,
                 P. O. Box 1776
                 Draper, UT 84020-1776
Phone: (801) 576-3174

Vermont
Attn: Counterdrug Coordinator
Address: Camp Johnson, GMA
                 Colchester, VT 05446-3004
Phone: (802) 654-0350

Virginia
Attn: Counterdrug Coordinator
Address: 600 E. Broad Street
                 Richmond, VA 23219-1832
Phone: (804) 775-9305

Washington
Attn: Counterdrug Coordinator
Address: Camp Murray
                 Tacoma, WA 98430-5063
Phone: (206) 512-8894

West Virginia
Attn: Counterdrug Coordinator
Address: 1740 Coonskin Drive
                 Charleston, WV 25311-1085
Phone: (304) 341-6425

Wisconsin
Attn: Counterdrug Coordinator
Address: 2400 Wright Street, P. O. Box 8111
                 Madison, WI 53708-81116
Phone: (608) 242-3540

Wyoming
Attn: Counterdrug Coordinator
Address: 5500 Bishop Blvd
                 Cheyenne, WY 82009-3220
Phone: (307) 772-5259

Drug Demand Reduction Administrators

Alabama
Attn: Drug Demand Reduction Administrator
Address: P. O. Box 3711
                 Montgomery, AL 36109-0711
Phone: (334) 213-7724

Alaska
Attn: Drug Demand Reduction Administrator
Address: P. O. Box 5800, Bldg 49000
                 Ft. Richardson, AK 99505-5800
Phone: (907) 428-6204

Arizona
Attn: Drug Demand Reduction Administrator
Address: 5636 E. McDowell Road
                 Phoenix, AZ 85008-3495
Phone: (602) 267-2341

Arkansas
Attn: Drug Demand Reduction Administrator
Address: Camp J.T. Robinson
                 Attn: DPT-MS-CD
                 North Little Rock, AR 72199-9600
Phone: (501) 212-5484

California
Attn: Drug Demand Reduction Administrator
Address: 9800 Goethe Road
             P.O. Box 269101
             Sacramento, CA 95826-9101
Phone: (916) 854-3309

Colorado
Attn: Drug Demand Reduction Administrator
Address: 6868 S. Revere Pkwy, Suite 158
             Englewood, CO 80112-6703
Phone: (303) 397-3091

Connecticut
Attn: Drug Demand Reduction Administrator
Address: 360 Broad Street
             Hartford, CT 06105-3795
Phone: (860) 493-2724

Delaware
Attn: Drug Demand Reduction Administrator
Address: First Regiment Road
             Wilmington, DE 19808-2191
Phone: (302) 326-7079

District of Columbia
Attn: Drug Demand Reduction Administrator
Address: 2001 E. Capital, SE
             Washington, D.C. 20003-1719
Phone: (202) 433-5221

Florida
Attn: Drug Demand Reduction Administrator
Address: P. O. Box 1008
             St. Augustine, FL 32085-1008
Phone: (904) 823-0167

Georgia
Attn: Drug Demand Reduction Administrator
Address: 1388 First, Bldg. 840
             Dobbins AFB, GA 30069-5007
Phone: (770) 919-3477

Guam
Attn: Drug Demand Reduction Administrator
Address: 622 E. Harmon IND Park Rd.
             Tamuning, GU 96911-4421
Phone: 011 (671) 647-2752

Hawaii
Attn: Drug Demand Reduction Administrator
Address: 3949 Diamond Head Road
             Honolulu, HI 96816-4495
Phone: (808) 733-4429

Idaho
Attn: Drug Demand Reduction Administrator
Address: 4736 Kennedy, Bldg T-927
             Boise, ID 83705-8135
Phone: (208) 422-6080

Illinois
Attn: Drug Demand Reduction Administrator
Address: 1301 N. MacArthur Blvd.
             Springfield, IL 62702-2399
Phone: (217) 785-3763

Indiana
Attn: Drug Demand Reduction Administrator
Address: 2002 South Holt Road
             Indianapolis, IN 46241-0326
Phone: (317) 247-3179

Iowa
Attn: Drug Demand Reduction Administrator
Address: 7700 NW Beaver Drive, Camp Dodge
             P.O. Box 269101
             Johnston, IA 50131-4643
Phone: (515) 252-4643

Kansas
Attn: Drug Demand Reduction Administrator
Address: 2722 South West Topeka Blvd.
             Topeka, KS 66611-1298
Phone: (913) 274-1380

Kentucky
Attn: Drug Demand Reduction Administrator
Address: 100 Minuteman Parkway
             Frankfort, KY 40601-6188
Phone: (502) 564-6278

Louisiana
Attn: Drug Demand Reduction Administrator
Address: Hq Bldg 35, Rm 251, Jackson Barracks
             New Orleans, LA 70146-0330
Phone: (504) 278-8555

Maine
Attn: Drug Demand Reduction Administrator
Address: Camp Keyes
             Augusta, ME 04333-0033
Phone: (207) 626-4334

Maryland
Attn: Drug Demand Reduction Administrator
Address: 13620 Meuse-Argonne Circle Rd.
             Reisterstown, MD 21136-4537
Phone: (410) 833-1660

Massachusetts
Attn: Drug Demand Reduction Administrator
Address: 25 Haverhill Road
             Reading, MA 01867-1999
Phone: (617) 994-0500

Michigan
Attn: Drug Demand Reduction Administrator
Address: 2500 So. Washington Avenue
             Lansing, MI 48917-5101
Phone: (517) 483-5813

Minnesota
Attn: Drug Demand Reduction Administrator
Address: 20 West 1211 Street
             St. Paul, MN 55155-2098
Phone: (612) 282-4149

Mississippi
Attn: Drug Demand Reduction Administrator
Address: 144 Military Drive
             Jackson, MS 39208-8860
Phone: (601) 354-6117

Missouri
Attn: Drug Demand Reduction Administrator
Address: 2302 Militia Drive
             Jefferson City, MO, 65101-1203
Phone: (573) 526-9307

Montana
Attn: Drug Demand Reduction Administrator
Address: 1100 North Main, P. O. Box 4789
             Helena, MT 59604-478
Phone: (406) 444-6909

Nebraska
Attn: Drug Demand Reduction Administrator
Address: 1300 Military Road
             Lincoln, NE 68508-1090
Phone: (402) 458-1132

Nevada
Attn: Drug Demand Reduction Administrator
Address: 4600 Alpha Avenue, #8212
             Reno, NV 89506-1276
Phone: (702) 677-5217

New Hampshire
Attn: Drug Demand Reduction Administrator
Address: State Military Reservation 4 Pembroke Rd
             Concord, NH 03301-5652
Phone: (603) 288-3364

New Jersey
Attn: Drug Demand Reduction Administrator
Address: 3650 Saylor Pond Road
             Fort Dix, NJ 08460-7600
Phone: (609) 562-0667

New Mexico
Attn: Drug Demand Reduction Administrator
Address: P. O. Box 5610
             Albuquerque, NM 87185-5610
Phone: (505) 846-7234

New York
Attn: Drug Demand Reduction Administrator
Address: 1 Air National Guard Road
             Scotia, NY 12302-9752
Phone: (518) 344-2056

North Carolina
Attn: Drug Demand Reduction Administrator
Address: 4105 Reedy Creed Road
             Raleigh, NC 27607-6410
Phone: (919) 664-6552

North Dakota
Attn: Drug Demand Reduction Administrator
Address: P. O. Box 5511, Fraine Barracks, Rd190
             Bismarck, ND 58502-5511
Phone: (710) 224-5271

Ohio
Attn: Drug Demand Reduction Administrator
Address: 2825 W. Dublin Granville Road
             Columbus, OH 43235-2789
Phone: (614) 889-7000

Oklahoma
Attn: Drug Demand Reduction Administrator
Address: 3501 Military Circle, NE
             Oklahoma City, OK 73111-4398
Phone: (405) 425-8354

Oregon
Attn: Drug Demand Reduction Administrator
Address: 1921 Turner Road, SE
             Salem, OR 97302-2099
Phone: (503) 945-3585

Pennsylvania
Attn: Drug Demand Reduction Administrator
Address: Fort Indiantown Gap, Bldg 9-7
             Annville, PA 17003-5002
Phone: (717) 861-8716

Puerto Rico
Attn: Drug Demand Reduction Administrator
Address: G. P. O. Box 9023786
             San Juan, PR 00902-3786
Phone: (787) 289-1455

Rhode Island
Attn: Drug Demand Reduction Administrator
Address: Command Readiness Center
             645 New London Avenue
             Cranston, RI 02920-3097
Phone: (401) 457-4139

South Carolina
Attn: Drug Demand Reduction Administrator
Address: 1 National Guard Road
             Columbia, SC 29201-4766
Phone: (803) 806-4402

South Dakota
Attn: Drug Demand Reduction Administrator
Address: 2823 West Main Street
             Rapid City, SD 57702-8186
Phone: (605) 399-6661

Tennessee
Attn: Drug Demand Reduction Administrator
Address: 3041 Sidco Drive
             Nashville, TN 37204-1502
Phone: (615) 313-0889

Texas
Attn: Drug Demand Reduction Administrator
Address: P. O. Box 5218, Bldg 10, Camp Mabry
             9001 North Interstate Highway 35
             Austin, Texas 78763-5218
Phone: (512) 406-6975

Utah
Attn: Drug Demand Reduction Administrator
Address: 12953 Minuteman Drive, P. O. Box 1776
             Draper, UT 84020-1776
Phone: (801) 576-3763

Vermont
Attn: Drug Demand Reduction Administrator
Address: Camp Johnson, GMA
             Colchester, VT 05446-3004
Phone: (802) 654-0440

Virginia
Attn: Drug Demand Reduction Administrator
Address: 600 E. Broad Street
             Richmond, VA 23219-1832
Phone: (804) 775-9175

Virgin Islands
Attn: Drug Demand Reduction Administrator
Address: RR 2 Bx 9925 Mannings Bay
             Kingshill, St. Croix, VI 00850-9764
Phone: (809) 773-8270

Washington
Attn: Drug Demand Reduction Administrator
Address: Camp Murray
             Tacoma, WA 98430-5063
Phone: (206) 512-8611

West Virginia
Attn: Drug Demand Reduction Administrator
Address: 1740 Coonskin Drive
             Charleston, WV 25311-1085
Phone: (304) 341-6460

Wisconsin
Attn: Drug Demand Reduction Administrator
Address: 2400 Wright Street, P. O. Box 8111
             Madison, WI 53708-81116
Phone: (608) 242-3548

Wyoming
Attn: Drug Demand Reduction Administrator
             Address: 5500 Bishop Blvd
             Cheyenne, WY 82009-3220
Phone: (307) 772-5957

Notes and References

PREFACE

1　personal communication: this is based on a discussion between the author and DEA officials at the DEA headquarters in Washington, D.C. on 19 May 2000. The DEA representatives declined to be quoted

CHAPTER 1

1　Plant S. *Writing on Drugs*. New York: Farrar, Straus, and Giroux, 1999
2　Grinspoon L, Bakalar JB. *Psychedelic Drugs Reconsidered*. New York: The Lindesmith Center, 1997, p 238
3　Sir William Osler, *Science and Immortality*, 1904
4　Siegel R. *Intoxication: Life in Pursuit of Artificial Paradise*. New York: Dutton, 1989
5　Random House Webster's Unabridged Dictionary, 2nd ed., Random House, New York, 1998
6　Weil A, Rosen W. *From Chocolate to Morphine: Everything You Need to Know About Mind-Altering Drugs*. Rev. ed. Boston: Houghton Mifflin, 1993
7　Kuhn C, Swartzwelder S, Wilson W. *Buzzed: The Straight Facts About the Most Use and Abused Drugs from Alcohol to Ecstasy*. New York: W.W. Norton, 1998
8　Grinspoon L, Bakalar JB., ibid, p 238
9　Inaba DS, Cohen WE, Holstein ME. *Uppers, Downers, All Arounders: Physical and Mental Effects of Psychoactive Drugs*. 3rd ed. Ashland, OR: CNS Publications, 1997
10　*Monitoring the Future Study. Trends in Prevalence of Various Drugs for 8th Graders, 10th Graders and High School Seniors*. Rockville, MD: National Institute on Drug Abuse; 1999

CHAPTER 2

1　Inaba DS, Cohen WE, Holstein ME. *Uppers, Downers, All Arounders: Physical and Mental Effects of Psychoactive Drugs*. 3rd ed. Ashland, OR: CNS Publications, 1997
2　Inaba DS, et al. ibid., p 142
3　Howard-Jones N. The origins of hypodermic medication. *Scientific American*, Jan, 1971
4　Musto DF. *The American Disease: Origins of Narcotic Control*. 3rd ed. New York: Oxford University Press, 1999, p 43
5　Lacey R, Danziger D. *The Year 1000: What Life Was Like at the Turn of the Millennium*. Back Bay Books, 1999
6　For a detailed review of this myth, see Grinspoon L. *Marihuana Reconsidered*. 2nd ed. Oakland, CA: Quick American Archives, 1994; Plant S. *Writing on Drugs*. New York: Farrar, Straus, and Giroux, 1999
7　Sherman C, Smith A. *Highlights: An Illustrated History of Cannabis*. Berkeley: Ten Speed Press, 1999
8　Gowin DR. *Bloom or doom*. In: T. Lyttle, ed. *Psychedelics Reimagined*. Brooklyn, NY: Autonomedia, 1999
9　Robinson R. *The Great Book of Hemp*. Rochester, VT: Park Street Press, 1996
10　Roffman RA. *Marijuana as Medicine*. Seattle: Madrona, 1982.
11　Moraes F. *The Little Book of Heroin*. Berkeley, CA: Ronin, 2000
12　Quoted in Bugliosi VT. *Drugs in America: The Case for Victory*. New York: Knightsbridge, 1991
13　Mantegazza P. *Sulle virtio igieniche e medicinale della Cocca, a sugli alimenti nervosi in generale*. Milan, Italy, 1859
14　Andrews G, Solomon D, eds. *The Coca Leaf and Cocaine Papers*. New York: Harcourt Brace Jovanovich; 1975
15　Shoenberg BS. Coke's the one. *South Med J*. 1988; 81:69-74
16　Kennedy J. *Coca Exotica: The Illustrated Story of Cocaine*. New York: Cornwall, 1985, p 75

17   Editorial. *JAMA* June 1900; 34: 1637

18   Musto DF. Ibid. p 44

19   Musto DF. Ibid. p 7

20   Grinspoon L, Bakalar JB. *Psychedelic Drugs Reconsidered.* New York: The Lindesmith Center, 1997, p 274

21   Evans Schultes R, Hofmann A. *Plants of the Gods: Their Sacred, Healing and Hallucinogenic Powers.* Rochester, Vermont: Healing Arts Press, 1992

22   Harner M. *The role of hallucinogenic plants in European witchcraft.* In: *Hallucinogens and Shamanism.* M Harner, ed. New York: Oxford University Press, 1972

23   Harris M. *Cows, Pigs, Wars, and Witches: The Riddles of Culture.* New York: Vintage, 1974

24   see, for example, publications such as *The Entheogen Law Reporter*, available from telr@cwnet.com

25   Evans Schultes R, Hofmann A. Ibid.

26   Grinspoon L, Bakalar JB., Ibid

27   Kast E. *Pain and LSD-25: A theory of attenuation of anticipation.* In D Solomon, ed. LSD: *The Consciousness-Expanding Drug.* New York: Putnam, 1966

28   Grinspoon L, Bakalar JB. Ibid

29   Lee MA, Shlain B. *Acid Dreams: The Complete Social History of LSD: The CIA, The Sixties, and Beyond.* New York: Grove Press, 1992

30   Bedford S. *Aldous Huxley: A Biography.* New York: Knopf, 1974 [quoted in Grinspoon and Bakalar, 1997]

31   Grinspoon L, Bakalar JB., Ibid

CHAPTER 3

1   Original letter may be viewed at: http://www.lindesmith.org/news/un.html

2   Quoted in: Musto DF. *The American Disease: Origins of Narcotic Control.* 3rd ed. New York: Oxford University Press, 1999, p 44

3   Jonnes, J. *Hep-Cats, Narcs, and Pipe Dreams: A History of America's Romance with Illegal Drugs.* Baltimore: Johns Hopkins Univ Press, 1996, p 25

4   Musto DF. *The American Disease: Origins of Narcotic Control.* 3rd ed. New York: Oxford University Press, 1999, p 93

5   Musto DF. Ibid. p 107

6   Musto DF. Ibid. p 220

7   Inaba DS, Cohen WE, Holstein ME. *Uppers, Downers, All Arounders: Physical and Mental Effects of Psychoactive Drugs.* 3rd ed. Ashland, OR: CNS Publications, 1997, p 20

8   Meyer Berger, reporter for *The New Yorker*, quoted in: Jonnes, J. Ibid., p 128

9   Musto DF. Opium, cocaine and marijuana in American history. *Scientific American*, July: 40-47, 1991

10   http://www.usdoj.gov/dea/concern/abuse/chap1/control/control.htm

11   Musto DF. Ibid. p 248

12   Reagan N. We must be intolerant of drug use. *USA Today* 1986; 8 Aug.

13   Taylor AH. *American Diplomacy and the Narcotics Traffic, 1900-1939: A Study in International Humanitarian Reform.* Durham, NC: Duke University Press, 1969

14   from Russell D. *Drug War: Covert Money, Power & Policy.* Camden, NY: Kalyx, 2000, p 600

15   from Donziger SR, ed. *The Real War on Crime: The Report of the National Criminal Justice Administration.* New York: HarperPerennial, 1996, p118

16   Hertzberg H. Comment. *The New Yorker*, Feb 7, 2000, p 31

17   estimated by the Center for International Policy; Rosenberg MJ. "Caribbean drug war slogs on." *Salt Lake Tribune*, Dec 17, 2000, p G2

18   based on data from Quinn JF. *Corrections: A Concise Introduction.* Prospect Heights, Illinois: Waveland Press, 1999; *Sourcebook of Criminal Justice Statistics 1996.* Washington, DC: U.S. Dept of Justice, 1997; Gilliard DK, Beck AJ. *Prisoners in 1997.* Washington, DC: U.S. Dept of Justice, 1998; Donziger SR, ed.

The Real War on Crime: The Report of the National Criminal Justice Administration. New York: HarperPerennial, 1996; Mauer M. *Americans Behind Bars: The International Use of Incarceration, 1992-1993*. Washington, DC: The Sentencing Project, 1994; Austin J. *An Overview of Incarceration Trends in the United States and Their Impact on Crime*. San Francisco: The National Council on Crime and Delinquency, 1994

19 quoted by Rosenberg MJ. "Caribbean drug war slogs on." *Salt Lake Tribune*, Dec 17, 2000, p G1

20 http://www.usdoj.gov/dea/concern/abuse/chap1/control/formal.htm

21 Kuhn C, Swartzwelder S, Wilson W. *Buzzed: The Straight Facts About the Most Use and Abused Drugs from Alcohol to Ecstasy*. New York: W.W. Norton, 1998

22 Katz, *Los Angeles Times*, 1 Mar 1998

23 http://www.usdoj.gov/dea/concern/abuse/chap1/penal/chart2.htm

24 http://www.usdoj.gov/dea/concern/abuse/chap1/penal/chart1.htm

CHAPTER 4

1   American Psychiatric Association. *Diagnostic and Statistical Manual of Mental Disorders*. 4th ed. Washington, DC: American Psychiatric Association, 1994

2   Inaba DS, Cohen WE, Holstein ME. *Uppers, Downers, All Arounders: Physical and Mental Effects of Psychoactive Drugs*. 3rd ed. Ashland, OR: CNS Publications, 1997, p 65

3   Ellenhorn MJ. *Ellenhorn's Medical Toxicology: Diagnosis and Treatment of Human Poisoning*. 2nd ed. Baltimore: Williams & Wilkins, 1997

4   Ellenhorn MJ. Ibid

5   Ellenhorn MJ. Ibid. p 327

6   Moraes F. *The Little Book of Heroin*. Berkeley, CA: Ronin, 2000

7   Ellenhorn MJ. Ibid

8   Kaku DA, Lowenstein DH. Emergence of recreational drug abuse as major risk factor for stroke in young adults. *Ann Intern Med* 1990; 113: 821-827

9   Wilkins JN, Conner BT, Gorelick DA. *Management of stimulant, hallucinogen, marijuana and phencyclidine intoxication and withdrawal*. Chap 5. Principles of Addiction Medicine. 2nd ed. Graham AW, Schultz TK, eds. Chevy Chase, MD: American Society of Addiction Medicine, 1998, pp 465-485

10 Lange WR, White N, Robinson N. Medical complications of substance abuse. *Postgrad Med* 1992; 92: 205-214

11 Wilford BB. Abuse of prescription drugs. *West J Med* 1990; 152:609-612

12 Seymour RB, Smith DE. Identifying and responding to drug abuse in the workplace: an overview. *Journal of Psychoactive Drugs 1990*; 22: 383-405

13 Eddy NB, Halbach H, Isbell H, Seevers MH. *Bull WHO 1965*; 32: 723

14 American Psychiatric Association, Ibid. p 181

15 Koob GF, Bloom FE. Cellular and molecular mechanisms of drug dependence. *Science 1988*; 242: 715-723

16 derived from: Hansen G, Venturelli P. *Drugs and Society*. 6th ed. Sudbury, MA: Jones and Bartlett, 2001

17 quoted in: Musto DF. *The American Disease: Origins of Narcotic Control*. 3rd ed. New York: Oxford University Press, 1999, p 69

18 Nowinski J. *Substance Abuse in Adolescents & Young Adults: A Guide to Treatment*. New York: W.W. Norton and Co., 1990

19 Prochaska JO, Norcross JC, DiClemente CC. *Changing for Good*. New York: William Morrow and Co., 1994

20 *Alcoholics Anonymous. Twelve Steps and Twelve Traditions*. New York: Alcoholics Anonymous World Services, Inc., 1981

21 Bovard J. The D.A.R.E. program has been ineffective. In: *Illegal Drugs*. CP Cozic, ed. San Diego: Greenhaven Press, pp 96-98

22 Bryce S. Fighting the battle for our minds. *Journal of Cognitive Liberties 2000*; 1: 23-33

CHAPTER 5

1 Potter BA, Orfali J. *Drug Testing at Work: A Guide for Employers*. Berkeley, CA: Ronin, 1998

2 American Civil Liberties Union. In Brief: Privacy in America: Workplace Drug Testing, 1996

3 Omnibus Transportation Employee Testing Act of 1991. Public Law 102-143, 102nd Congress, October 28, 1991

4 Department of Health and Human Services. *Mandatory guidelines for federal workplace drug testing programs*. Federal Register 1988;53 (April 11): 11,970-89

5 Nuclear Regulatory Commission. *Fitness-for-duty programs*. Federal Register 1989;54 (June 7):24,468-508

6 Swotinsky R, Smith D. *The Medical Review Officer's Manual: MROCC's Guide to Drug Testing*. Boca Raton, FL: OEM Press, 1999. – This is the standard text by the Medical Review Officer Certification Council, an excellent review of the issues involved in drug testing of the NIDA-5 drugs

7 English A., Matthews M., Extravour K, et al. *State Minor Consent Statutes: A Summary*. San Francisco, CA: National Center for Youth Law for Continuing Education in Adolescent Health, April 1995

8 much of this section is based on the very straightforward and helpful summary of this issue in: Potter BA, Orfali J. *Pass the Test: An Employee Guide to Drug Testing*. Berkeley, CA: Ronin, 1999

9 Potter BA, Orfali J. *Pass the Test: An Employee Guide to Drug Testing*. Berkeley, CA: Ronin, 1999

10 for a review of hair testing, see: Cone EJ, Welch MJ, Babecki MG (eds.) *Hair Testing for Drugs of Abuse: International Research on Standards and Technology*. National Institute on Drug Abuse. NIH Publication No. 95-3727. Rockville, MD: Superintendent of Documents, U.S. Government Printing Office, 1995.

11 for addresses, please see Self-Help Resources: Drug Identification

12 American College of Occupational and Environmental Medicine. *Medical Review Office Drug and Alcohol Testing Advanced Course: 2001*. Arlington Heights, IL: ACOEM

13 Substance Abuse and Mental Health Services Administration. *Urine Specimen Collection Handbook for Federal Workplace Drug Testing Programs*. DHHS Publication No. (SMA)96-3114, 1996

14 Judson, BA, Himmelberger DU, Goldstein A. Measurement of urine temperature as an alternative to observed urination in narcotic treatment programs. *Am J Drug Alcohol Abuse* 1979; 6:197

15 Peron, NB, Ehrenkranz JRL. Fake urine samples for drug analysis: hot but not hot enough. *JAMA* 1988; 259: 841

16 Cone, EJ, Lange R, Darwin WD. In vivo adulteration: excess fluid ingestion causes false-negative marijuana and cocaine urine test results. *J Anal Toxicol* 1998; 22:460-73

17 Neb. Rev. Stat. Section 48-1909

18 Tex. Health and Safety Code Ann. Section 481.133

19 Perez-Reyes M., Diguiseppi S, Mason AP, Davis KH. Passive inhalation of marijuana smoke and urinary excretion of cannabinoids. *Clin Pharmacol Ther* 1983;34:36-41

20 Law B, Mason PA, Moffat AC, et al. Passive inhalation of cannabis smoke. *J Pharm Pharmacol* 1984;36: 578-81

21 Cone, EJ, Johnson RE, Darwin M, et al. Passive inhalation of marijuana smoke: urinalysis and room air levels of delta THC. *J Anal Toxicol* 1987;11:89-96

22 Siegel RK, ElSohly MA, Plowman T, et al. Cocaine in herbal tea. *JAMA* 1986;255:40

CHAPTER 6

1 Aldridge S. *Magic Molecules: How Drugs Work*. Cambridge, UK: Cambridge University Press, 1998

2 *Punch*, 14 July, 1855

3 for an excellent review of the concept of mind, see Pinker S. *How the Mind Works*. New York: W.W. Norton, 1997; for a good explanation of notion that "mind" does not exist, see Blackmore S. *The Meme Machine*. New York: Oxford University Press, 1999

4 Koob GF, Bloom FE. Cellular and molecular mechanisms of drug dependence. *Science* 1988; 242: 715-723

5 Jackson TW, Hornfeldt CS. Seizure activity following recreational LSD use in patients treated with lithium and fluoxetine. *Vet Hum Toxicol* 1991; 33: 387

6 Grinspoon L, Bakalar JB. *Psychedelic Drugs Reconsidered*. New York: The Lindesmith Center, 1997, pp 240-243

7 Kuhn C, Swartzwelder S, Wilson W. *Buzzed: The Straight Facts About the Most Use and Abused Drugs from Alcohol to Ecstasy*. New York: W.W. Norton, 1998, p 208

8 Fester U. *Secrets of Methamphetamine Manufacture: Including Recipes for MDA, Ecstasy, and Other Psychedelic Amphetamines*. 5th ed. Port Townsend, WA: Loompanics, 1999

9 Henderson GL. Designer drugs: past history and future prospects. *J Forens Sci* 1988; 33: 569-575

10 Langston JW, Irwin I. MPTP: current concepts and controversies. *Clin Neuropharmacol* 1986; 9: 485-507

11 Langston JW, Palfreman J. *The Case of the Frozen Addicts*. New York: Vintage, 1996

12 Buchanan JF, Brown CR. 'Designer drugs'. A problem in clinical toxicology. *Med Toxicol Adverse Drug Exp* 1988; 3: 1-17

13 Marnell T, ed. *Drug Identification Bible*. 3rd ed. Denver: Drug Identification Bible, 1997

14 The most prolific of these chemists is Dr. Alexander Shulgin, who invented more than 200 phenethylamines and a great number of tryptamine hallucinogens. His personal and chemical explorations are described in great detail in *PIHKAL: A Chemical Love Story*, and *TIHKAL: The Continuation*, both by Shulgin A, Shulgin A. Berkeley: Transform Press, 1991, 1997.

15 Inaba DS, Cohen WE, Holstein ME. *Uppers, Downers, All Arounders: Physical and Mental Effects of Psychoactive Drugs*. 3rd ed. Ashland, OR: CNS Publications, 1997, p 52

16 Smith H. *Cleansing the Doors of Perception*. Putnam, 2000, p 20

17 Art Kleps, quoted in: Norberg S. *Confessions of a Dope Dealer*. San Francisco: North Mountain Press, 2000.

18 Musto DF. Opium, cocaine and marijuana in American history. *Scientific American*, July: 40-47, 1991

CHAPTER 7

1 Report of The U.N. Office for Drug Control and Crime Prevention, January 2001

2 Substance Abuse and Mental Health Services Administration, 1999

3 National Household Survey on Drug Abuse Main Findings, 1997

4 *Partnership for a Drug-Free America. More children are using drugs*. In: *Illegal Drugs*. CP Cozic, ed. San Diego: Greenhaven Press, pp 16-19; also see www.drugfreeamerica.org/pats.html

5 Davis H, Baum C, Graham DJ. Indices of drug misuse for prescription drugs. *Int J Addict* 1991; 26: 777-795

6 Substance Abuse and Mental Health Services Administration. 1997 National Household Survey on Drug Abuse Main Findings, 1999

7 Wink W. Getting off drugs: the legalization option. *Friends Journal*, Feb, 1996

8 many of these are taken from a list in Kuhn C, Swartzwelder S, Wilson W. *Buzzed: The Straight Facts About the Most Use and Abused Drugs from Alcohol to Ecstasy*. New York: W.W. Norton, 1998, p 275-304.

9 Duke SB. *Legalizing drugs would reduce crime*. In: *Illegal Drugs*. CP Cozic, ed. San Diego: Greenhaven Press, pp 115-117

10 Adint V. *Drugs and Crime*. New York: Rosen, 1997

11 Lowry TP. The psychosexual aspects of the volatile nitrites. *Journal of Psychoactive Drugs* 14: 77-79.

12 Reported in: *The Entheogen Law Reporter*, winter 1996/1997, #13, p 126

13 Young LA, Young LG, Klein MM, Klein DM, Beyer D. *Recreational Drugs*. New York: Berkley Books, 1977

14 Vanderhoff BT, Mosser KH. Jimson weed toxicity: management of anticholinergic plant ingestion. *Am Fam Phys* 1992; 46: 526-530

15 Andrews S. *Herbs of the Northern Shaman: A Guide to Mind-Altering Plants of the Northern Hemisphere*. Port Townsend, WA: Loompanics, 2000

16 Andrews S: ibid.

17 Young LA, et al. Ibid.

18 Kuhn C, Swartzwelder S, Wilson W. *Buzzed: The Straight Facts About the Most Use and Abused Drugs from Alcohol to Ecstasy*. New York: W.W. Norton, 1998, p 121

19 Kelly K. *The Little Book of Ketamine*. Berkeley, CA: Ronin, 1999.

20 Andrews S: ibid.

21 Young LA, et al. Ibid., p 171

22 quoted in: Shulgin A, Shulgin A. *PIHKAL: A Chemical Love Story*. Berkeley: Transform Press, 1991

23 for an up-to-date review of the rapidly-growing interest in this substance, see http://salvia.lycaeum.org/

24 Valdes LJ. Salvia divinorum and the unique diterpene hallucinogen, Salvinorin (divinorin) *A. J. Psychoactive Drugs* 1994; Jul;26(3):277-283

25 Valdes LJ, et al. Divinorin A, a psychotropic terpenoid, and divinorin B from the hallucinogenic Mexican mint Salvia divinorum. *Journal of Organic Chemistry* 1984; 49: 4716-4720.

26 Ortega, A. et al. Salvinorin, a new trans-neoclerodane diterpene from Salvia divinorum (Labiatae). *Journal of the Chemical Society Perkins Transactions*. 1982; 2505-2508.

27 Siebert DJ. Salvia divinorum and salvinorin A: new pharmacologic findings. *Journal of Ethnopharmacology.* 1994; June;43(1):53-56.

28 DeKorne J. *Psychedelic Shamanism: The Cultivation, Preparation and Shamanic Use of Psychotropic Plants*. Port Townsend, WA: Breakout Productions, 1994

AMPHETAMINES

1   *TIME*, April 2, 2001, p 34

2   Plant S. *Writing on Drugs*. New York: Farrar, Straus, and Giroux, 1999

3   Eisner B. *Ecstasy: The MDMA Story*. 2nd ed. Berkely, CA: Ronin, 1994, p 127

4   Weil A, Rosen W. *From Chocolate to Morphine: Everything You Need to Know About Mind-Altering Drugs*. Rev. ed. Boston: Houghton Mifflin, 1993

5   Young LA, Young LG, Klein MM, Klein DM, Beyer D. *Recreational Drugs*. New York: Berkley Books,1977

6   Inaba DS, Cohen WE, Holstein ME. *Uppers, Downers, All Arounders: Physical and Mental Effects of Psychoactive Drugs*. 3rd ed. Ashland, OR: CNS Publications, 1997, p 103

7   Swotinsky R, Smith D. *The Medical Review Officer's Manual*. Beverly Farms, MA: OEM Press, 1999

8   Beebe DK, Walley E. Smokable methamphetamine ("Ice"): an old drug in a different form. *Am Fam Phys* 1995; 92: 449-453)

9   Marnell T, ed. *Drug Identification Bible*. 3rd ed. Denver: Drug Identification Bible, 1997, p 539

10 Plant S. Ibid.

11 Kristen G, Schaefer A, von Schlichtegroll A. *Fenetylline: therapeutic use, misuse and/or abuse. Drug Alcohol Depend* 1986; 17: 259-271

12 Gurtner H. Aminorex and pulmonary hypertension. *Cor Vasa* 1985; 27: 160-171

13 Brewster ME, Davis FT. Appearance of aminorex as a designer analog of methylaminorex. *J Forens Sci* 1991; 36:587-592

14 Young R. Aminorex produces stimulus effects similar to amphetamine and unlike those of fenfluramine. *Pharmacol Biochem Behav* 1992 May 42:1 175-8

15 Woolverton WL, Massey BW, Winger G, Patrick GA, Harris LS. Evaluation of the abuse liability of aminorex. *Drug Alcohol Depend* 1994 Dec 36:3 187-92

16 Report of the International Narcotics Control Board, 1995

17 Chait LD, Uhlenhuth EH, Johanson CE. The discriminative stimulus and subjective effects of d-amphetamine, phenmetrazine and fenfluramine in humans. *Psychopharmacology* (Berl) 1986; 89:3 301-6

18 Ellenhorn MJ. *Ellenhorn's Medical Toxicology: Diagnosis and Treatment of Human Poisoning*. 2nd ed. Baltimore: Williams & Wilkins, 1997, p 341

19 American Psychiatric Association. *Diagnostic and Statistical Manual of Mental Disorders*. 4th ed. Washington, DC: American Psychiatric Association, 1994, p 210

20 *TIME*, April 2, 2001, p 37

21 Allcott JV, Barnhart RA, Mooney LA. Acute lead poisoning in two users of illicit methamphetamine. *JAMA* 1987; 258: 510-511

22 Associated Press "Meth labs a hazard to police, emergency workers, government warns." *Salt Lake Tribune*, Nov 17, 2000.

23 taken from a Special Report: *Drugs on American Streets*. Plymouth, MN: Publishers Group, 1999

24 Fester U. *Secrets of Methamphetamine Manufacture: Including Recipes for MDA, Ecstasy, and Other Psychedelic Amphetamines*. 5th ed. Port Townsend, WA: Loompanics, 1999

25 Kennedy K. "Meth mania: even cops duck for cover." *Salt Lake Tribune*. June 28, 1999

26 Witkin JM, Ricaurte GA, Katz JL. Behavioral effects of N-methylamphetamine and N,N-dimethylamphetamine in rats and squirrel monkeys. *J Pharmacol Exp Ther* 1990; 253: 466-474

27 Young LA, Young LG, Klein MM, Klein DM, Beyer D. *Recreational Drugs*. New York: Berkley Books, 1977

28 http://www.usdoj.gov/dea/concern/abuse/chap4/stimula/methylph.htm

29 Sekine H, Nakahara Y. Abuse of smoking methamphetamine mixed with tobacco: II. The formation mechanism of pyrolysis products. *J Forensic Sci* 1990; 35: 580-590

30 Swotinsky R, Smith D. Ibid.

31 Musshoff F. Illegal or legitimate use? Precursor compounds to amphetamine and methamphetamine. *Drug Metab Rev* 2000; 32: 15-44

32 Inaba DS, et al. Ibid. p 57

33 Kuhn C, Swartzwelder S, Wilson W. *Buzzed: The Straight Facts About the Most Use and Abused Drugs from Alcohol to Ecstasy*. New York: W.W. Norton, 1998, p 211

34 http://www.usdoj.gov/dea/concern/abuse/chap4/stimula/amphetam.htm

BARBITURATES

1 Hawks RL, Chiang CN. Examples of specific drug assays: In: Hawks RL, Chiang CN (eds), *Urine Testing for Drugs of Abuse*. (NIDA Research Monograph 73.) Rockville, MD: Department of Health and Human Services, 1986. p 109

2 http://www.usdoj.gov/dea/concern/abuse/chap3/depress/barbit.htm

3 Young LA, Young LG, Klein MM, Klein DM, Beyer D. *Recreational Drugs*. New York: Berkley Books, 1977, p 35

4 Young LA, et al. Ibid. p 37

5 Humphry D. *Final Exit: The Practicalities of Self-Deliverance and Assisted Suicide for the Dying*. 2nd ed. Bantam Doubleday Dell, 1997

6 Swotinsky R, Smith D. *The Medical Review Officer's Manual*. Beverly Farms, MA: OEM Press, 1999, p 89

7 Hawks RL, Chiang CN. Ibid.

8 Ellenhorn MJ. *Ellenhorn's Medical Toxicology: Diagnosis and Treatment of Human Poisoning*. 2nd ed. Baltimore: Williams & Wilkins, 1997

CATHINONE

1 Inaba DS, Cohen WE, Holstein ME. *Uppers, Downers, All Arounders: Physical and Mental Effects of Psychoactive Drugs*. 3rd ed. Ashland, OR: CNS Publications, 1997, p 111

2 Young R, Glennon RA. Cocaine-stimulus generalization to two new designer drugs: methcathinone and 4-methylaminorex. *Pharmacol Biochem Behav* 1993 May 45:1 229-31

3 http://www.usdoj.gov/dea/concern/abuse/chap4/stimula/khat.htm

4 Young R, Glennon RA. Discriminative stimulus effects of S(-)-methcathinone (CAT): a potent stimulant drug of abuse. *Psychopharmacology* (Berl) 1998 Dec 140:3 250-6

5 Kalix P. Cathinone, a natural amphetamine. *Pharmacol Toxicol* 1992 Feb 70:2 77-86

6 http://www.usdoj.gov/dea/concern/abuse/chap4/stimula/methcath.htm

7 Carrell S. Methcathinone: the next drug epidemic? *Emerg Med News* 1993;15: 1-24

8 Goldstone MS. 'Cat': methcathinone—a new drug of abuse. *JAMA* 1993; 269:2508

COCAINE

1   Quoted in Bugliosi VT. *Drugs in America: the case for victory.* New York: Knightsbridge, 1991

2   Oyler J, Darwin WD, Cone EJ. Cocaine contamination of United States paper currency. *J Anal Toxicol* 1996; 20: 13-216.

3   Sacher AN. Inequalities of the drug war: legislative discrimination on the cocaine battlefield. *Cardozo Law Review* 19:1149-1200, 1997

4   Martensen RL. From papal endorsement to Southern vice: the cultural transit of coca and cocaine. *JAMA* 1996; 276:1615

5   based on reports in *Telegraph, Vanity Fair, USA Today,* and many other publications.

6   Report of International Narcotics Control Board, 1995

7   *Boston Globe,* March 21, 1994

8   Weil A. "The new politics of coca." *The New Yorker,* May 15, 1995, 70-80

9   Weil A, Rosen W. *From Chocolate to Morphine: Everything You Need to Know About Mind-Altering Drugs.* Rev. ed. Boston: Houghton Mifflin, 1993

10 Harris J. *Drugged Athletes: The Crisis in American Sports.* New York: Four Winds Press, 1987, p 128

11 http://www.usdoj.gov/dea/concern/abuse/chap4/stimula/cocaine.htm

12 based on: Bouknight LG, Bouknight RR. Cocaine: a particularly addictive drug. *Postgrad Med* 1988; 83(4):115-118, 121-124, 131

13 from: "U.S. Drug Enforcement Administration." *Los Angeles Times,* Dec 20, 1994, p. A21

14 Marnell T, ed. *Drug Identification Bible.* 3rd ed. Denver: Drug Identification Bible, 1997, p 440

15 Romach MK, et al. Attenuation of the euphoric effects of cocaine by the dopamine D1/D5 antagonist ecopiam. *Archives of General Psychiatry* 1999;56: 1101-1106

16 Kuhn C, Swartzwelder S, Wilson W. *Buzzed: The Straight Facts About the Most Use and Abused Drugs from Alcohol to Ecstasy.* New York: W.W. Norton, 1998, p 210

17 Jatlow P, Elsworth JD, Bradberry CW, et al. Cocaethylene: a neuropharmacologically active metabolite associated with concurrent cocaine-ethanol ingestion. *Life Sci* 1991; 48:1787-94

18 Grant BF, Harford TC. Concurrent and simultaneous use of alcohol with cocaine: results of national survey. *Drug Alcohol Depend* 1990;25:97-104

19 Keegan A. Cocaine plus alcohol. A deadly mix. *NIDA Notes* 1991; 6(2):18-19

20 Ambre J. The urinary excretion of cocaine and metabolites in humans: a kinetic analysis of published data. *J Anal Toxicol* 1985;9:241-5

21 ElSohly MA. Urinalysis and casual handling of marijuana and cocaine. *J Anal Toxicol* 1991;15:46

22 Cone EJ, Kato K, Hillsgrove M. Cocaine excretion in the semen of drug users. *J Anal Toxicol* 1996;20:139-40.

23 Roberts J, Greenberg M. Cocaine washout syndrome. *Ann Intern Med* 2000; 132: 679

24 Gawin FH, Kleber HD. Abstinence symptomatology and psychiatric diagnosis in cocaine abusers. *Archives of General Psychiatry* 1986; 43: 107-113.

25 Gold M. Founder of 800-Cocaine Toll-Free national Hotline for US cocaine users and victims, 1983. Reported in: Moffitt A, Malouf J, Thompson C. *Drug Precipice.* Sydney, Australia: University of New South Wales Press, 1998

26 Isner JM, Chokshi SK. Cocaine and vasospasm. *New Engl J Med* 1989; 321:1604-6

27 Foltin RW, Fischman MW, Pedroso JJ, Pearlson GD. Marijuana and cocaine interactions in humans: cardiovascular consequences. *Pharmacol Biochem Behav* 1987; 28: 459-464

28 from: Pascual-Leone A, Dhuna A, Anderson DC. Longterm neurological complications of chronic, habitual cocaine abuse. *Neurotoxicology* 1991; 12: 393-400

29 Inaba DS, Cohen WE, Holstein ME. *Uppers, Downers, All Arounders: Physical and Mental Effects of Psychoactive Drugs.* 3rd ed. Ashland, OR: CNS Publications, 1997, p 95

30 Ellenhorn MJ. *Ellenhorn's Medical Toxicology: Diagnosis and Treatment of Human Poisoning.* 2nd ed. Baltimore: Williams & Wilkins, 1997

31 Bunn WH, Giannini AJ. Cardiovascular complications of cocaine abuse. *American Family Phys* 1992; 46:769-773

DMT

1 Quoted in: Stafford P. *Psychedelics Encyclopedia.* 3rd ed. Berkeley, CA: Ronin, 1992, p 310

2 Weil AT, Davis W. Bufo alvarius: a potent hallucinogen of animal origin. *Journal of Ethnopharmacology* 1995; 41:1-8

3 Stafford P. *Psychedelics Encyclopedia.* 3rd ed. Berkeley, CA: Ronin, 1992

4 Meyer P. Apparent communication with discarnate entities induced by dimethyltryptamine (DMT). In: T Lyttle, ed. *Psychedelic Monographs and Essays,* Vol. 6. Boyton Beach, FL: PM&E Publishing Group, 1993

5 http://www.usdoj.gov/dea/concern/abuse/chap5/dmt.htm

6 Much of the history in this chapter is derived from the very interesting review of the subject by W. Davis, *The Clouded Leopard: Travels to Landscapes of Spirit and Desire.* Vancouver: Douglas & McIntyre, 1998

7 Lyttle T, Goldstein D, Gartz J. Bufo toads and bufotenine: fact and fiction surrounding an alleged psychedelic. *Journal of Psychoactive Drugs* 1996; 28: 267-289.

8 "It could have been an extremely grim fairy tale," *Discover* 12, 1986, reported in: Lyttle T. Misuse and legend in the "toad licking" phenonmenon. *International Journal of the Addictions* 1993; 28: 521-538

9 Allen A. Toadies. *History Today* 1994; 44(8): 50-52.

10 Horgan J. Bufo abuse: a toxic toad gets licked, boiled, teed up and tanned. *Scientific American,* Aug 1990, pp 26-27

11 Carillo C. "Toads take a licking from desperate druggies." *The New York Post,* Jan 31, 1990, p 4

12 Most A. *Bufo alvarius: Psychedelic Toad of the Sonoran Desert.* New Mexico: Venon Press, 1984

13 Davis W. Ibid.

14 Stamets P. *Psilocybin Mushrooms of the World.* Berkeley, CA: Ten Speed Press, 1996

15 http://www.usdoj.gov/dea/concern/abuse/chap5/psilocy.htm

16 Renfroe C, Messinger TA. Street drug analysis: an eleven-year perspective on illicit drug alteration. Seminar on Adolescent Medicine 1: 247-258, 1985

17 Boys F. *Poisonous Amphibians and Reptiles.* Springfield IL: Thomas, 1959; Marki F, Axelrod J, Witkop B. Dehydrobufotenine: a novel type of trycyclic serotonin metabolite from Bufo marinus. *J Am Chem Soc* 1961; 83: 3341.

18 Davis W, Weil A. Identity of a New World psychoactive toad. *Ancient Mesoamerica* 1992; 3: 51-59

19 Ellenhorn MJ. *Ellenhorn's Medical Toxicology: Diagnosis and Treatment of Human Poisoning.* 2nd ed. Baltimore: Williams & Wilkins, 1997

FLUNITRAZEPAM

1 Layton C. Flunitrazepam. In: *The 5 Minute Toxicology Consult.* RC Dart, ed. pp 386-387. Philadelphia: Lippincott Williams & Wilkins, 2000

2 http://www.usdoj.gov/dea/pubs/rohypnol/rohypnol.htm

3 Ellenhorn MJ. Ellenhorn's *Medical Toxicology: Diagnosis and Treatment of Human Poisoning.* 2nd ed. Baltimore: Williams & Wilkins, 1997

4 Swotinsky R, Smith D. *The Medical Review Officer's Manual: MROCC's Guide to Drug Testing* Boca Raton, FL: OEM Press, 1999, p 90

5 Heyndrickx B. Fatal intoxication due to flunitrazepam. *J Anal Toxicol* 1987; 11: 278.

GHB

1 Nordenberg T. The death of the party. All the rave, GHB's hazards go unheeded. *FDA Consum* 2000; 34:14-19.

2 O'Mathúna D. Gamma-hydroxybutyrate (GHB) for bodybuilding. *Alternative Medicine Alert* 2000; 3: 140-142

3   D'Alessandro D. "Your attention please." *The Sporting News.* Jan 10, 2000: 44

4   Zvosec DL, et al. Adverse events, including death, associated with the use of 1,4-butanediol. *N Engl J Med* 2001; 344: 87-94

5   Orphan Medical Inc. Xyrem® NDA for narcolepsy symptoms submitted by Orphan Medical. www.orphan.com/press_release_detail.cfm?ID=117

6   Fowkes SW. GHB Report to the California Legislature. http://www.ceri.com/report.htm

7   Tunnicliff G. Sites of action of gamma-hydroxybutyrate (GHB)—A neuroactive drug with abuse potential. *J Toxicol Clin Toxicol* 1997; 35: 581-590

8   Smith KM. Drugs used in acquaintance rape. *J Am Pharm Assoc* 1999; 39: 519-525

9   Schwartz RH. Gamma-hydroxy butyrate. *Am Fam Physician* 1998; 57: 2078, 2081

10   Scharf MB, et al. Pharmacokinetics of gammahydroxy-butyrate (GHB) in narcoleptic patients. *Sleep* 1998; 21: 507-514.

11   Henry, GL. Coma and altered states of consciousness. In: Tintinalli JE, Krome RL, Ruiz E, eds. *Emergency Medicine: A Comprehensive Study Guide.* 3rd ed. New York: McGraw-Hill, 1992

12   Office of Applied Studies: Substance Abuse and Mental Health Services Administration Drug Abuse Warning Network 1992-1996. Unpublished Data 1996

13   Rambourg-Schepens MO, Buffet M, Durak C. Gamma Butyrolactone Poisoning and its Similarities to Gamma Hydroxybutyric Acid: Two Case Reports. *Veterinary and Human Toxicology* 1997; 39:4: 234-235

14   Hernandez M, et al. GHB-induced delirium: A case report and review of the literature of gamma hydroxybutyric acid. *Am J Drug Alcohol Abuse* 1998; 24: 179-183

15   Lane RB. Gamma hydroxy butyrate (GHB). *JAMA* 1991; 265: 2959

16   CDC: Gamma Hydroxy Butyrate Use - New York and Texas, 1995-1996. *Morbidity and Mortality Weekly Report* 1997; 46:13: 281-283

17   http://trendydrugs.org/deathlist0700.html

18   Chin MY, Kreutzer RA, Dyer JE. Acute poisoning from β-hydroxybutyrate in California. *West J Med* 1992; 156: 380-384

19   Chin RL, Sporer KA, Cullison B. Clinical Course of Gamma-Hydroxybutyrate Overdose. *Annals of Emergency Medicine* 1998; 31:6: 716-722

20   Li J, Stokes SA, Woeckener A. A Tale of Novel Intoxication: Seven Cases of Gamma-Hydroxybutyric Acid Overdose. *Annals of Emergency Medicine* 1998; 31:6: 723-728

21   Li J, Stokes SA, Woeckener A. A Tale of Novel Intoxication: A Review of the Effects of Gamma-Hydroxybutyric Acid with Recommendations for Management. *Annals of Emergency Medicine* 1998; 31:6: 729-736

IBOGAINE

1   Ellenhorn MJ. *Ellenhorn's Medical Toxicology: Diagnosis and Treatment of Human Poisoning.* 2nd ed. Baltimore: Williams & Wilkins, 1997, p 935

2   Mash DC, Kovera CA, Buck BE, Norenberg MD, Shapshak P, Hearn WL, Sanchez-Ramos J. Medication development of ibogaine as a pharmacotherapy for drug dependence. *Ann N Y Acad Sci* 1998; 30: 274-292

3   Goutarel R. Pharmacodynamics and therapeutic applications of Iboga and Ibogaine. In: T Lyttle, ed. *Psychedelic Monographs and Essays*, Vol. 6. Boyton Beach, FL: PM&E Publishing Group, 1993

4   Glick SD, Maisonneuve IS. Mechanisms of antiaddictive actions of ibogaine. *Ann N Y Acad Sci* 1998; 844: 214-26

5   Molinari HH, Maisonneuve IM, Glick SD. Ibogaine neurotoxicity: a re-evaluation. *Brain Res* 1996; 737:255-62

6   Ellenhorn MJ. Ibid

LSD

1   Lee M, Shlain B. *Acid Dreams: The Complete Social History of LSD: The CIA, The Sixties, and Beyond.* New York: Grove Press

2   quoted, with slight paraphrase, in: Cloud C. *Acid Trips and Chemistry.* Berkeley, CA: Ronin, 1999

3   http://www.nida.nih.gov/Infofax/lsd.html

4   National Household Survey on Drug Abuse (NHSDA)

5   Fester U. *Practical LSD Manufacture.* 2nd ed. Port Townsend, WA: Loompanics, 1997

6   this illustrative example is provided by Weil A, Rosen W. *From Chocolate to Morphine: Everything You Need to Know About Mind-Altering Drugs.* Rev. ed. Boston: Houghton Mifflin, 1993, p 95

7   Young LA, Young LG, Klein MM, Klein DM, Beyer D. *Recreational Drugs.* New York: Berkley Books, 1977, p 129

8   Schick JFE, Smith DE. An analysis of the LSD flashback. *Journal of Psychedelic Drugs* 1970; 3: 13-19

9   Weiss RD, Greenfield SF, Mirin SM. Intoxication and withdrawal syndromes. In: SE Hyman, ed. *Manual of Psychiatric Emergencies.* pp 217-227. Boston, MA: Little, Brown, & Co., 1994

10 http://www.usdoj.gov/dea/concern/abuse/chap5/lsd.htm

11 Strassman RJ. Adverse reactions to psychedelic drugs: a review of the literature. *Journal of Nervous and Mental Disease* 1984; 172: 577-595.

12 Mirin SM, Weiss RD. Substance abuse and mental illness. In: RJ Frances, SI Miller, eds. *Clinical Textbook of Addictive Disorders.* pp 271-298. New York, NY: Guilford Press, 1991

13 Wilkins JN, Conner BT, Gorelick DA. Management of stimulant, hallucinogen, marijuana and phencyclidine intoxication and withdrawal. Chap 5. *Principles of Addiction Medicine.* 2nd ed. Graham AW, Schultz TK, eds. pp 465-485. Chevy Chase, MD: American Society of Addiction Medicine, 1998

MARIJUANA

1   Iversen, LL. *The Science of Marijuana.* London: Oxford University Press, 2000, p 18

2   Roffman RA. *Marijuana as Medicine.* Seattle: Madrona, 1982. An excellent and readable account of the history of marijuana use and its medicinal values.

3   Margolis J, Clorfene R. *A Child's Garden of Grass.* 1969

4   Australian Drug Intelligence Assessment, quoted in: Moffitt A, Malouf J, Thompson C. *Drug Precipice.* Sydney, Australia: University of New South Wales Press, 1998

5   http://www.usdoj.gov/dea/concern/abuse/chap6/hashish.htm

6   http://www.usdoj.gov/dea/concern/abuse/chap6/hashoil.htm

7   In the Matter of Marihuana Rescheduling Petition, Docket 86-22 opinion, Recommended Ruling, Findings of Fact, Conclusions of Law, and Decision of Administrative Law Judge, September 6, 1988. Washington, DC: Drug Enforcement Agency; 1988

8   quoted in Grinspoon L, Bakalar J. *Marihuana, the Forbidden Medicine.* New Haven, Conn Yale University Press, 1993

9   Grinspoon L, Bakalar J. *Marihuana, the Forbidden Medicine.* New Haven, Conn Yale University Press, 1993

10 Grinspoon L, Bakalar JB. Marihuana as medicine: a plea for reconsideration. *JAMA* 1995; 273: 1875-1876

11 In the Matter of Marihuana Rescheduling Petition Docket 86-22, Affidavit of Daniel Dansac, M.D. Washington, DC: Drug Enforcement Agency; 1987

12 Hanasono GK, Sullivan HR, Gries CL, Jordan WH, Emmerson JL. A species comparison of the toxicity of nabilone, a new synthetic cannabinoid. *Fundam Appl Toxicol* 1987; 9: 185-197

13 Doblin R, Kleiman MAR. Marihuana as anti-emetic medicine: a survey of oncologists' attitudes and experiences. *J Clin Oncol* 1991; 9: 1275-1290.

14 Editorial. Therapeutic Marijuana Use Supported While Thorough Proposed Study Done *JAMA* 1999; 281

15 Grinspoon L. Bakalar JB. Ibid.; 1987

16 Grinspoon, L, Bakalar, JB. Ibid; 1987

17 Russell D. *Drug War: Covert Money, Power & Policy.* Camden, NY: Kalyx, 2000, p 602

18 National Center of Addiction and Substance Abuse, 1998, reported in *Special Report: Drugs on American Streets*. Plymouth, MN: Publishers Group, 1999

19 as told to the author, August 2000

20 Iversen, LL. *The Science of Marijuana*. London: Oxford University Press, 2000

21 *TIME*, March 5, 2001, p 18, based on International Narcotics Control Board data

22 NORML is located at 1001 Connecticut Ave., N.W., Suite 710, Washington, D.C. 20036, ph 202-483-5500, fax 202-483-0057. It has a prominent web site containing news of marijuana research, use, and laws: www.norml.org.

23 Editorial. *The Lancet*. 1995; 346: 1241

24 Marnell T, ed. *Drug Identification Bible*. 3rd ed. Denver: Drug Identification Bible, 1997

25 Roffman RA., Ibid.

26 Kuhn C, Swartzwelder S, Wilson W. *Buzzed: The Straight Facts About the Most Use and Abused Drugs from Alcohol to Ecstasy*. New York: W.W. Norton, 1998, p 126

27 Leirer VO, Yesavage JA, Morrow DG. Marijuana carry-over effects on aircraft pilot performance. *Aviat Space Environ Med* 1991; 62: 221-227

28 Marshall CR. The active principle of Indian Hemp: a preliminary communication. *Lancet* 1897; i:225-238

29 Huestis MA, Mitchell JM, Cone EJ. Urinary excretion profiles of 11-nor-delta-9-tetrahydrocannabinol-9-carbolylic acid in humans after single smoked doses of marijuana. *J Anal Toxicol* 1996;116: 1433-7

30 Ellis GM, Mann MA, Judson BA, et al. Excretion patterns of cannabinoid metabolites after last use in a group of chronic users. *Clin Pharmacol Ter* 1985; 38: 572-578

31 Dakis CA, Potlash ALC, Annito W, et al. Persistence of urinary marijuana levels after supervised abstinence. *Am J Psychiatry* 1982; 22: 445-454

32 Wilkins JN, Conner BT, Gorelick DA. Management of stimulant, hallucinogen, marijuana and phencyclidine intoxication and withdrawal. In: *Principles of Addiction Medicine*, 2nd ed. Graham AW, Schulz TK, eds. Chap 5. Chevy Chase, MD: American Society of Addiction Medicine, 1998

33 http://www.usdoj.gov/dea/concern/abuse/chap6/marijuan.htm

34 Iversen, ibid, p 46

35 Grinspoon, L, Bakalar, JB. Ibid; 1987, p 182

36 Rubin V, Comitas L. *Ganja in Jamaica: A Medical Anthropological Study of Chronic Marijuana Use*. The Hague: Mouton, 1975

37 *The Lancet* 1995; Nov 11: 1241

MDMA

1 Eisner B. *Ecstasy: The MDMA Story*. 2nd ed. Berkeley, CA: Ronin, 1994

2 Kuhn C, Swartzwelder S, Wilson W. *Buzzed: The Straight Facts About the Most Used and Abused Drugs from Alcohol to Ecstasy*. New York: W.W. Norton, 1998

3 Joseph M. *Ecstasy: Its History and Lore*. London: Carlton Books, 2000

4 Jeremy Bigwood, quoted in: Stafford P. *Psychedelics Encyclopedia*. 3rd ed. Berkeley, CA: Ronin, 1992

5 Glennon RA. MDMA-like stimulus effects of alpha-ethyltryptamine and the alpha-ethyl homolog of DOM. *Pharmacol Biochem Behav* 1993; 46: 459-462

6 Stafford P. *Psychedelics Encyclopedia*. 3rd ed. Berkeley, CA: Ronin, 1992

7 Ellenhorn MJ. *Ellenhorn's Medical Toxicology: Diagnosis and Treatment of Human Poisoning*. 2nd ed. Baltimore: Williams & Wilkins, 1997, p 347

8 Cloud, J. *The Lure of Ecstasy, TIME* 2000; June 5: 62-68

9 quoted in Cloud, J. *The Lure of Ecstasy, TIME* 2000; June 5: 62-68

10 "Flood of ecstacy a new challenge for customs." *Salt Lake Tribune*, Aug 26, 2000, p A6

11 http://www.usdoj.gov/dea/concern/abuse/chap5/dom.htm

12 Kuhn C, et al. Ibid.

13 Wolff K, Hay AWM, Sherlock K, Conner M. Contents of 'Ecstasy'. *Lancet* 1995; 346:1100-1105

14 Giroud C, Augsburger M, Rivier L, Mangin P, Sadeghipour F, Varesio E, Veuthey JL, Kamalaprija P. 2C-B: a new psychoactive phenylethylamine recently discovered in Ecstasy tablets sold on the Swiss black market [see comments]. *J Anal Toxicol* 1998 Sep 22:5 345-54

15 Wolfe TR, Caravat EM. Massive dextromethorphan ingestion and abuse. *Am J Emerg Med* 1995; 13: 174-176

16 Kuhn C, et al. Ibid.

17 Marnell T, ed. *Drug Identification Bible*. 3rd ed. Denver: Drug Identification Bible, 1997, p 559

18 Bronson ME, Jiang W, DeRuiter J, Clark CR. A behavioral comparison of Nexus, cathinone, BDB, and MDA. *Pharmacol Biochem Behav* 1995; 51: 473-475

19 Peroutka SJ. 'Ecstasy': a human neurotoxin? *Arch Gen Psychiatry* 1989; 416:191

20 Ricaurte C, Bryan G, Strauss L, et al. Hallucinogenic amphetamine selectively destroys serotonin nerve terminals. *Science* 1985; 229:986-988

21 Ricaurte GA, Gorno LS, Wilson MA, et al. (+/-)-3,4-Methylenedioxymethamphetamine selectively damages central serotonergic neurons in nonhuman primates. *JAMA* 1988; 260:51-55

22 Hatzidimitriou G, McCann UD, Ricaurte GA. Altered serotonin innervation patterns in the forebrain of monkeys treated with (±)3,4-methylenedioxymethamphetamine seven years previously: factors influencing abnormal recovery. *Journal of Neuroscience* 1999; 19:5096-5107.

23 Randall T. Ecstasy-fueled 'rave' parties become dances of death for English youths. *JAMA* 1992; 268: 1505-1506

24 Morano RA, Spies C, Walker FB, Plank SM. Fatal intoxication involving etryptamine. *J Forensic Sci* 1993; 38: 721-725

Methaqualone

1 Ziemer M. *Quaaludes*. Berkeley Heights, NJ: Enslow, 1997

2 The Week. *National Review*, Dec 8, 1972, p 1332

3 quoted in Ziemer, p 41

4 http://www.usdoj.gov/dea/concern/abuse/chap3/depress/glute.htm

5 Angelos SA, Meyers JA. The isolation and identification of precursors and reaction products in the clandestine manufacture of methaqualone and mecloqualone. *J Forensic Sci* 1985; 30: 1022-1047

6 Havier RG, Lin R. Deaths as a result of a combination of codeine and glutethimide. *J Forens Sci* 1985; 30: 563-566

7 Hogshire J. *Pills-A-Go-Go: A Fiendish Investigation into Pill Marketing, Art, History and Consumption*. Venice, CA: Feral House, 1999

8 Luck RE, Montgomery WS. Glutethimide withdrawal syndrome—the ethics of supply and demand. *Aust NZ J Med* 1992; 22: 708

9 Ellenhorn MJ. *Ellenhorn's Medical Toxicology: Diagnosis and Treatment of Human Poisoning*. 2nd ed. Baltimore: Williams & Wilkins, 1997

Opiates

1 Booth M. *Opium: A History*. New York: St. Martins Griffin, 1996

2 http://www.usdoj.gov/dea/concern/abuse/chap2/narcotic/natural.htm

3 Roche D. "The potent perils of a miracle drug." *TIME*, Jan 8, 2001

4 Romagnoli A, Keats AS. Comparative respiratory depression to tilidine and morphine. *Clin Pharmacol Ther* 1975; 17: 523-528

5 Van Boven M, Daenens P, Bruneel N. A death case involving tilidine. *Arch Toxicol* 1976; 36: 121-125

6 *Dorlands Illustrated Medical Dictionary*, 27th, Philadelphia: W.B. Saunders Co., 1988

7 Peclet C, Rousseau JJ, Rousseau M. Anileridine intoxication. *Bull Int Assoc Forens Toxicol* 1981; 16: 27-28

8   Gillespie TJ, Gandolfi AJ, Davis TP, Morano RA. Identification and quantification of alpha-methylfentanyl in post mortem specimens. *J Anal Toxicol* 1982; 6: 139-142

9   Marcovici M, O'Brien CP, McLellan AT, Kacian J. A clinical, controlled study of l-alpha-acetylmethadol in the treatment of narcotic addiction. *Am J Psychiatry* 1981; 138: 234-236

10   Karp-Gelernter E, Wurmser L, Savage C. Therapeutic effects of methadone and 1-alpha-acetylmethadol. *Am J Psychiatry* 1976; 133: 955-957

11   Segal R, Everson A, Sellers EM, Thakur R. Failure of acetylmethadol in treatment of narcotic addicts due to nonpharmacologic factors. *Can Med Assoc J* 1976; 115:1014-1016

12   Crowley TJ, Macdonald MJ, Wagner JE, Zerbe G. Acetylmethadol versus methadone: human mood and motility. *Psychopharmacology* (Berl) 1985; 86: 458-63

13   Section 291.501: Methadone in the maintenance treatment of narcotic addicts. Part 310: New drugs. Recodification of Methadone Regulations. Title 21: Food and Drugs. Federal Register 1977;42:46, 698-710. Methadone guidelines are also available from the FDA by telephone at 301-295-8020

14   McNeely J. Methadone is an effective treatment for heroin addiction. In: *Illegal Drugs*. CP Cozic, ed. San Diego: Greenhaven Press, pp 91-95

15   Buchanan JF, Brown CR. 'Designer drugs'. A problem in clinical toxicology. *Med Toxicol Adverse Drug Exp* 1988; 3: 1-17

16   Inaba DS, Cohen WE, Holstein ME. *Uppers, Downers, All Arounders: Physical and Mental Effects of Psychoactive Drugs*. 3rd ed. Ashland, OR: CNS Publications, 1997

17   Report of International Narcotics Control Board, 1997

18   Moraes F. *The Little Book of Heroin*. Berkeley, CA: Ronin, 2000

19   Martin M, Hecker J, Clark R, Frye J, Jehle D, Lucid EJ, Harchelroad F. China White epidemic: an eastern United States Emergency Department experience. *Ann Emerg Med* 1991; 20: 158-164

20   Henderson GL, Harkey MR, Jones AD. Rapid screening of fentanyl (China White) powder samples by solid-phase radioimmunoassay. *J Anal Toxicol* 1990; 14: 172-175

21   Hibbs J, Perper J, Winek CL. An outbreak of designer drug-related deaths in Pennsylvania [see comments]. *JAMA* 1991; 265: 1011-1013

22   Cone EJ, Welch P, Paul BC, et al. Forensic drug testing for opiates: III. Urinary excretion rates of morphine and codeine following codeine administration. *J Anal Toxicol* 1991;15:161-6

23   Cone EJ, Welch P, Mitchell JM, et al. Forensic drug testing for opiates: I. Detection of 6-acetylmorphine in urine as an indicator of recent heroin exposure; drug and assay considerations and detection times. *J Anal Toxicol* 1996;20:541-6

24   Unnithan S, Strang J. Poppy tea dependency. *Br J Psychiatry* 1993; 163:813-814

25   Kaplan R. Poppy seed dependence. *Med J Aust* 1994; 161: 176

26   Swotinsky R, Smith D. *The Medical Review Officer's Manual*. Beverly Farms, MA: OEM Press, 1999, p 85

27   Holtdorf K. *Ur-ine Trouble*. Scottsdale AZ: Vandalay Press, 1998.

28   Selavka CM. Poppy seed ingestion as a contributing factor to opiate-positive urinalysis results: the Pacific perspective. *J Forensic Sci* 1991;36:685-96

29   Findlay JW, Butz RF, Welch RM. Codeine kinetics determined by radioimmunoassay. *Clin Pharmacol Ther* 1977; 22:439

30   Inaba DS, et al. Ibid. p 57

31   NIH Consensus Conference. Effective Medical Treatment of Opiate Addiction. *JAMA*. 1998; 280: 1936-1943. Full bibliography is available at http://www.nlm.nih.gov/pubs/cbm/heroin_addiction.html.

32   Moraes F. *The Little Book of Heroin*. Berkeley, CA: Ronin, 2000

33   Kuhn C, Swartzwelder S, Wilson W. *Buzzed: The Straight Facts About the Most Use and Abused Drugs from Alcohol to Ecstasy*. New York: W.W. Norton, 1998, p 174

34   Wodak A. Managing illicit drug use. A practical guide. *Drugs* 1994; 47: 446-457

35   Kosten TR. Current pharmacotherapies for opioid dependence. *Psychopharmacol Bull* 1990; 26: 69-74

36 Moraes F. Ibid

37 Ellenhorn MJ. *Ellenhorn's Medical Toxicology: Diagnosis and Treatment of Human Poisoning.* 2nd ed. Baltimore: Williams & Wilkins, 1997

38 Chamberlain RT. *Methadone: In-Service Training and Continuing Education AACC/TDM.* Washington, DC: American Association for Clinical Chemistry, Inc., 1989;10(9):5-17

PCP

1 http://www.usdoj.gov/dea/concern/abuse/chap5/pcp.htm

2 Lue LP, Scimeca JA, Thomas BF, Martin BR. Pyrolytic fate of piperidinocyclohexanecarbonitrile, a contaminant of phencyclidine, during smoking. *J Anal Toxicol* 1988 Mar-Apr 12:2 57-61

3 Kuhn C, Swartzwelder S, Wilson W. *Buzzed: The Straight Facts About the Most Use and Abused Drugs from Alcohol to Ecstasy.* New York: W.W. Norton, 1998, p 93

4 Cook CE, Brine DR, Jeffecote AR. Phencyclidine deposition after intravenous and oral doses. *Clin Pharmacol Ther* 1982;31:625-34

5 Simpson GM, Khajawall AM, Alatorre E, et al. Urinary phencyclidine excretion in chronic abusers. *J Toxicol Clin Toxicol* 1982;19:1051-9

6 Levine BS, Smith ML. Effects of diphenhydramine on immunoassay of phencyclidine in urine. *Clin Chem* 1990;36:1258

7 Swotinsky R, Smith D. *The Medical Review Officer's Manual.* Beverly Farms, MA: OEM Press, 1999

8 Tennant FS, Rawson RA, McCann M. Withdrawal from chronic phencyclidine dependence with desipramine. *American Journal of Psychiatry* 1981; 138:845-847

9 Weiss CJ, Millman RB. Hallucinogens, phencyclidine, marijuana, inhalants. In: RJ Frances, MI Sheldon, eds. *Clinical Textbook for Addictive Disorders.* pp 147-170. New York, NY: Guilford Press, 1991

10 Altura BT, Quirion R, Pert CB, Altura BM. Phencyclidine ("angel dust") analogs and sigma opiate benzomorphans cause cerebral arterial spasm. *Proc Natl Acad Sci U S A* 1983; Feb 80:3 865-869

11 American Psychiatric Association. *Diagnostic and Statistical Manual of Mental Disorders.* 4th ed. Washington, DC: American Psychiatric Association, 1994, p 260

12 Ellenhorn MJ. *Ellenhorn's Medical Toxicology: Diagnosis and Treatment of Human Poisoning.* 2nd ed. Baltimore: Williams & Wilkins, 1997

13 Valentine JL, Owens SM. Antiphencyclidine monoclonal antibody therapy significantly changes phencyclidine concentrations in brain and other tissues in rats. *J Pharmacol Exp Ther* 1996; 278: 717-724

14 Valentine JL, Mayersohn M, Wessinger WD, Arnold LW, Owens SM. Antiphencyclidine monoclonal Fab fragments reverse phencyclidine-induced behavioral effects and ataxia in rats. *J Pharmacol Exp Ther* 1996; 278: 709-716

Peyote

1 Keller WJ, Yeary RA. Catecholamine metabolism in a psychoactive cactus. *Clin Toxicol* 1980; 16: 233-243

2 Neal JM, Sato PT, Howald WN, McLaughlin JL. Peyote alkaloids: identification in the Mexican cactus Pelecyphora aselliformis Ehrenberg. *Science* 176: 1131-1133, 1972

3 Prescott WH. *History of the Conquest of Mexico.* 3 vols. Boston: Phillips, Sampson and Co., 1855

4 de Sahagún, Fr B. *Historia general de las cosas de Nueva España.* Vol 3. Mexico City: Pedro Robredo, 1938, p 118

5 Ibid, p 240

6 Leonard I. Peyote and the Mexican inquisition. *American Anthropologist* 44: 324-326, 1942

7 García Fr B. *Manual para administrar los santos sacramentos etc.* Mexico City: Rivera, 1760

8 Roseman T. *The Peyote Story.* Hollywood, CA: Wilshire Book Co., 1963

9 Heffter A. Ueber Pellote. Ein Beitrage zu pharmakologischen Kenntnis der Cacteen. *Archiv für experimentalle Pathologie und Pharmakologie* 1894; 34: 65-86

10   Anderson EF. *Peyote: the divine cactus.* 2nd ed. Tucson, AZ: University of Arizona Press, 1996

11   Howard JH. The mescal-bean cult of the central and southern plains: an ancestor of the peyote cult? *American Anthropologist* 1957; 59: 75-87,

12   Stafford P. *Psychedelics Encyclopedia.* 3rd ed. Berkeley, CA: Ronin, 1992

13   Mount G. *The Peyote Book: A Study of Native Medicine.* 3rd ed. Cottonwood, CA: Sweetlight, 1993

14   Mount G. Ibid.

15   Bullis RK. Swallowing the scroll: legal implications of the recent Supreme Court peyote cases. *Journal of Psychoactive Drugs* 1990; 22: 325-332

16   the ruling is: City of Boerne v. Flores (1997) 521 U.S. 507

17   People v. Guerrero (No. 0001-91) Superior Court of Guam. This ruling is unpublished but available for review at at www.alchemind.org.

18   a good discussion of this issue is presented in: Boire RG. Religious defense under RFRA still alive in federal court. *Journal of Cognitive Liberties* 2000; 1: 55-57

19   quoted by Boire RG. Mescaline, peyote, and the law. In: Gottlieb A. *Peyote and Other Psychoactive Cacti.* Berkeley: Ronin, 1997

20   *The Entheogen Law Reporter,* #14, spring 1997, p 146

21   Calabrese JD. Spiritual healing and human development in the Native American Church: toward a cultural psychiatry of peyote. *Psychoanalytic Review* 1997; 84: 237-255

22   Huttlinger KW, Tanner D. The peyote way: implications for Culture Care theory. *J Transcult Nurs* 1994; 5: 5-11

23   Crosby DM, McLaughlin JL. Cactus alkaloids. XIX. Crystallization of mescaline HCl and 3-methoxytyramine HCl from Trichocereus pachanoi. *Lloydia* 1973; 36: 416-418.

24   Mack RB. Marching to a different cactus: peyote (mescaline) intoxication. *North Carolina Med J* 1986; 47: 137-138

25   http://www.usdoj.gov/dea/concern/abuse/chap5/peyote.htm

26   Beauvais F, LaBoueff S. Drug and alcohol abuse intervention in American Indian communities. *Int J Addict.* 1985; 20:139-71.

27   Albaugh, BJ, Anderson PO. Peyote in the treatment of alcoholism among American Indians. *American Journal of Psychiatry* 1974; 131: 1247-1251

28   Blum K, Futterman SL, Pascarosa P. Peyote, a potential ethnopharmacologic agent for alcoholism and other drug dependencies: possible biochemical rationale. *Clin Toxicol* 1977; 11:4 459-72

29   quoted in: Mount G. Ibid., p 81

30   Schwarz RH. Mescaline: a survey. *Amer Fam Phys* 1988; 37: 122-124

31   Dorrance DL, Janiger O, Teplitz RL. Effect of peyote on human chromosomes. Cytogenetic study of the Huichol Indians of Northern Mexico. *JAMA* 1975; 234:299-302

32   Mount G. *The Peyote Book: A Study of Native Medicine.* 3rd ed. Cottonwood, CA: Sweetlight, 1993

33   Hashimoto H, Clyde VJ, Parko KL. Botulism from peyote. *New Engl J Med* 1998; 339: 203-204

34   quoted in: Mount G. Ibid., p 81

35   Nolte KB. Fatal peyote ingestion associated with Mallory-Weiss laceration. *Western Journal of Medicine* 1999; 170: 328

36   Lyman JL, Mohler SR. The airline passenger undergoing withdrawal or overdose from narcotics or other drugs. *Aviat Space Environ Med* 1985; 56: 451-456

37   Ellenhorn MJ. *Ellenhorn's Medical Toxicology: Diagnosis and Treatment of Human Poisoning.* 2nd ed. Baltimore: Williams & Wilkins, 1997

Index

2-AG 332
222 372
2C-B 77, 104, 154, 198, 341, 343
3C-BZ 153
3C-E 153
2C-F 154
2C-G 154
2C-G-3 154
2C-G-4 154
2C-G-5 154
2C-G-N 154
2C-H 154
2C-I 155
2C-N 155
2C-O-4 155
2C-P 155
2C-SE 155
2C-T 155
    2C-T-2 155
    2C-T-4 155
    2C-T-7 155
    2C-T-8 155
    2C-T-9 155
    2C-T-13 155
    2C-T-15 155
    2C-T-17 155
    2C-T-21 155
4-D 155
5-hydroxytryptamine (5-HT) 141
4-MA 153
6-monoacetylmorphine (6-MAM) 375

absenteeism 110
AC&C 372
Acapulco Gold 322
acetaminophen 345, 361
acetic acid 362
acetic anhydride 26, 362
acetone 144, 211, 212, 233, 244, 249, 252
acetorphine 77, 195, 369
acetoxypiperidine 198

acetyl-alpha-methylfentanyl 76, 195, 366
acetylcholine 273
    receptor 139
acetyldihydrocodeine 77, 195, 369
acetylmethadol 76, 195
acid-heads 104
Acorus calamus 181
activated charcoal 93
ADAM 340
Adderall 122
addiction 12, 20, 28, 58, **95-101**
addictive personality 98
Administrative Law Judge 75
adrenaline 123, **139-140**, 203, 246
AEM 154
Aeschylus 43
AET 195, 266
Afghanistan 31, 67, 324, 371
Africa 31, 52, 231, 232
African Americans 69
Agave 398
AIDS 245, 326
air pollution 115
air traffic controller 110
Airo Indians 265
AL 154
Alberta 181
alcohol 8, 12, 27, 28, 32, 57, **177-178,** 194
    dehydrogenase 289
Alcoholics Anonymous 100, 409
ALEPH 153
    ALEPH-2 153
    ALEPH-4 153
    ALEPH-6 153
    ALEPH-7 153
Alfenta 365
alfentanyl 79, 195, 365
Algeria 52
Alka-Seltzer Plus 216
alkylphoxysulfonate 120
Alles, Gordon 203

allylbenzene 144
allylprodine 76, 195, 369
Aloisio, Monica 404
Alpert, Richard 51, 265
alpha-aminopropriophenone 195
alpha-endopsychosin 143
alpha-ethyltryptamine 77, 266
alpha-methylfentanyl 76, 195, 366
alpha-methylthiofentanyl 76, 366
alphacetylmethadol 76, 195
alphameprodine 76, 195, 369
alphamethadol 76, 195
alphaprodine 79, 195, 369
alprazolam 279, 378
aluminum 211
Amanita
    muscaria 6, 43, 139, **178-179**
    phalloides 273
Amazon 37, 156
American Coalition 61
American Home Products 208
American Medical Association 52, 327
American Psychiatric Association 89, 96
American Revolution 180
Americans with Disabilities Act (ADA) 113
aminohexaphen 195
aminorex 78, 195, 207
aminoxaphen 78
amma-hydroxy-butyric acid 287
ammonia 193, 244
ammonium chloride 219
amnesia 276, 296, 317
amobarbital 79, 195, 226
Amogel PG 123
amotivational syndrome 335
amphetamine 11, 79, 94, 112, 195,
  203-221, 251, 339
    d-amphetamine 204
    l-amphetamine 204
    psychosis 218
amphetaminil 216
Amsterdam 404
amulet 7
amyl nitrate 178, 273
amytal 226
Anadenantherea peregrina 265
ananda 332
anandamide 332

Andes 38, 241
anhedonia 217
anhydro-ecgonine methyl ester (AEME) 254
anhydrous ammonia 212
anileridine 79, 195, 365
animals 177
Anolor 300 122
Anslinger, Harry J. 36, 61
Anti-Drug Abuse Act 67
Anti-Saloon League 28
anti-war protests 53
anticonvulsants 223
anxiety 351
Apocynaceae 301
appetite suppressant 339
aprobarbital 223
Arab 231
arachidonic acid 332
arachidonylglycerol (2-AG) 332
Arco-Lase Plus 122
Areca catechu 179
areca palm tree 179
Argyreia nervosa 184
ARIADNE 154
Ariocarpus fissuratus 395
Ariocarpus retusus 395
Aristotle 43
Arizona 269, 329, 402, 405
Artane 193
asarone 182
ASB 154
ascorbic acid 219
aspergillosis 335
Aspergillus 335
aspirin 13, 27, 123, 325, 390
assassin 32
Assyrians 44
asthma 188, 203
Atapryl 122
ataxia 354
atelectasis 91
Atharva-Veda 30
Athens 43, 44
athletes 105
Atlanta 40, 42
atrial fibrillation 295
atropine 185, 188, 298, 306
attention deficit disorder (ADD) 206

attention deficit hyperactivity
    disorder (ADHD) 204, 206
Attorney General 74
Aurorex 349
Australia 268, 290, 342, 354, 360
autopsy 93, 175
Axocet 122
axon terminals 135
ayahuasca 104, 179
Aymara 38
Aztec 188
        civilization 395
        people 6, 23, 271

B 154
baby boom 63, 310
Bacon, Francis 190
baking soda 213, 244, 253, 291
bambalacha 36
Banisteriopsis caapi 179
barbital 223
barbiturate 11, 16, 102, **222-230**,
    325, 351, 390
barbituric acid 223
bark 143
Barry, Marion 247
basal ganglia 152, 292, 332
base 249
Basel 309
Bashilange 30
basulca 246, 249
batu 206
Baudelaire, Charles 12, 31, 35
Bayer 26
Bayer, Adolph Von 223
BD 289
BDB 146, 343, 347
Beatles 310
beatniks 37, 63
BEATRICE 153
Bedouins 184
beef 194
beer 57, 178, 183
Belgium 44, 344, 365
belladonna 183
bellatal 122
Belushi, John 352

Benadryl 388
Bennett, William 102
bennies 11
benzaldehyde 144
benzanthrene 334
benzedrine 11, 204
benzene 185, 398
benzethidine 76, 195, 369
benzocaine 255
benzodiazepine 390
benzodiazepines 73, 225, 279
benzoyl-ecgonine 254, 255
benzphetamine 216
benzpyrene 334
benzylfentanyl 195, 366
benzylmethyl ketone 79
benzylmorphine 77, 195, 369
Bergman, Robert 408
Berkeley 51, 345
beta-D 155
betacetylmethadol 76, 195, 369
betameprodine 76, 195, 369
betamethadol 76, 195, 369
betaprodine 76, 195, 369
betel leaf 179
betel nuts 179
bezitramide 79, 196, 369
bhang 30
Bible 6, 46, 103, 401
binge 254, 255
Biphetamine 122
birch 178
birth 135
BIS-TOM 153
black drop 20
Black Panthers 52
black tar 372
bleach 283
blitz 204
blood potassium balance 295
blood testing 115
blood-brain barrier 131
blotter 311
Blue Myrtle 406
Blues Brothers, The 352
blunt 322
BOB 154
BOD 154

body dysphoria 102
body packing 175
body stuffers 175
BOH 154
BOHD 154
Bohemian 63
Boissard 35
Bolivia 65, 177, 243, 246, 248, 251
BOM 154
bone marrow 189
Bordeaux 39
Boston 233
botulism 409
brain 22, 131, 244
   abscess 92
   stem 132
Bravo, H.H. 397
Brazil 191
Britain 184
British Columbia 272
British Empire 24
Bromo 343
bromobenzene 387
Brompton's Cocktail 123, 247
bronchitis 188, 334
bronchopleural fistula 91
Brontex 123
Brooklyn College 351
Broom 180
Broward County 352
Browning, Elizabeth Barrett 35
Bruce, Lenny 95, 381
brujos 183
buds 323
Buffalo, Mary 400
Bufo
   alvarius 269
   bufo bufo 274
   gargarizans 274
   marinus 266, 274
   vulgaris 274
bufogenin 267
bufotenine 77, 131, 196, **266-274**
bufotoxin 267
Bupap 122
bupivacaine 255
buprenorphine 364
Bureau of Indian Affairs 402

Burma 210
Burroughs, William 50, 97, 226, 377
Bush, George W. 71, 247, 328
butabarbital 223, 352
butalbital 123, 223
butane 185, 186
butanediol 289
butorphanol 141
button 393
Bwiti cult 301

Caen, Herb 49
caffeine 12, 14, 123, **180-181**,
   210, 231, 234, 251, 345
Calamus 181
calcium 38
   hydroxide 291
   morphenate 362
Cali 282
California 27, 53, 165, 173, 205, 211,
   269-272, 282, 288, 290, 311, 322,
   329, 340, 405
California Institute of Integral Studies 340
California Poppy 182
Cambodia 371
Canada 33, 71, 323, 342, 372, 402
cancer 50, 321
candidiasis, systemic 92
candyflipping 344
cane toad 274
cannabidiol (CBD) 327, 330
cannabidiolic acid (CBDA) 330
cannabinoids 331
cannabinol (CBN) 331
Cannabis 30, 34, **319-336**
   indica 321, 330
   ruderalis 330
   sativa 321, 330
Canton River 24
Capac, Manco 241
capital 123
Captagon 207
Caqueta 248
Carbex 122
carbon dioxide 293
carbon monoxide 334
carcinogens 192

cardamom 20
carfentanil 79, 196, 366
Caribbean 69, 266
carisoprodol 43
cartels 248
Carter, Jimmy 65, 328
casadein 35
Casanova 9
Castaneda, Carlos 183
cataract surgery 291
Catha edulis 231, 233
cathinone 78, 104, 196, **231-237**
Catholic Eucharist 401
catmint 182
catnip 182
caudate nucleus 152
cedar 22, 408
cellulitis 92
cellulose 34
cerebellum 133, 186, 305, 332
cerebral cortex 133
cerebral mucormycosis 92
cerebrospinal fluid 292
cetacaine 255
chain-of-custody form (COC) 116
chasing the dragon 370
chaute 395
chautle 395
chelerythrine 182
Chemical Diversion and Trafficking Act 213
chemical warfare 310
Chemical Warfare Service 48, 339
chemical weapons 48
chemotherapy 327
Cherokee Indian 268
Chicago 27
Chichimecas 395
Chico and the Man 352
Chihuahua 396
childbirth 31, 291, 396
Chile 36
China 6, 23-31, 57, 180-183, 203,
    267, 321, 325
China White 145, 371
chippers 99
chitin 274
chloral hydrate 316
chlorodyne 35

chloroform 185, 211
chlorpheniramine 352
chlorpromazine 327
chocolate 154, 180
cholecystokinin 158
Christ, Jesus 401
Christian 400
    Sabbath 401
Christianity 304
Christmas
    drinks 189
    tree 46
chromium 234
    salts 233
chrysanthemum pattern 265
Church of the Awakening 404
Church of the Toad of Light 270
Church of the Tree of Life 404
Churchill 204
CIA 48, 339
Cicero 43, 44
cigarette 23, 192
cigarillos 23
cigars 23, 192
cimetidine 279
cimora 191
cinnamon 20
Civil War 26, 33, 165
clandestine labs 151, 205, 207, 211
Claviceps purpurea 44
Clayton, Richard 101
Clear Choice 120, 122
Cleaver, Eldridge 52
Clinton, Oklahoma 409
Clinton, William Jefferson 69, 328
clobenzorex 216
clonidine 94, 374, 378
clonitazene 76, 196, 369
Clorox 252
cloves 179
Cobain, Kurt 282
coca 37, 193, **239-261**
    leaves 196
    paste 246
Coca-Cola 40, 42, 242
cocaethylene 254
cocaine 11, 16, 28, 37, 112, 123, 194,
    196, **239-261**

freebase 149
hydrochloride 123, 242, 244, 247
metabolites 112
psychosis 41
sulfate 249
codeine 26, 78, 196, 352, **360**
methylbromide 77, 196
6-glucuronide 375
N-oxide 77, 196
Codex Vindobonensis 272
Codimal PH 123
coffee 15, 38, **180-181**, 203, 228, 241
cohoba 265
cold turkey 379
Cold War 310
Coleman camper fuel 212
Coleridge, Samuel Taylor 35
Coleus 182
blumei 182
pumila 182
Colic Mixture 35
Colima 395
collection booth 117
Colombia 65, 176, 243, 248-249, 282, 363
Colorado 405
Colorado River Toad 143, 269
Columbus, Christopher 21, 191, 265
coma 219, 225, 235, 284, 287, 294,
297-298, 350, 389
Comanche 399
Communist Revolution 25
Compassionate IND 326
Compassionate Use Act 329
Comprehensive Crime Control Act 67
Comprehensive Drug Abuse Prevention
and Control Act 63
Comprehensive Methamphetamine
Control Act 213
compulsive behavior 12
Comtrex 183
condoms 175
confirmatory test 118
Congo 301
conquistadors 23, 37, 395
Constantinople 19
Constitution 33
contact high 160
Controlled Substances Act (CSA) 9, 10,
62-76, 195, 271, 393, 403

Controlled Substances Analogue
Enforcement Act 145
Controlled Substances Trafficking
Prohibition Act 85
Convention of Psychotropic Substances 280
convulsions 179
coolants 185, 186
Cora 396
cornstarch 251
corruption 29
Cortés, Hernán 395
cortex 132, 292, 314
Coryphantha macromeris 183, 394
cotton 32, 33
fever 92
cough suppressants 26
couriers 174, 175
CPM 155
crack 81, 94, 166, 233, **239-261**
cranberry juice 215, 388
crank 207
bugs 218
crazy bread 31
creatine 121
creatinine 121
Cree Indian 181
Crusades 44
crystal 205
lab 249
Cuba 272
custody and control form (CCF) 116
cyanide 185, 334
gas 211
cyclohexamine 78, 196
cyclohexanone 387
cyprenorphine 77, 196, 369
cytisine 398
Cytisus scoparius 180
cytochrome P450-246 157, 347
cytosine 180
CZ-74 69

DACA 63
Dallas 233
Damiana 182
dance-club 287
DanceSafe 345
DARE 101

darnel 31
Darvon 167, 368
date rape 280, 288
Datura 6, 44, 46, **182-184**, 397
        stramonium 182
Dauphiné 44
Davy, Humphrey 189
de Bellay, Griffon 301
de Quincey, Thomas 18, 20
DEA 143, 187, 214, 232, 340, 345, 362
Declaration of Independence 33
decocainized coca 125
Deconsal C 123
deer 268
Delacroix, Eugene 35
Delay, Jean 49
delirium 227
delta 140
delta wave 293
delta-9-tetrahydrocannabinol (THC) 35,
   322, 330
Delysid 309
Demerol 10, 151, 352
dendrites 135
Department of Commerce 64
Department of Defense Authorization Act 66
Department of Justice 64
Department of Transportation (DOT) 111
deprenyl 216, 349
Depression, The Great 325
depression 28
Descartes, René 134
designer drugs 68, 368
desomorphine 77, 196, 369
DESOXY 155
desoxyephedrine 206
Desoxyn Gradumet 122
DET 196, 266
Detoxify Carbo Clean 122
Detroit 233
Detroit Red 36
devil's
        apple 6, 182
        herb 184
        weed 6, 34, 182
Dexatrim 216
dexedrine 122
dexfenfluramine 215
dextroamphetamine 204, 207, 208

dextromethamphetamine 206
dextromethorphan 72, 183, 345
dextromoramide 76, 196, 369
dextropropoxyphene 196, 365, 368
        bulk 79
Dextrostat 122
Diabismul 123
diacetylmorphine 26, 362
diampromide 76, 196, 369
Diana, Princess of Wales 244
diarrhea 179, 333, 360, 377
diazepam 279
Dickens, Charles 20
Didrex 122
diethyl ether 244
diethylamide 309
diethylamine 311
diethylthiambutene 76, 196, 369
diethyltryptamine (DET) 77, 196, 266
difenoxin 76, 196, 369
dihydrocodeine 79, 196, 369
dihydrokawain 186
dihydromethysticin 186
dihydromorphine 77, 196, 369
dihydroyangonin 186
dilated pupils 139
Dilaudid 364
dimenoxadol 76, 196, 369
dimepheptanol 76, 196, 369
Dimetane 183
        DC 123
        DX 123
dimethoxy-amphetamine 77, 153, 196
dimethoxy-4-ethylamphetamine 77, 196
dimethoxy-phenethylamine 77, 198
dimethyl-amphetamine (DMA) 78, 198,
   213-216
dimethyl-thiambutene 76, 196, 369
dimethyl-tryptamine (DMT) 78, 196, 265
dioxaphetyl butyrate 76, 196, 369
diphenhydramine 388
diphenoxylate 79, 196, 369, 377
dipipanone 76, 196, 369
dipropyl-tryptamine 266
dirty basing 244
dishwashing detergents 120
Disney, Walt 399
distillation 177

divinorin C 190
dizziness 179
Djibouti 231
DM 183
DMA 146, 153, 196, 343
    methyl 154
DMCPA 153
DME 155
DMMDA 153
DMMDA-2 153
DMPEA 155
DMT 196, 265, 274, 314
    5-hydroxy-DMT 266, 274
    5-MeO-DMT 269
    5-methoxy-DMT 131, 265
    phosphoryloxy-N,N-DMT 274
DOAM 153, 343
DOB 77, 153, 341, 343
DOBU 153, 343
DOC 153
DOEF 153
DOET 11, 77, 146, 153, 196, 341-343
Dogbane 301
DOI 153
Dolophine 224, 367
DOM (STP) 77, 146, 152-153, 196, 314, 341
DON 153
Doña Ana (Doñana)183, 394
Donnatal 122, 226
donor 117
doop 8
Doors of Perception 399
Doors, The 399
dopamine 97, 137, 138-139, 152, 192,
    217, 253-254, 274, 292, 346
DOPR 153, 343
Doriden 351
Dow Chemical Company 339
downers 11, 224
DPT 266
Dr. Brown Sedative Tablets 35
Drano 283
dreams 27
dronabinol 196, 327
droog 8
drotebanol 77, 196, 369
drug
    anticancer 9

automatism 224
czar 102
definition 8
name
        chemical 11
        generic 11
        popular 11
        street 11
        trade 11
    origin 5
    over-the-counter 9
    potency 8
    prescription 9, 14
    psychoactive 12
    recreational 13
    trade 173
    war 56
Drug Abuse Control Amendments 63, 402
Drug Abuse Resistance Education 101
Drug Abuse Warning Network (DAWN) 167,
    381
Drug Enforcement Administration (DEA) 9,
    64-78, 311, 326
Drug Free Workplace Act 111
Drug, Medicalization, Prevention,
    and Control Act 329
Drug Services Research Survey (DSRS) 168
Drug-Induced Rape Prevention
    and Punishment Act 281
dry mouth 139
Duchess of Windsor 209
ducks 268
Duisberg, Carl 26
Dumas 35
Duramorph 123
Dutch 8
Dwaleberry 184
DXM 183
dynorphin 141
dysphoria 141
dystonia musculorum deformans 291

E 155, 344
EA-1475 339
Ebers Papyrus 184
ECG 295
ecgonine 196

methyl ester 254, 255
Echinopsis pachanoi 191, 394
Ecstasy 16, 166, 288, 340
ecstasy 6
Ecuador 191, 394
Edgewood 339
 Arsenal 48
Edinburgh 365
Edison, Thomas A. 39
EEE 153
EEG 161, 296
EEM 153
Egypt 6, 9, 31, 32, 44, 231
Eighteenth Amendment 60
Eisner, Bruce 341
Eldepryl 122, 349
electroencephalograph (EEG) 296
elemicin 190
elephants 365
Eleusian 103
 Mysteries 44
Eleusis 43
Eli Lilly 35, 48, 203, 367
Eliminator 122
Elk Hair 400
Ellis, Havelock 35
embalming fluid 325
EME 153
Emergency Department 93, 219, 246,
 284, 297, 298, 350
EMM 153
emphathogen 340
emphysema 334
employee health care 110
Endabuse 303
endocarditis 92
endogenous opioids 141
endophthalmitis 92
endorphin 138, 141, 373
enforcers 174
England 24, 33, 180
enkephalin 137
entheogens 46
Epená 193
Ephedra 151, 184, 203
 nevadensis 184
ephedrine 78, 151, 184, 203, **211-234**, 345

ephedrone 232
epidural abscess 92
epilepsy 296
epinephrine 138, 140, 274
Epsom salts 213, 233
Equador 38
erectile dysfunction 335
ergonovine 311
ergot 44, 45, 48, 309
ergotamine 311
Erythroxylum
 coca 241
 ipadu 241
 novogratense 241
 truxillense 241
Escobar, Pablo 243
Esgic 122
 Plus 122
esophagus 130
ethanol 250
ether 211, 213, 244, 387
Ethiopia 180, 231
ethyl 2-furoate 193
ethyl ether 144
ETHYL-J 155
ETHYL-K 155
ethylamphetamine 216
 N-ethylamphetamine 78, 198
ethylmethylthiambutene 76, 196, 369
ethylmorphine 78, 196, 369
etonitazene 76, 196, 369
etorphine 77, 79, 196, 365, 369
etoxeridine 76, 196, 369
euphoria 14, 233, 373, 378
Eve 343
Exodus 6, 181
Experimental Agents 339
eyelashes 115

F-2, F-22 153
famprofazone 216
Fang 30
Fantasia 399
Farnsworth, Dr. 52
fasting 160
Fayed, Dodi 244
FBI 51, 52, 328

FDA 204
Federal Aviation Administration (FAA) 111
Federal Bureau of Narcotics 61
Federal Highway Administration (FHWA) 111
Federal Railroad Administration (FRA) 111
Federal Register 75
Federal Sentencing Reform Act 67
Federal Transit Administration (FTA) 111
FedEx 85
Fen-Phen 209
fencamine 216
fenethylline 78, 196, 207, 216
fenfluramine 209
fenproporex 216
fentanyl 10, 79, 130, 141, 151, 196,
  365-366
        beta-hydroxy-3-methylfentanyl 76,
            195, 366
        beta-hydroxyfentanyl 76, 195, 366
fermentation 177
fetus 95
fever 235
fibromyalgia 291
Final Exit 225
fingernails 115
Fioricet 122-123
Fiorinal 123
Fiortal 123
firs 178
flake 250, 252
Flamingo Park 351
flashback 160, 275, 315
FLEA 153
Florentino 272
Florida 266, 280, 282, 290
flower children 54
flowers 143
flumazenil 284
flunitrazepam 78, 140, 279
fluoxetine 279, 348
flush and rush 374
Food and Drug Administration (FDA) 64,
  73, 287
Food, Drug and Cosmetic Act 63
Ford, Betty 88
Ford, Henry 57
formaldehyde 325

France 44, 191, 287, 291, 360
Franklin, Benjamin 20, 380
free radicals 291
freebase 244
freon 185, 193
Freud, Sigmund 40, 192
frontal cortex 374
frothing agent 189
fungal
        cerebritis 92
        meningitis 92
fungi 143
furanose dihydro 289
furethidine 76, 196, 369
furfenorex 216
furosemide 121

G-3 153
G-4 153
G-5 153
G-N 153
GABA 138, **140**, 225, 283, 287, 292
Gabon 301, 304
Galen, Claudius 34
Gallup poll 66
gambling industry 115
gamma-amino-butyric acid 140, 287
gamma-butyrolactone 289
gamma-DOM 153
gamma-hydroxybutyrate 78, 196, 287
GANESHA 153
gangs 174, 387
Ganja 323
Gaoni, Y. 35
Garcia, Jerry 380
Garden of Eden 19
Garland, Judy 207
gas chromatography/mass spectrometry
  (GC/MS) 112, 333
gas frolics 189
gas gangrene 92
gasoline 12, 185, 325
gastrointestinal tract 130
Gates, Daryl 101
gateway theory 15
Gautier 35
GBL 287, 289

GCS 294
Genesis 103
Georgia 42, 290
German violinists 267
Germany 31, 48, 281, 352
GHB 11, 16, 78, 103, 196, **285-298**, 344, 406
Ghost Dance 399
ginger 181
Ginsburg, Allen 49, 265, 398
Glasgow Coma Scale (GCS) 294
glass 206
glaucoma 327
global economy 177
glue 12
glutamate 140, 387
glutaraldehyde 120
glutethimide 79, 196, 351
glycine 143
God 6, 396
Goering, Hermann 205
gonorrhea 92
Gore, Al 246
Gould, Stephen Jay 326
Granada 189
grandfather 22
Grant, Cary 48
Grant, Ulysses S. 39
grapefruit juice 407
grass 31
Grateful Dead 380
Great Britain 71, 233
Greece 6, 33, 43, 44, 103, 184
Greek 8
green dragon 182
Greer, George 340
greyback beetles 268
growth hormone 287
Guam 405
Guardia, Fiorello La 62
Guaviare 248
Gugliotta, Tom 289
gun scrubber 212
gunpowder 267
gyms 103

Hadrian 43
Hague, The 29
hair testing 115
Haiti 265
Halcion 225, 279
Haldol 219, 390
hallucinations 218-219, 231, 235, 389
hallucinogen 178, 183, 266, 306, 310
    definition 46
haloperidol 219, 390
Halstead, William 41
Hammer of Witches 45
Hand of Death 224
Hannibal 19
Harlem 36
harmala alkaloids 273
harmine 347
Harris, Marvin, 45
Harrison, Francis Barton 59
Harrison Narcotic Act 59, **60-63**, 362
Harvard 52
    Center for Personality Research 51
    University 52
hash oil 325
hashish 12, 30, 31, 32, **321-324**, 336
hashishiyya 32
hatchet cactus 395
Hawaii 165, 184, 206, 322
Hay Fever Association 40
head rush 347
Health and Human Services (HHS) 73
Health Canada 342
health clubs 103
Health Inca Tea 125
HealthTech Pre-Cleanse Formula 122
Hearst, William Randolph 34, 61
Heaven's Gate 224
Hebrew University 332
Heffter, Arthur 398
Helen of Troy 19
Hells Angels 207
hemorrhagic shock 291
hemp 31-33, 321-331
Henbane 183, 184
Henderson, Gary 145

hepatitis, viral 92, 245, 370
    A 92
    B 92
    C 91, 92
    D 92
herbal extract 213
Hernandez, Francisco 271
heroin 11, 28, 36, 77, 196, 362
Heroin Signature Program 362
Hierba de la Pastora 190
Hierba de la Virgen 190
High Times Magazine 270
hikuri 396
Himalayas 30
hip 27
hippies 28
hippocampus 133, 292, 332
Hippocrates 19
histamine 374
Hitler, Adolph 48, 204
HIV 91, 92, 321, 370
Hoffman-La Roche 279
Hofmann, Albert 44, 47, 128, 271, 309
Holiday, Billie 36
Holland 323, 329
Holmes, Sherlock 20
Holy Fire 44
homebake 372
homeopathic 9
Homer 19, 182
homochelidonine 182
homosexual 179
honey 20
Hong Kong 25
hookah 23
Hooper's Anodyne 29
hops 185
hordenine 395
HOT-2 155
HOT-7 155
HOT-17 155
hotbox 253
HTLV-1 92
HTLV-2 92
huffing 185
Hugo, Victor 35
Huichol Indians 395, 396
Human Be-in 53, 341

humulene 185
Humulus lupulus 185
Huntington's Chorea 291
Huxley, Aldous 43, 47, 50, 54, 399
Hydrangea 185
    paniculata grandiflora 185
hydrazine 311
hydriolic acid 213
hydrochloric acid 211, 244, 249
hydrocodone 79, 196, **363**
hydrogen chloride 211, 212
hydrogen sulfide 189
hydromorphinol 77, 197, **369**
hydromorphone 79, 197, **364**
hydroponics 324
hyoscyamine 185, 188
Hyoscyamous niger 184
hyperactivity 219
Hypnos 25, 27
hypodermic needle 26
hypothalamus 133
hypoxic cell injury 291

Ibiza 288
ibogaine 11, 78, 104, 133, 197, **299-306**
ibotenic acid 178
ice 145, 206
IDNNA 153
illusion 314
IM 155
Immobilizer 365
immunoassay 118, 120
Imodium 378
impotence 347
Inca Empire 37, 241
IND 291, 326
Independence 33
India 6, 23, 24, 30, 43, 103, 183, 184, 323, 325, 351
Indian Religious Crime Code 399
Indiana 232
Indocybin 271
indole 149, 273, 408
    ring 156
Indonesia 23, 189
infant deformity 95
Infantol 123

infection
    bone and joint 92
Infumorph 123
inositol 242
insecticides 213
insects 143
insomnia 185, 287, 293, 333, 351, 377
Institute of Medicine 328
International Opium Commission 29
Internet 119, 166, 179, 187, 190, 211, 289
intravenous drug use 91, 92
intubation 294
Inuit 15
inverse tolerance 159
Investigational New Drug *see* IND
iodine 212
    gas 211
IP 155
Iran 30, 371
Iraq 5
Ireland 31
IRIS 153
iron 38
irregular heartbeat 139
Isfahan 30
Islam 180, 304
isocarboxazid 349
isomethadone 79, 197, 369
isopropanol 211
isoquinolines 373
Italy 291

J 155
Jake 60
Jamaica 325
Jamaican ginger extract 60
James, William 189
Jamestown 33
Japan 31, 205, 206
Jefferson, Thomas 33
jerky eyes 235
Jerome of Brunswick 20
Jerusalem 332
JFK Airport 176
Jimson weed 182
Johns Hopkins 41, 349
Johnson, President Lyndon 53

joint 15, 322
Joint Resolution American Indian
    Religious Freedom 403
Jones, John 97
Junkie 377
junkies 104
juvenile 174

K-Head 187
K-Hole 187
K-Land 187
Kadian 123
kappa 141, 304
kava kava 186
kawain 186
Kennedy, John F. 52, 53
Kennedy, Robert 53
Kentucky 101, 364
Kenya 231
kerosene 212, 246, 325
Kerouac, Jack 50
Kesey, Ken 49, 53
Ketajet 187
Ketalar 187
ketamine 141, 187, 190, 345
Ketaset 187
ketobimidone 76, 197, 364, 369
Ketter 187
Kevorkian, Jack 226
khat 193, *231-235*
    paste 232
Kickapoos 402
kindling 159
King George III 33
King Henry VIII 33
King James I 33
Kiowa 400
Kipling, Rudyard 27
Klear 119
kola nut 40
Koller, Karl 39
Korea 205, 206
Korean War 166
Kraepelin, Emil 41
kupuri 396

La Paz 246
La Rocha 280
LAAM 197, 366
Laborit, Henri 287
lactose 149, 213, 242, 251
Lancet 334
Landis, Carole 224
Laos 210
larches 178
Lasix 121
Latin 9
laudanum 19, 20, 28, 360
laughing gas 189
laundry detergent 291
Le Club des Hachichins 35
lead acetate 211
Leary, Timothy 51, 159
Leaves of Grass 181
Lebanon 324
levo-alphacetylmethadol (LAAM) 79, 197
levoamphetamine 204
levomethorphan 79, 197, 369
levomoramide 76, 197, 369
levophenacylmorphan 76, 197, 369
levorphanol 79, 197, 369
Lewin, Louis 398
Librium 225, 378
Liddy, G. Gordon 52
lidocaine 149, 242, 251-255
LIFE Magazine 271
Life Skills Training (LST) 101
limbic
        cortex 139
        system 133, 141
lime 37
linen 32
liquid ecstasy (Liquid X) 289
liquor 178
Lithuania 34
liver 22, 157, 273
        damage 91
living rock 395
Lobelia 188
lobeline 188
locoweed 182
locus ceruleus 314, 374
Lomotil 377
London 31, 288

lookouts 174
lophophine 155
Lortab 363
Los Angeles 288
Lotsof, Howard 303
Love Drug 351
LSD 8, 46-53, 68, 78, 130, 197,
    307-317, 344
        LSD-25 49, 309
        LSD-49 314
Luce, Claire Booth 48
Luce, Henry 48
Lucy in the Sky with Diamonds 310
luftwaffe 204
lung cancer 191
lupuline 185
lysergic acid 144, 184, **309**, 311
lysergic acid amide 188
LyserSaüre Diäthylamid 309
Lyttle, Tom 269

M 155
Ma Huang 15, 184, 203
mace 189
maceration pit 249
macromerine 183, 394
MADAM-6 153
Magic Mushroom 271
magnesium hydroxide 291
mailbox 85
Maine 364
MAL 155
malaria 92, 351
Malaysia 281, 371
Malaysian acacia tree 179
Malcolm X 36
Malleus Maleficorum 45
Mama Coca 38
Manco Capac 37
mandatory minimums 68
Mandragora officinarum 188
mandragorine 188
mandrake 183, 188
Mandrax 351
Manerix 349
Manhattan 173
manna 6

mannitol 149, 213, 242, 251
Mantegazza, Paolo 39
MAO 156, 349
mappine 77, 197
mara'akame 396
Marcaine 255
Marco Polo 30
Marcus Aurelius 43
María Juana 31
Marihuana Tax Act 35, 62, 325-327
marijuana 21, 30, 37, 62, 78, 112, 143,
    197, **319-336**
        metabolite 112, 119
Marinol 35, 123, 327
Marplan 349
Mary Jane's Super Clean 120
Maryland 48, 339
Massachusetts 33, 211
maté 180
Maui 322
Mayan civilization 267
Mazatec 190, 272
        Indians 182
MBDB 341
Mbiri 304
McBeal, Ally 208
McCaffrey, Barry 69
McCarthy, Joseph 61
McFate, Yale 402
McMillan, Trevor 71
MDA 11, 77, 146, 153, 190, 197, **339-343**
        5-methoxy-MDA 146, 343
        N-ethyl MDA 77
        N-hydroxy MDA 77
MDAL 153
MDBU 153
MDBZ 153
MDCPM 153
MDDM 153
MDE 77, 153, 197
MDEA 77, 146, **341-345**
MDHOET 153
MDIP 153
MDM 343
MDMA 11, 16, 77, 94, 102-104, 149, 153,
    166, 189, 197, 232, 282, 288, **337-350**
MDMC 153
        intermediate 79, 197

MDMEO 153
MDMEOET 153
MDMP 155
MDOH 153
MDPEA 155
MDPH 155
MDPL 153
MDPR 153
ME 155
mechanical ventilation 294
Mechoulam, R. 35
mecloqualone 78, 146, 197
MEDA 153
Medellín 243
Medical Review Officer (MRO) 124, 216
Medigesic 122
meditation 160
MEE 153
mefenorex 216
melanin 115
MEM 153
memory 291
Mendocino 322
meningitis, candidal 92
Menninger, Karl A. 408
menstrual
        cramps 327
        cycles 335
MEPEA 155
meperidine 10, 79, 139, 151, 197-198,
    365-367
mephobarbital 223
Merck 339
        Merck, Sharpe and Dohme 26
mercuric chloride 211
Mescal 398
        Button 398
Mescalero Apaches 398
mescaline 46-50, 78, 143, 154, 183, 191,
    197, 341, **393**
mesocarb 216
mesolimbic 253
Mesopotamia 19
META-DOB 154
META-DOT 154
metazocine 79, 197, 369
meth labs 63, 211
methadone 79, 94, 197, 224, 247, **366**

maintenance programs 368
methamphetamine 11, 68, 79, 112, 197, **204-215**, 232-233, 339, 345
 N-cyanomethyl-methamphetamine 215
 N-methamphetamine (MA) 213
methanol 185, 252
methaqualone 78, 102, 197, **349-357**
methcathinone 78, 165, 197, **232-235**
methohexital 223
methoxyamphetamine 77, 199
methyl-4-(3-pyridyl) benzoate 254
methyl-amine 211
methyl-aminorex 78, 145-146, 197, 207
methyl-cathinone 78
methyl-desorphine 77, 197, 369
methyl-dihydromorphine 77, 197, 369
methyl-DOB 154
methyl-fentanyl 76, 145-146, 197, **366**
methyl-J 155
methyl-K 155
methyl-MA 154
methyl-MMDA-2 154
methyl-morphine 26
methyl-phenidate 79, 197, **206-208**, 215
methyl-thiofentanyl 76, 197, **366**
methylene-dianaline 354
methylenedioxy-amphetamine 77, 151, 339
 N-hydroxy-3,4-methylenedioxy
  -amphetamine 77, 197
methylenedioxy-methamphetamine *see* MDMA
methylenedioxy-N-ethylamphetamine 77, 197
methysticin 186
Metopon 79, 197, 369
Metzner, Ralph 340
Mexican inquisition 396
Mexico 6, 23, 51, 182, 183, 187-190, 210, 248, 266-269, 282, 322, 363, 371, 393, 396
Miami 248, 282
 Vice 243
Miami Beach 351
Michigan 232, 288
midbrain 132-133, 292
Middle Ages 31
midwives 45
migraine 32, 325
Milk of Magnesia 291
minimal brain dysfunction (MBD) 204

Minneapolis 292
Minnesota 101
miscarriage 95
Miss Universe 208
MMDA 154, 190, 341
 MMDA-2 154
 MMDA-3a 154
 MMDA-3b 154
MME 154
moclobemide 349
molasses 372
Moluccas 189
Monase 77, 197
monoamine oxidase (MAO) 156, 273, 349
monomethylpropion 78
Monroe, Marilyn 208, 225
Montezuma 271
Mooney, James 400
moramide-intermediate 79, 197, 369
Moreau, Jacques-Joseph, 35
Morgan, J.P. 60
Mormon 184, 203
 tea 203
morning glory 184, 188
Morocco 31
morpheridine 76, 197, 369
Morpheus 25, 27
morphine 24-28, 79, 197, 352, **360**
 3-glucoronide 375
 methylbromide 77, 197
 methylsulfonate 77, 197
 N-oxide 77, 197
Moscow 187, 232
Moses 181
Most, Albert 270
moth larvae 265
mothballs 266
motorcycle gangs 232
MP 155
MPM 154
MPP+ 145
MPPP 76, 146, 197, 367
MPTP 145, 151
MRO (Medical Review Officer) 124
Mrs. Winslow's Soothing Syrup 29
MS-Contin 123, 361
MS/L 123
MS/S 123

MSG 213
MSIR 123
MSM 212
mu opiate receptor 140
mucous membrane 130
mules 175
multiple sclerosis 321
Murderer's Berry 184
muriatic acid 212, 233
muscarine 178
    receptor 139
muscimol 178
muscle twitching 139
muscling 129
Myanmar 210
mycelium 272
Myristica fragrans 189
myristicin 190, 341
myrophine 77, 197, 369
Myrtillocactus geometrizan 406

N-methyl-D-aspartate (NMDA) 304, 388
nabilone 79, 197, 327
NAC *see* Native American Church
Nahuatl 398
nail polish 289
Nairobi 231
nalbuphine 141, **364**
naloxone 141, 298, **364**
naltrexone 364, 379
Napoleon 31
Napoleonic Wars 23
narcolepsy 204, 291-293
narcotic 13, 19, 28, 58, 359
        fruit 189
Narcotics Anonymous 101
Narcotics Control Act 63
Narcotics Manufacturing Act 63
Nardil 349
National Drug Abuse Treatment Unit
    Survey (NDATUS) 168
National Formulary 35
National High School Senior Survey 167
National Household Survey
    on Drug Abuse 109, 310, 328

National Institute of Drug Abuse *see* NIDA
National Institute of Mental Health (NIMH) 53
National Organization for the Reform
    of Marijuana Laws *see* NORML
National Wholesale Druggists' Association 59
Native American Church (NAC) 103, 104, 393
Native American Free Exercise of Religion Act 403
Native Americans 22, 178, 188
Naturally Klean Herbal Tea 122
Navaho 402
Navaholand NAC 402
NDA International, Inc. 303
NEA 146
neanderthal 5
Nebraska 119, 122
necrotizing cystitis 354
needle-exchange programs 92
Nembutal 122, 225, 226
Neo-American Church 404
Nepal 324
nepenthe 19
Nepeta cataria 182
Nerval 35
Netherlands 329, 344, 406
neuromodulators 138
neurosine 35
neurotransmitter 93, 136
New England 33
New Jersey 53
New Mexico 405
New Orleans 27
New York 27, 53, 173, 187, 211, 233,
    248, 297, 344, 351, 405
New Zealand 372
newsprint 34
NEXUS 77, 146, 198, 347
Nicaragua 67
nicocodeine 77, 198, 369
nicomorphine 77, 198, 369
Nicot, Jean 191
Nicotiana tabacum 191
nicotine 97, 138, 180, 192, 253
    receptors 304
NIDA 73, 109, 112, 166, 247, 303, 368
Nieman, Albert 39
nitrite 119
nitrous oxide 189
Nixon, Richard 64

NMDA 143, 304, 387
nocturnal myoclonus 291
noracymethadol 76, 198, 369
noradrenaline 292
norcocaine 254
norcodeine 375
norephedrone 198
norepinephrine 138-140, 151, 254, 274, 346
noribogaine 305
norlevophanol 76, 198, 369
normethadone 76, 198, 369
NORML 330
        Foundation 330
normophine 77, 198, 369
norpipanone 76, 198, 369
North Africa 233, 359
North Carolina 101
Novocain 255
Nuclear Regulatory Commission (NRC) 111
nucleus accumbens 97, 133, 152, 254, 304, 374
Nucofed 123
nutmeg 20, 179, 189

O-methyl-transferase 269
Oaxaca 188, 190, 272
Obetrol 11
ODCCP 344
Odyssey 19, 182
Office of National Drug Control Policy see ONDCP
Office of Strategic Services see OSS
Ohio River Valley 21
Ohio State University 351
Oklahoma City 400
Oklahoma Territory 400
Olmec 268
Olmey's lesions 191
OMS 123
ONDCP 69, 102
One Day Cough Cure 35
Operation Libertador 69
opiate 19, 102, 112, **357-382**
        metabolites 112
        overdose 93
        receptor 93
opioid 10
opium 7, 10, 22, 194, 198, 357-382
        dens 27

extracts 78
fluid 78
granulated 78
gum 359
poppy 19, 27, 198
powder 78, 359
raw 78, 359
tincture of 78
Opium Poppy Control Act 63
Opium War 25
Optimil 351
Oracle of Delphi 184
Oramorph SR 123
Oregon 173, 405
organized crime 173, 178, 210, 344
Orphan Medical Inc. 292
ORTHO-DOT 154
ortho-toluidine 354
O'Shaughnessy, W. B. 34
Osler, William 325
Osmond, Humphry 47
OSS 339
overdose 28, 219
oxycodone 79, 198, 364
OxyContin 364
oxygen 189
oxymorphone 79, 198, **369**

P 155
P2P 79, 198, 211
Pacaps 122
Pacific Islanders 15
Pacific Islands 187
Pacific Ocean 186
pain 50
paint thinner 12, 212
Pakistan 324, 371
Pan-Indian movement 402
Pandora 103
Papaver somniferum 359
paper 34
para-fluorofentanyl 76, 198, 366
Paracelsus 8, 19
parachute 281
paragoric 123, 360
parahexyl 78, 198
paranoia 218, 231-234, 276

psychosis 207
parepectolin 123
Parest 351
Paris 31, 39
    Exposition 301
Parke-Davis 35-39, 187, 232, 385
Parker, Charlie 36
Parker, Quanah 400
Parkinson's Disease 139, 146, 193, 218, 235, 291, 367
Parnate 349
parole 80
parolees 105, 116
Partnership Attitude Tracking Study (PATS) 167
Partnership for a Drug Free America 102
pasta 249
patent medicines 27, 57
Paul, Ramón 265
Paxil 141
PCC 79, 198, 386-387
PCDEA 386
PCE 78, 198, 386
PCP 79, 103, 112, 140-141, 187, 190, 198, 273, **385**
PCPy 78, 198, **386**
PE 155
PEA 155
Pediacof 123
Pelcyphora aselliformis 394
pellets 176
Pemberton, John S. 40
Pen Tsao Ching 30
penal code 174
penis 130, 247
    gangrene 92
Pennsylvania 119, 122
Pentagon 404
pentamethylene dibromide 387
pentazocine 141
pentobarbital 79, 198, **223-226**, 352
pep pills 11
PEPAP 77, 198, 367
pepper 387
Percocet 364
Percodan 364
Persephone 43
Persian Brown 371
Peru 36, 65, 176, 191, 243-248, 394

PET 161
pethidine 79, 198, **367**
    hydroxypethidine 76, 197, **367**
    intermediate-A 79, 198, **367**
    intermediate-B 79, 198, **367**
    intermediate-C 79, 198, **367**
peyote 11, 50, 78, 103-104, 143, 191-194, 198, **391-410**
    false 183, 395
Peyote of God 397
Peyote of the Goddess 397
Peyote Road 400
Peyote Way Church of God 404
peyotero 394, 406
peyotillo 394
péyotl 395
phantasticant 47
phantom limb pain 327
pharmacists 58
PharmChek 116
PharmChem 116, 408
phenadoxone 77, 198, 369
phenampromide 77, 198, 369
phenanthrenes 373
phenaphen 123
phenazocine 79, 198, 369
phencyclidine 79, 112, 198, **385**
    ethylamine analog of 78, 198
    pyrrolidine analog of 78, 198
    thiophene analog of 78, 199
phendimetrazine 208
phenelzine 349
Phenergan VC 123
phenethylamine 152-154, 183
phenmetrazine 79, 198, 208
phenobarbital 223, 226, 227, 352
phenomorphan 77, 199, 369
phenoperidine 77, 199, 369
phentermine 209
phentolamine 219
phenyl-2-propanone *see* P2P
phenylacetone 79, 198, 215
phenylalkylamines 152
phenylcyclohexylamine 79, 199
    N-ethyl-1-phenylcyclohexylamine 78
phenylisopropylamine 11
phenylmagnesium bromide 387
phenylpropanolamine 216

pesticides 193
Philadelphia 26, 145
Philippines 29
phlebitis 92
Phoenix, River 382
pholcodine 77, 199, 369
phosgene 311
phosphane gas 211
photo developer 213
PHP 78, 198
PHPD 316
phrenilin 122
physostigmine 298
Pilgrims 33
pillula 9
pilots 105, 111
piminodine 79, 199, 369
Pindar 43
Pine Ridge Reservation 402
pinpoint pupils 94, 131, 234
pipe 22, 23, 192
pipeline workers 111
Piper chavica betel 179
Piper methysticum 186
piperidine 188, 387
piperidinocyclohexanecarbonitrile 79, 198
piperidyl benzilate
        N-ethyl-3-piperidyl benzilate 78,
        197, 254
        N-methyl-3-piperidyl benzilate 78,
        198, 254
piritramide 77, 199, 369
Piso's Cure 35
Plato 43
PMA 77, 146, 199, 342, 345
pneumomediastinum 91
pneumothorax 91
Poe, Edgar Allan 35
poison 6, 8, 19
Poison Control Centers 297
Poland 34
Polo, Marco 32
Poly-Histine CS 123
Polynesian 184
Pope Innocent VIII 32
Pope Leo XIII 39
Pope Paul VI 402
poppers 179

poppy 7, 359
        straw 198, 359
pork 194
Posse Comitatus 66
post-hallucinogen perceptual disorder *see* PHPD
pot 322
potassium
        chloride 226
        cyanide 387
        dichromate 233
        hydroxide 291
        permanganate 234, 249
potatoes 38
potiguaya 322
pre-employment screen 115
pregnant 95
Preludin 208
prenylamine 216
Presidential Executive Order 13
Presley, Elvis 224, 352
Prevention Dimension 101
Priestly, Joseph 189
Primatene Tablets 216
primordia knots 272
Prinze, Freddie 352
prison 13
prisoners 116, 130
procaine 213, 252, 255
professional drivers 105
proheptazine 77, 199, 369
Prohibition 60, 178
Project MK-Ultra 339
promethazine 123
propane 185, 186
propanolol 219
propellant 186, 189
properidine 77, 199, 369
propionoxypiperidine 197
propiophenone 78
propiram 77, 199, 369
Proposition 200 329
Proposition 215 329
propoxyphene 167, 368
propynyl 155
prostitution 175
protopine 182
Prozac 141, 279, 315, 348
Pryor, Richard 244
psalms 30

pseudoephedrine 184, 211, 212
psilocin 78, 156, 199, 274
Psilocybe
  azurescens 274
  cubensis 271
  cyanescens 270
  mexicana 270
psilocybin 50-51, 63, 78, 131, 156, 182, 190, 199, **263-276**, 408
psychedelics 13
psychoanalysis 40, 41, 49
psycholytic 46
psychopharmacology 310
psychotomimetic 46
Psychotria viridis 179
public health 10
Puerto Rico 248
pulmonary
  edema 91
  embolism 91
  fibrosis 91
  hypertension 207
  talcosis 91
Pure Food and Drug Act 43, 58
Purkinje cells 305
putamen 152
Putumayo 248
pyramidal cell 133
pyridine 120, 372
pyridinium chlorochromate 120
pyrrolidine 78, 199

Quaalude 351-352
quadrinal 122
Quechua Indian 179
Queretaro 397
Quick Flush Capsules and Tea 122
Quick Tabs 122

racemethorphan 79, 199, 369
racemoramide 77, 199, 369
racemorphan 79, 199, 369
radiation exposure 291
railroad workers 111
Rajneesh, Bhagwan Shree 340
Russia 34, 187, 231-232

Ram Dass, Baba 52
Ramadan 233
raphe cells 141
Rave, John 400
raves 103, 288, 290
Ready-Clean 122
Reagan, Nancy 66
Reagan, Ronald 13, 111, 328
Rebagliati, Ross 333
rectum 175, 247
red phosphorous 211-212
religion 6
Religious Freedom Restoration Act (RFRA) 404
REM (dreaming) sleep 293
remifentanil 79, 199, **366**
Renaissance 45
Repan 122
    CF 122
reptilian brain 133
Research and Special Programs Administration (RSPA) 111
resin 323, 331
Restoril 279, 378
retina 214
rhabdomyolysis 350
RICO 63
Rig-Veda 43
right-bundle branch block 295
Rio Grande River 393, 406
Ritalin 15, **206-207**, 216
ritonavir 349
Rivea corymbosa 188
RNS suppositories 123
roached out 282
Roadman 400
Robert Wood Johnston Foundation 167
Robitussin 183, 345
    A-C 123
    DAC 123
robo dosing 183
rocks 245, 252
Rohypnol 104, 140, 279
Rollins, Sonny 36
Roman 32, 34
Rome 33, 184
Rosengarten and Company 25
Roxanol 123, 361
rum-runners 61

rye 309
Ryna
        C 123
        CX 123

S(-)-alpha-aminopropiophenone 234
sabbat 45
Sacramento 210
safrole 190
sagebrush 408
Sahagún, Bernardino de 395
saliva 116, 138, 179, 242
salivation 333
salt 120
Salt Lake City 211, 289
Salvia divinorum 190
salvinorin A 190
San Antonio 173
San Francisco 27, 49, 53-57, 288, 341,
    385, 398
San Jose 145
San Pedro 191, 394, 406
Sandoz 48, 53, 271, 309
sanguinarine 182
Santo Daime Doctrine 179
sanyassins 340
saponification 291
satanic mass 32
Saturday Night Live 352
SB 155
Scheherazade 31
schizophrenia 46, 49, 139, 218
Schultes, Richard Evan 46-47
scopolamine 185, 188
Scotch 15
screening test 118
Scrooge 20
seashells 37
secobarbital 79, 199, **223-226**
Seconal 122, **224-226**
Sedapap 122
sedatives 223
selegiline 122
semen 125, 255
Sernyl 385
Sernylan 385
serotonin 137, 138, 141, 254, 274, 314, 346

Sertürner, Friedrich 24, 25
Seville 23
shabu 165, 206
Shakespeare 32, 182
shampoo 115
Shanghai 25, 29
Shanidar 5
Shaw, Artie 37
Sheffield University 347
Shen-Nung 30
Shermans 387
Shiva 30
shroom 272
Shulgin, Alexander T. 154, 339
shy bladder 117
Siberian shamans 268
Sierra Madre Occidental 396
sigma opiate receptor 140
sigma-2 304
Silk Route 23
sinsemilla 323, 331
skin popping 129
skunk 323
slamming 129
slang words 168
sleeping pill 223
Sleepy Grass 311
small intestine 130
Smith, Bob 100
Smithsonian Institution 400
smoke 22
smoking 22
Smoking Opium Exclusion Act 58
smuggling 29, 329
snorting 130, 244
SNR 123
social norms 104
sodium
        bicarbonate 244
        bisulfide 387
        chromate 233
        dichromate 233-234
        hydroxide 211-212, 233, 291, 398
        pentothal 226, 316
solvent 12
        sniffing 185
Soma 6, 43, 103, 123, 178
Somalia 231

Somnus 25
Sonoran Desert 269
Sophocles 43
Sophora secundiflora 398
Sopor 351
Sorcerer's Cherry 184
South America 23, 37-38, 175
South Carolina 119
Soviet Union 48, 204, 231-232, 310
Spain 23, 29, 37, 281, 360
Spanish Conquest 38
Spectrum 343
speed 11, 205
        bugs 218
        freaks 54, 205, 216
speedball 205, 370
sperm counts 335
spinal abscess 92
spirit 6
splash 205
spores 272
spotters 174
Squibb Company 35
Squire's Extract 35
Sri Lanka 371
St. Anthony 44
St. Anthony's Fire 44
St. Louis 27
St. Peter 191
St. Petersburg 232
stand-down 124
Stanford University 344
Starr County 406
stereotyped movements 218
Stevens, Calvin 187
Stevenson, Robert Louis 41
Stipa robusta 311
Stoll, Werner 309
stomach 22, 130
STP 77, 341
street terms 168
striatum 292
stroke 95, 235
Stropharia cubensis 270
strychnine 147, 213, 312
Students Taught Awareness and Resistance
  (STAR) 101
Stuff, The 122

Sublimaze 365
substance abuse, definition 89
Substance Abuse and Mental Health
  Services Administration 166
substantia nigra 292
succinylcholine 226
Sudafed 211
sudden death syndrome 157, 347
sudden infant death syndrome (SIDS) 95
sudden sniffing death 186
Sufenta 365
sufentanil 79, 199, **365**
Sufi 31
Suicide Machine 226
sulfur trioxide 311
sulfuric acid 144, 211-212, 233-234,
  246-249, 398
Sumerians 19
Summer of Love 54
Sun God 37
Sunami 395
supernatural 7
Supreme Court
        of California 403
        of Oregon 403
        of United States 403
sustantia nigra 146
sweat 138, 139, 333
        testing 116
Sweet Flag 181
Switzerland 309, 345, 380
synapse 136
synaptic cleft 136
synesthesia 313
synhexyl 78, 199
syphilis 92
syringe 28, 165
Syrup Lobelia 35
Syrup Tolu Compound 35

TA 154
tabernacle 181
Tabernanthe iboga 78, 199, **301**
TAC 123, 246
tackle 33
Tagamet 279
talbutal 223

talcum powder 251
talk therapy 310
T'ang Dynasty 23
Tanganyika 183
Tao 31
tar 334
Tarahumara 103, 396, 400
tardive dyskinesia 291
TASB 155
Tatewari 396
taxiing 354
TB 155
TCP 78, 199, 386
TCPy 78, 199, 386
TE 155
tea 24, 36, 180-183, 193, 241
tears 138
Telemachus 19
temazepam 279, 378
Temperance Movement 29, 40
Tenake 122
Teonanacatl 6, 271
Tepecano 396
tequila 398
Terrible Tuesdays 348
terrorists 32
Test Free 122
Test Pure 122
tetanus 92
tetracaine 123, 246
tetrahydrocannabinol *see* THC
Texas 119, 122, 173, 183, 282, 290, 297,
    393, 403, 406
        Border Patrol 282
        Department of Public Safety 406
        mountain laurel 398
Thailand 187, 210
thalamus 133
THC 78, 112, 119, 199, 143, **333**
THC Terminator Drink 122
thebacon 77, 199, 369
thebaine 79, 199, 360
Thebes 364
        papyrus 19
thenylfentanyl 199, **366**
theophylline 210, 223
therapeutic ratio 224
Thai Sticks 323

thiamylal 223
thiofentanyl 77, 199, **366**
thiopental 223
Thorazine 390
THP 386
tickborne relapsing fever 92
tickets 312
tilidine 77, 199, **365**
TIM 155
TIME magazine 48
TM 155
TMA 154, 190, 199
        TMA-2 154, 182
        TMA-3 154
        TMA-4 154
        TMA-5 154
        TMA-6 154
TME 155
TMMDA-2 154
TMPEA 155
toad kissers 269
toady 267
tobacco 12, 14, 15, 23, 38, 191, **241**
TOET 154
toking 335
toluene 144, 185-186, 212, 233-234
TOM 154
TOMSO 154
Toontown 288
Toronto 342
toxicology screen 93
toxin 8
TP 155
TPCP 78, 199
trans-beta-methylstyrene 215
tranylcypromine 349
Treaty of Nanking 25
tremors 235
Trexan 379
Triaminic 123, 216
triazolam 279
trichloroethane 212
Trichocereus
        pachanoi 191, 394
        peruvianus 394
trifluoracetic acid 311
trihexylphenidyl 193
trimeperidine 77, 199, **367**

trimethoxy-amphetamine 77, 199
trimethoxy-phenethylamine 408
Triptolemus 43
TRIS 155
      T-TRIS 155
truck drivers 109
tryptamines 156
TSB 155
Tsuwiri 395
tuberculosis 26, 92
      meningitis 92
Tuinal 122
Tupi Indians 179
Turkey 360, 371
turmeric 179
Turnera diffusa 182
Tussar
      2 123
      SF 123
Tussi-Organidin NR 123
Twain, Mark 27
Tylenol with codeine 123

U waves 295
U4Euh 145
ultra-rapid detox 379
United Nations 56, 64
      Commission on Narcotic Drugs 280
      Office for Drug Control
         and Crime Prevention 344
United States 10-12, 29, 33, 40, 48-50, 102,
  166, 173, 192, 231, 243, 310, 321, 393
      Coast Guard (USCG) 111
      Congress 326
      Court of Appeals 75
      Customs 233
      Pharmacopeia 326
      Pharmacopoeia 35
      Postal Service 84
University of California at Santa Barbara 340
uppers 11, 224
UPS 85
urban gangs 103
UrinAid 120
urine 219, 254, 268, 388
      testing 115
Urine Luck 120

Utah 203, 403
Utravol 35

vagina 45, 130, 175, 247
Valium 167, 225, 228, 279, 316, 352,
  390, 410
Valley of the Dolls 224
Vassar 351
Vatican 39
Vedas 30, 43
venom 267
ventral tegmentum 139, 374
ventricular ectopy 295
Venus 343
verbal response 294
vermis 305
Vespucci, Amerigo 37
Vetelar 187
veterinary 35
Vicks Inhaler 122, 206
Vicodin 363
Victoria, Queen 34
Vietnam War 63-64, 166, 187, 205
Vin Tonique Mariani 39
vinegar 215, 362, 388
vines 143
violinists 267
Virginia 33, 364
      Company 33
virola 193
Visine 283
      eye drops 120
vitamin B 122, 149
vitamin B12 189
vitamin C 215, 219, 382, 388
vitreous humor 115
vodka 178
Volstead Act 60
vomiting 179
Von Bayer, Adolph 223
Von Fleishl, , Ernst 40

waka 186
Wal-Mart 213
Wales 33
Wallace, Bob 345

wallbangers 354
Walters, John 102
War for Free Trade 25
Washington 173
Washington, D.C. 233, 247
Washington, George 33
Washo 402
Wasson, Gordon 46, 271
Watergate 52
Watson, J.W. 42
Watts, Alan 161
wavy caps 270
Weather Underground 52
Weil, Andrew 160
whippets 189
White House 53
        Office of National Drug Control
        Policy *see* ONDCP
white sage 22
Whitman, Walt 181
Whizzies 119
Wilde, Oscar 12, 35
Wiley, H.W. 57
Wilson, Bill 100
Wilson, John 399, 400
windowpane 311
wine 23
Wisconsin 232
witch 45, 270
witchcraft 45
Witch's Berry 184
witness consciousness 341
Wizard of Oz 207
wood pulp 34
wool 32
Wordsworth, William 35
World Health Assembly 303
World Health Organization (WHO) 207
wound botulism 92
Wounded Knee massacre 399
Wright, Alder 26
Wright, Hamilton 29

Xanax 225, 279, 378
xylocaine 255, 371
Xyrem 292

yagé 179
yangonin 186
Yangtze 25
Yaqui 396
Yemen 231
yerba del diablo 6
yin 31
yoga 161
yopo tree 265
Young, Francis L. 326
yuppie drug 242

Zapotecs 188
Zoff, Leo 340
Zoloft 141
Zulu 30
Zumarraga, Juan de 395